Metabolic Encephalopathies

Therapy and Prognosis

Fondazione Pierfranco e Luisa Mariani
viale Bianca Maria 28
20129 Milan, Italy

Telephone: +39 (2) 795458 & 796356
Fax: +39 (2) 76009582

Metabolic Encephalopathies

Therapy and Prognosis

Postgraduate Course of the Pierfranco e Luisa Mariani Foundation, Milan
Milan State University, 1–3 March 1994

Edited by
Stefano Di Donato
Rossella Parini
Graziella Uziel

Mariani Foundation Paediatric Neurology series: 4
Series editor: Maria Majno

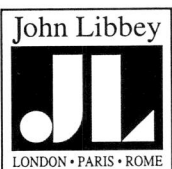

John Libbey
LONDON · PARIS · ROME

British Library Cataloguing in Publication Data

Metabolic Encephalopathies
Therapy and Prognosis
   Mariani Foundation Paediatric Neurology series: Vol. 4
   I. Di Donato, S. II. Series
618.928

ISSN: 0969-0301
ISBN: 0 86196 489 6

Published by

John Libbey & Company Ltd, 13 Smiths Yard, Summerley Street, London SW18 4HR, England.
Telephone: 0181-947 2777: Fax 0181-947 2664
John Libbey Eurotext Ltd, 127 Avenue de la République, 92120 Montrouge, France.
John Libbey - C.I.C. s.r.l., via Lazzaro Spallanzani 11, 00161 Rome, Italy

© 1995 John Libbey & Company Ltd. All rights reserved.
Unauthorised duplication contravenes applicable laws.

Printed in Great Britain by Biddles Ltd, Guildford, UK

Contents

Chapter 1	Recent insights into metabolic disorders *Stefano Di Donato*	1
Chapter 2	Fatty acid oxidation disorders *Graziella Uziel, Franco Taroni and Stefano Di Donato*	11
Chapter 3	Mitochondrial encephalomyopathies *Carlo Antozzi, Graziella Uziel, Caterina Mariotti, Marco Rimoldi, Stefano Di Donato and Massimo Zeviani*	25
Chapter 4	Lactic acidaemia: clinical diagnosis, treatment, and prognosis *Darryl C. De Vivo and Christine K. Wade*	37
Chapter 5	Hyperphenylalaninaemia: therapy and follow-up *Enrica Riva, Isabella Basile, Diego Luotti and Giacomo Biasucci*	51
Chapter 6	Genotype/phenotype correlation in phenylketonuria *Irma Dianzani, Luisa de Sanctis, Sergio Giannattasio, Carla Alliaudi, Maria Sartore, Carlo Dionisi Vici, Alberto Burlina, Massimo Burroni, Francesco Papadia, Gianfranco Sebastio, Vito Guzzetta, Ersilia Marra, Clara Camaschella and Alberto Ponzone*	61
Chapter 7	Diagnosis of metabolic disorders with acute neonatal onset *Florence Poggi-Travert, Marco Spada, Thierry Billette de Villemeur, Philippe Hubert, Christiane Charpentier, Daniel Rabier, Pierre Kamoun and Jean-Marie Saudubray*	71
Chapter 8	Multisystem involvement in lysinuric protein intolerance: a study on 20 Italian patients *Giancarlo Parenti, Barbara Incerti, Maria Rosaria Larocca, Carla Borrone, Maja Di Rocco, Rossella Parini, Irma Dianzani, Alberto Ponzone, Pietro Strisciuglio, Domenico Sperli, Carlo Dionisi Vici, Gianfranco Rizzoni and Generoso Andria*	85
Chapter 9	Variable clinical presentation is a characteristic feature of late-onset hyperammonaemias *Rossella Parini, Carlo Corbetta, Antonio Bastone and Mario Salmona*	91

Chapter 10	Treatment of organic acidurias *Alberto B. Burlina*	103
Chapter 11	Lysosomal storage diseases *Rosanna Gatti*	111
Chapter 12	Enzyme replacement therapy for Gaucher's disease types 1, 2 and 3 *Mario Carrozzi, Manuela Zanatta, Aldo Scabar and Bruno Bembi*	121
Chapter 13	Peroxisomal disorders: classification, diagnosis and treatment *Ruud B.H. Schutgens, Peter G. Barth, Björn M. van Geel and Ronald J.A. Wanders*	129
Chapter 14	Four cases of rhizomelic chondrodysplasia punctata: heterogeneity and variability *Ubaldo Caruso*	141
Chapter 15	Neuroradiological findings in metabolic diseases of the central nervous system *Mario Savoiardo, Ludovico D'Incerti and Elisa Ciceri*	145
Chapter 16	Neuropsychological development of children with metabolic diseases *Roberto Militerni, Antonella Gritti, Monica Ghezzi and Giancarlo Parenti*	157
Chapter 17	Multicentric study of a group of Italian patients with metabolic diseases *Paola Vizziello, Roberto Militerni, Olimpia Caropreso, Andrea Pasqui, and Ermellina Fedrizzi*	167
Chapter 18	From communicating to the family to communicating with the family: the process and its discontinuity *Graziella Fava Vizziello*	179
Chapter 19	Children with chronic disease and their family: a psychoanalytical point of view *Danièle Brun*	187
Chapter 20	Genetic counselling and prenatal diagnosis *Faustina Lalatta*	195

Chapter 1

Recent insights into metabolic disorders

Stefano Di Donato

Division of Biochemistry & Genetics, Istituto Nazionale Neurologico Carlo Besta, via Celoria 11, 20133 Milan, Italy

Introduction

Inborn errors of metabolism are genetic disorders due to the deficiency of specific enzymes involved in the catabolism of amino acids, carbohydrates, lipids, and nucleic acids. In the majority of these diseases the direct metabolic effects of the enzyme deficiency are an accumulation of metabolites upstream of the site of action of the enzyme involved, and a defect in the metabolic pathway downstream of that site. Early diagnosis is important because treatment may prevent acute metabolic attacks and mental retardation, epilepsy, severe brain damage, or death. Early diagnosis is also a prerequisite for optimal genetic counseling. Nowadays, the biochemical and genetic tools available, in addition to careful clinical examination, generally allow rapid diagnosis. Usually, as a first step, the diagnostic procedures include the analysis of body fluids, tissue specimens or cultured cells from the patient, in order to identify the principal biochemical pathway involved in the disease; the following step is the analysis of blood or cultured cells to determine the enzyme defect; the final step is the study of nuclear DNA (nDNA) or mitochondrial DNA (mtDNA) to unravel the mutation(s) causing the disease. These analyses can be done in advanced medical institutions for the more common metabolic disorders, making the diagnostic procedures relatively simple to the keen clinician.

However, the relationships between genomic mutations and the biochemical and clinical phenotypes are far from being understood. Several factors contribute to our ignorance of this essential step, i.e. how the mutant genotype affects the biochemical phenotype and, in turn, how the enzyme defect is translated into the clinical phenotype. First, different mutations at the same gene locus go along with variable abnormalities at the protein level, including enzyme inactivation, decreased enzyme stability, or changes in the kinetic properties of the enzyme. Second, enzymes are frequently expressed as different tissue-specific isoforms, and the control of gene expression varies from tissue to tissue. Third, mutations may not only affect the particular enzyme activity which is coded for by the corresponding gene, but can cause more general derangements of that biochemical pathway, as well as more generalized metabolic effects (think of organic or lactic acidoses of infancy, where local cellular acidosis can block ATP synthesis, or end in the activation of neuronal death through glutamate receptor stimulation). Lastly, the information we collect on the patient's biochemical and molecular status comes from the analysis of cells which may not be primarily involved in the disease process, as exemplified by the current analysis of mitochondrial genes and gene products in leucocytes or fibroblasts from patients with signs and symptoms of central nervous system pathology.

New sophisticated techniques of molecular genetics and cellular biology (*in vitro* and *in vivo*) allow functional studies that may help to elucidate some of the unsolved topics. These studies are important because they have changed our previous attitude toward inborn errors of metabolism, from a diagnostic approach which included morphological, biochemical and molecular tools, to a pathophysiological appoach designed to improve our understanding of the disease-causing metabolic changes. The ultimate goal of such studies is to establish a rationale for therapy. Functional investigations in metabolic diseases include the following:

(1) the study of the correlation between the mutant genotype and the clinical phenotype;

(2) the study of the local expression of a mutation in cells directly involved in the pathology;

(3) the search for new genes causing metabolic disorders.

Studies on genotype/phenotype relationships

In most genetic metabolic diseases there is a rough correlation between the degree of enzyme deficiency and the degree of clinical involvement. Mutations giving rise to 'null activity' of enzymes involved in important biochemical pathways are generally incompatible with life; mutations associated with 1 to 10 per cent residual enzyme activity cause a severe disease with early onset; mutations involved with residual enzyme activities of 10 per cent or more cause a disease with later onset and mild-to-moderate clinical involvement. However, there are several exceptions, and in many diseases it is unclear how genomic mutations affect enzyme activity. The understanding of these issues is crucial to define the pathogenicity of a point mutation or a deletion in a genomic sequence, and to establish a correct nosography (think of genotypic heterogeneity *vs* phenotypic heterogeneity, i.e. the different phenotypic expression of allelic mutants), and to set a rationale for therapy. Accordingly, we need studies directed at solving these problems.

Some of these studies can be performed *in vitro* by transfecting recipient cells (possibly devoid of the particular function to be studied) with expression vectors carrying different copies of the disease-causing gene, including the wild type gene, the gene with the likely pathogenic mutation, and the gene with other ancillary mutations or polymorphisms. Other studies, especially those directed to the study of mutations affecting genes either expressed in tissues not available for direct molecular analysis, such as the brain, or involved in embryonic and fetal development, frequently need an *in vivo* approach.

In vitro studies

Carnitine palmitoyltransferase deficiency

Carnitine palmitoyltransferase II (CPT II) deficiency, is one of the more common genetic defects of mitochondrial β-oxidation in man (Di Donato, 1994). CPT II deficiency is also a prototype of genetic defects of β-oxidation because it presents clinically, with two principal phenotypes: an early-onset disease characterized by hypoketotic hypoglycaemia, liver failure, cardiomyopathy, and sudden death, and a late-onset disease of the young adult with recurrent episodes of muscle pain, rabdomyolysis, and myoglobinuria, triggered by prolonged exercise, cold, or fever (Demaugre *et al.*, 1991; Taroni *et al.*, 1992, 1993). In both diseases the activity of CPT II in fibroblasts and skeletal muscle is decreased to 10 to 20 per cent of the mean value of controls, though enzyme activity tends to be lower in the infantile form (Demaugre *et al.*, 1990). In patients with either clinical phenotype, kinetic studies show normal affinity of the mutant enzyme for the physiological substrates, but V_{max} values are drastically reduced; also, in both diseases biochemical studies show normal synthesis and reduced steady-state levels of the protein, indicating decreased stability of the protein (Taroni *et al.*, 1992, 1993). Therefore, it is not apparent from these studies why CPT II mutants present with such distinct clinical phenotypes. Molecular studies in patients with either the classical infantile or the adult presentation took advantage of the cloning of the cDNA encoding full-length human CPT II (Finocchiaro *et al.*, 1991). Both patients carried three missense mutations in a homozygous form at the CPT II locus. Notably, a Val368Ile and a Met674Val substitutions were present in both phenotypes; the patient with early onset, however, had an Arg631Cys additional mutation, while the adult patient carried a Ser113Cys mutation. To unravel the molecular basis of the different presentations, recipient Cos cells were transfected with transient expression vectors carrying either the wild type cDNA for CPT II, or cDNAs holding a single mutation, or the different mutations in association. Studies of enzyme activities in recipient transfected cells showed the following: the Arg368Ile and the Met674Val mutations, expressed either as a single mutant or in association, were associated with normal catalytic activity; the Arg631Cys mutation decreased enzyme activity to 30 per cent of the controls' value; the Ser113Cys mutation decreased activity to 42 per cent of the controls' value (Taroni *et al.*, 1992, 1993). Therefore, the Arg631Cys resulted in the pathogenic mutation in the infantile form, while the Ser113Leu substitution was the pathogenic mutation in the adult form. When the Arg631Cys mutation was expressed in association with the silent Arg368Ile and Met674Val polymorphisms, enzyme activity significantly fell from 31 per cent to 15 per cent; by contrast, when the two polymorphisms were expressed in association with the Ser113Lys mutation the decrease in activity was not statistically significant. The conclusion from these studies was that subtle differences in enzyme activity have a precise molecular background (Taroni *et al.*, 1992, 1993). Further studies on β-oxidation flux, showed that the Arg631Cys mutation not only drastically decreased CPT II activity, but was associated with a defect of both 3-hydroxyacylCoA dehydrogenase and 3-ketothiolase; by contrast, the Ser113Lys mutation only affected CPT II activity. These observations suggest that the carboxy- terminal mutation in CPT II (Arg631Cys), can induce structural changes in the supramolecular organization of the membrane-bound β-oxidation system which, in turn, might cause a further decrease in the β-oxidation flux (Taroni *et al.*, 1994, unpublished). A methodological bias in these studies is that recipient Cos cells used in transfection experiments have endogenous CPT activity. The availability of cells lacking specific enzymes helped in overcoming these problems. Cells from the yeast *saccaromyces cerevisiae* do not express CPT II activity, and were used in experiments that allowed the measurement of the precise biochemical outcome of the different mutations (F. Taroni & P. Cavadini, unpublished observations).

Fumarase deficiency

An alternative way to study the biochemical outcome of mutations is to make use of spontaneous mutants, as in the case of a study of human fumarase deficiency. Fumarase deficiency is a rare human disease clinically characterized by neonatal encephalopathy with seizures, acidosis, and early death; pathologically there is evidence for neurodevelopmental abnormalities, including areas of heterotopia in the brain and cerebellum; biochemically both mitochondrial and cytosolic isoforms of fumarase are absent (Gellera *et al.*, 1990). To analyse the effects of mutations on the biochemical phenotype, we took advantage of a yeast cell line, identified by Tzagaloff at Colombia University, which lacked both yeast fumarase isoforms (yeast FUM⁻) (Wu & Tzagaloff, 1987). An expression vector for yeast cells carrying wild type and mutant human fumarase cDNAs was constructed, and transfected into yeast FUM⁻ cells allowing the identification of the biochemical consequences of the mutations in the human FUM gene (Gellera *et al.*, 1994).

Glutaric aciduria type II

Human spontaneous mutants can also be instrumental in such studies. Glutaric aciduria type II (GA II), a devastating infantile disorder characterized by acidosis, hypoglycaemia, coma and early death, is due to the deficiency of either enzyme electron transfer flavoprotein (ETF), or ETF-coenzyme-Q-oxidoreductase (ETF-QR) (Christensen *et al.*, 1984; Frerman & Goodman, 1984; Di Donato,

1994). ETF is a heterodimeric enzyme composed by an α- and a β-subunit, and some of the GA II patients with ETF deficiency have mutations in the gene coding the α-subunit, while others have mutations in the gene encoding for the β-subunit (Frerman & Goodman, 1984; Loehr *et al.*, 1990; Yamaguchi *et al.*, 1990). Two Japanese brothers had severe glutaric aciduria type II (Yamaguchi *et al.*, 1990). Western blot analysis of cell extracts from the two siblings showed the absence of the β-ETF subunit. Molecular analysis of the β-ETF gene (Finocchiaro *et al.*, 1993) proved that both patients were compound heterozygotes: the maternal allele carried an A→G transition at nucleotide 518, causing a missense mutation at codon 164; the paternal allele carried a G→C transversion at the first nucleotide of the intron donor site, downstream of an exon that is skipped during the splicing event (Colombo *et al.*, 1994). The cells of the patients, lacking ETF activity, showed lowered β-oxidation of fatty acid to roughly 15 per cent of controls. After transfection with an expression vector carrying the wild-type cDNA for the β-ETF subunit, mutant cells recovered a normal β-oxidation flux (Colombo *et al.*, 1994).

Myopathy and cardiomyopathy associated with a mutation in the tRNA^{leu} mtDNA gene

A particular version of cellular studies, useful for the analysis of diseases due to mtDNA mutations, is the construction of mitochondrial cybrids between an immortalized cell line devoid of wild type mtDNA (but carrying its own nDNA) and cells from patients, enucleated by exposure to cytochalasin (but carrying their own mtDNA) (King *et al.*, 1992). The new cell line obtained should be suitable for testing the effect of the mitochondrial DNA mutation at the biochemical level, thus allowing the direct study, in a 'clean' molecular environment, of the cellular expression of a specific DNA genotype. We used this technique to study the physiometabolic effects of a mitochondrial DNA heteroplasmic mutation, the A→G^{3260} transition in the gene encoding tRNA^{leu}, associated with maternally inherited myopathy and cardiomyopathy (Mimyca) (Zeviani *et al.*, 1991). Although this mutation fulfilled the requirements for a mutation of mtDNA to be pathogenic (i.e. the mutation was heteroplasmic, it affected a conserved nucleotide with relevant functional properties, segregated with the disease, and the percentage of mutant *vs* wild-type genome directly correlated with the pathological phenotype), there was no direct way to test its pathogenicity since it affected a tRNA gene and was variably heteroplasmic in the patient's cells. To eliminate the possible influence of the autochthonus nuclear genome we fused myoblast-derived cytoplast from one patient with Mimyca with a human tumoral cell line deprived of mtDNA (ρ^0). The presence and amount of the mutant G^{3260} *vs* wild-type mtDNA were measured by a recently developed technique that allows accurate quantification of mutant and wild-type DNA in point mutation-associated diseases (solid-phase minisequencing) (Suomalainen *et al.*, 1993). We obtained fusion cell clones expressing different amounts of mutant *vs* wild-type mtDNA, and measured in these cell lines several indexes of mtDNA-related respiratory capacity, including oxygen consumption, complex I and complex IV specific activities, and lactate production. We found that clones with a high proportion of mutant tRNA^{leu} had all mitochondrial respiratory indexes markedly abnormal, as compared to those containing homoplasmic wild-type mtDNA, possibly because of impaired mitochondrial protein synthesis (Mariotti *et al.*, 1994). Therefore, the A→G^{3260} transition in the gene encoding tRNA^{leu} was *de facto* responsible for the mitochondrial dysfunction.

In vivo studies

CPEO plus with multiple mtDNA deletions and CNS involvement

Some tissues, including the brain, are unavailable for direct biochemical and molecular analysis, and require indirect techniques of assay such as NMR spectroscopy (Penn *et al.*, 1992) or PET scans that can reveal subtle changes in the energy potential and metabolism of discrete brain areas, thus explaining central nervous system involvement in the pathology. An example comes from the study of a 66-year-old lady with chronic progressive external ophthalmoplegia, distal musclar weakness and wasting, signs and symptoms of cerebellar dysfunction, mild dementia, and ragged-red fibres in the muscle biopsy. Molecular genetic analysis of a muscle biopsy showed the presence of multiple deletions of mtDNA, but biochemical analysis of the respiratory chain failed to disclose mitochondrial abnormalities (Galassi *et al.*, 1994). Therefore, it was not possible to establish in this patient a correlation between the molecular findings and the expected biochemical abnormality; also, no insights into the possible basis of central nervous system pathology could be inferred by the analysis of muscle biopsy. Notably, NMR analysis of the brain and cerebellum showed marked atrophy of mid-brain, basal ganglia and the cerebellum. Phosphorus magnetic resonance spectroscopy *in vivo* demonstrated increased ADP concentrations, with a corresponding decrease in the phosphorylation potential. The spectroscopic abnormalities were selectively distributed to different neuronal populations, suggesting an uneven distribution of mutant and wild-type DNA. In this case, only NMR spectroscopy could demonstrate abnormal mitochondrial metabolism in the brain, thus explaining the presence of the brain and cerebellar symptoms in a patient carrying molecular lesions in skeletal muscle (Galassi *et al.*, 1994).

Transgenic mice as tools for the study of neurodevelopmental pathology

As mentioned in the introduction to this chapter, some genes encode for proteins expressed only during embryonic development; therefore both gene transcripts and gene products may not be amenable for biochemical and molecular analysis in mature tissues. In this case, we need an *in vivo* approach in the developing organism, in order to understand the pathophysiology of the corresponding inherited disease. Transgenic mice, either carrying extra copies of the mutant genes or knocked out for the wild-type gene, are particularly informative for these studies. However, genes causing early neurodevelopmental abnormalities, such as those recently identified for Kallmann syndrome on chromosome X and for lyssencephaly on chromosome 17, generally encode for structural protein, trophic factors, or molecules with pathfinding properties, not involved in metabolic disorders. Accordingly, these genetic diseases will not be treated here.

The study of the local expression of a mutation in cells directly involved in pathology

Since organs are composed of cell lineages with different embryonic origins and differentiation, it is important to understand which cell or which cell compartment is specifically involved in the disease process. In mitochondrial encephalomyopathies (Zeviani *et al.*, 1991; Shoffner & Wallace, 1992), the relationships between the distribution and expression of abnormal mtDNA and the focal cellular biochemical consequences are complex and probably heterogeneous (Hammans *et al.*, 1992). Notably, in these diseases, the more frequently affected tissues are the brain, skeletal muscle, and heart, probably because they are highly dependent on respiration for their function and activity. In mitochondrial encephalomyopathies the effects of both point mutations and deletions can be studied at the single cell level, through the powerful techniques of *in situ* hybridization, *in situ* PCR, and immunocytochemistry. The distribution of the mutant and wild type mtDNAs, of their transcripts, and of the correlated protein products, can be identified, thus giving important insights in the cellular pathogenesis of the disease.

Kearns–Sayre syndrome (KSS) and chronic progressive ophthalmoplegia (CPEO)

Patients with Kearns–Sayre syndrome are characterized clinically by progressive external ophthalmoplegia (PEO), heart block, retinal degeneration, and additional signs and symptoms such as short stature, ataxia, weakness, dementia, and increased CSF protein; ragged-red fibres are typically seen in muscle biopsies (Zeviani *et al.*, 1988). At the molecular level, these patients harbour large-scale deletions of mtDNA; however, Southern blot analysis of mtDNA shows that wild-type mtDNA and deleted mtDNA coexist in the same biopsy specimen (a phenomenon called heteroplasmy). Accordingly, histoenzymatic analysis of muscle shows scattered citochrome-c-oxidase (COX) negative fibres, in a milieu of COX-positive fibres, suggesting that the biochemical effects of the mutation have an uneven distribution. It is not clear, however, whether COX-negative fibres represent islands of the muscle fibres where only mutant mtDNA occurs, or whether mutant and wild-type mtDNA coexist, in the same fibres. In the latter case the presence of COX-negative fibres, should result from the fact that the ratio between mutant and wild-type mtDNA exceeds the threshold beyond which wild-type mtDNA can complement mutant mtDNA. In a molecular study of disease, Moraes *et al.* (1992) accurately measured the amount of wild-type mtDNA and mtRNA, the amount of deleted mtDNA and deleted mtRNA, and the levels of nuclear-encoded and mitochondrial-encoded subunits of COX in single muscle fibres from the patients and an adequate number of controls. Even though the distribution of wild-type and deleted mtDNA within muscle fibres varied among patients who harboured large deletions, COX deficiency was found to be consistently associated with a substantial decrease in wild-type mtDNA. Moreover, in some patients wild-type and deleted mtDNA were codominant, with the threshold ratio of deleted *vs* wild-type mtDNA necessary to cause a specific respiratory chain malfunction depending on the site of the deletion. Notably, since the mitochondria that harbour mtDNA deletions encompassing COX subunits need complementation not only of tRNAs, but also of COX mRNAs, for normal COX activity to occur, fibres containing mostly these type of deletions were COX-negative even in the presence of relatively abundant wild-type mtDNA. This and other studies (Shoubridge *et al.*, 1990; Hammans *et al.*, 1992; Moraes *et al.*, 1992) were instrumental in understanding the molecular pathogenesis of Kearns–Sayre disease and chronic progressive external ophthalmoplegia (CPEO), two diseases caused by sporadic mtDNA deletions.

Myoclonus epilepsy with ragged-red fibres (MERRF)

Similarly to KSS and CPEO, studies on the focal cellular expression of mutant genomes were performed in a maternally inherited disease, myoclonus epilepsy with ragged-red fibres (MERRF) (Boulet *et al.*, 1992). MERRF is clinically characterized by myoclonus, generalized seizures, myopathy, ataxia and mild dementia; an A→G transition mutation at nucleotide 8344 in the mtDNA gene encoding for tRNA^{lys} is present in most pedigrees with the disease (Shoffner *et al.*, 1990), though a few families harbour a different mutation at nucleotide 8356 in the same gene (Zeviani *et al.*, 1993). In skeletal muscle from MERRF patients the proportion of mutant genomes was greater than 80 per cent of total mtDNA and the activity of COX was decreased. Studies in myoblasts showed that translation was severely depressed in homoplasmic mutant clones but normal in heteroplasmic clones. Approximately 15 per cent of wild-type mtDNA restored mRNA translation and COX activity to near normal levels. These studies demonstrated that the tRNA^{lys} mutation is a functionally recessive mutation that can be rescued by intraorganellar complementation with a small proportion of wild-type mtDNA. This conclusion can explain the steep threshold for expression of the MERRF clinical phenotype. Furthermore, this study showed that the vast majority of myoblasts in culture, derived from the satellite population in the muscle biopsy, were homoplasmic for the mutation, so that the overall population of mutant mtDNA was similar in myoblasts and in differentiated muscle. This finding suggests that the ratio of mutant *vs* wild-type mtDNA in skeletal muscle is determined either in ovum or during early development (Boulet *et al.*, 1992).

The search for new genes causing metabolic disorders

Some of the recently discovered mitochondrial disorders are associated with alterations of mtDNA and respiratory chain dysfunctions due to putative mutations in the nuclear genome: they include qualitative alterations, i.e. multiple large-scale deletion of mtDNA, and quantitative alterations, i.e. tissue-specific depletion of mtDNA. The non-maternal mode of inheritance rules out the possibility of a transmissible *cis* mutation of mtDNA, pointing to a defect of a transacting nucleus-coded factor, which can ultimately damage the mtDNA molecule (Zeviani & Tiranti, 1993).

Autosomal dominant chronic progressive ophthalmoplegia (AD-CPEO)

AD-CPEO is a disease with adult onset characterized by proximal weakness and wasting, sensorineural hypoacusia, progressive ophthalmoplegia and additional signs and symptoms such as bilateral cataract, tremor, ataxia and sensory-motor peripheral neuropathy (Zeviani *et al.*, 1989; Servidei *et al.*, 1991. In skeltal muscle of the affected patients, Southern blot analysis in skeletal muscle of the affected patients shows the presence of heterogeneous mtDNA species, due to multiple deleted michochondrial genomes coexisting with the wild-type genome (Servidei *et al.*, 1991; Zeviani *et al.*, 1990); the total amount (wild-type plus mutated) of mtDNA is greater than in normal skeletal muscle. Therefore the crucial anomaly in this disease is the presence of qualitative and quantitative abnormalities of mtDNA, probably caused by a mutation in the nuclear genome. The disease-gene involved should arguably have an important role in the normal, physiological communication between the two genomes in order to guarantee proper and correct mtDNA replication. Several studies were planned to identify the disease gene for AD-CPEO, including linkage studies and studies directed to the identification of candidate genes (Zeviani & Tiranti, 1993). Our knowledge of the set of nuclear genes implicated in mtDNA replication is still incomplete, although the human mtDNA-specific γ-DNA polymerase has been recently purified. Another important component of the mtDNA replicative system is a single-stranded mtDNA binding protein (mtSSB) (VanTuyle & Pavco, 1985): its likely function is 'to smooth up' the pathway to the γ-DNA polymerase by thoroughly coating the displaced H strand during replication (VanTuyle & Pavco, 1985; Zeviani & Tiranti, 1993). Since the region between the origin of H-strand replication and the origin of L-strand replication (i.e. the region which is actually coated by mtSSB during replication) was preferentially affected by deletions in AD-CPEO patients, we devised the possibility that the gene encoding human SSB could be a candidate gene in this disease. As a first step, the full-length cDNA encoding SSB from *Xenopus laevis* was cloned (Tiranti *et al.*, 1991); subsequently, taking advantage of the high sequence conservation of SSB in evolution, the corresponding human cDNA was cloned and the corresponding gene mapped to human chromosome 7 (Tiranti *et al.*, 1993). Although mutations of this gene were not found in patients with AD-CPEO, this investigation proved that genetic-molecular studies of human spontaneous mutation, are a major source of new information for the understanding of basic biological phenomena such as the control of mtDNA replication.

Acknowledgements

This work was partially supported by the grant 'Mitochondrial diseases' from ARIN (Associazione per la Promozione delle Ricerche Neurologiche, Milan), and the grant 'Mitochondrial respiration in degenerative disorders of adult age' of Ministero della Sanità (Rome). The data presented in this paper are largely due to the work of Gaetano Finocchiaro, M.D., Cinzia Gellera, M.S., Franco Taroni, M.D. and Massimo Zeviani, M.D., Division of Biochemistry & Genetics, Istituto Nazionale Neurologico Carlo Besta, Milan, Italy.

References

Boulet, L., Karpati, G. & Shoubridge, E.A. (1991): Distribution and threshold expression of the tRNA[lys] mutation in skeletal muscle of patients with myoclonic epilepsy and ragged-red fibers. *Am. J. Hum. Genet.* **51**, 1187–1200, 199253–1059.

Christensen, N., Kolvraa, S. & Gregersen, N. (1984): Glutaric aciduria type II: evidence for a defect related to the electron transfer flavoprotein or its dehydrogenase. *Pediatr. Res.* **18**, 663–667.

Colombo, I., Finocchiaro, G., Garavaglia, B., Garbuglio, N., Yamaguchi, S., Frerman, F.E., Berra, B. & Di Donato, S. (1994): Mutations and polymorphisms of the gene encoding the β-subunit of electron transfer flavoprotein in three patients with gluratric acidemia type II. *Hum. Mol. Genet.* **3**, 429–435.

Demaugre, F., Bonnefont, J.P., Cepanec, C., Scholte, J., Saudubray, J.M. & Leroux, J.P. (1990): Immunoquantitative analysis of carnitine palmitoyltransferase I and II defects. *Pediatr. Res.* **27**, 497–500.

Demaugre, F., Bonnefont, J.P., Colonna, M., Cepanec, C., Leroux, J.P. & Saudubray, J.M. (1991): Infantile form of carnitine palmitoyltransferase II deficiency with hepatomuscular symptoms and sudden death. Physiopathological approach to carnitine palmitoyltransferase II deficiency. *J. Clin. Invest.* **87**, 859–864.

Di Donato, S. (1994): Disorders of lipid metabolism affecting skeletal muscle: carnitine deficiency syndromes, defects in the catabolic pathway, and Chanarin diseases. In: *Myology*, 2nd edn., eds. A.G. Engel & C. Franzini-Armstrong, pp. 1587–1609. New York: McGraw-Hill.

Finocchiaro, G., Colombo, I., Garavaglia, B., Gellera, C., Valdameri, G., Garbuglio, N. & Di Donato, S. (1993): cDNA cloning and mitochondrial import of the β-subunit of the human electron transfer flavoprotein. *Eur. J. Biochem.* **213**, 1003–1008.

Frerman, F.E. & Goodman, S.I. (1984): Deficiency of electron transfer flavoprotein or electron transfer flavoprotein: ubiquinone oxidoreductase in glutaric aciduria type II fibroblasts. *Proc. Natl Acad. Sci. USA* **82**, 4517–4520.

Galassi, G., Sintini, M., Rimoldi, M., Zeviani, M., Bastardi, C., Tavani, F., Iotti, S. *et al.* (1994): Mitochondrial encephalomyopathy associated with multifocal neuronal atrophy: clinical, MRI and ^{31}P-MRS studies. *J. Neurol.* abstr, in press.

Gellera, C., Uziel, G., Rimoldi, M., Zeviani, M., Laverda, A., Carrara, F. & Di Donato, S. (1990): Fumarase deficiency is an autosomal recessive encephalopathy affecting both the mitochondrial and the cytosolic enzymes. *Neurology* **40**, 495–499.

Gellera, C., Di Donato, S. & Taroni, F. (1994): Molecular study of fumarase deficiency. *Neurology* **44 (Suppl. 2)**, A209.

Hammans, S.R., Sweeney, M.G., Wicks, D.A.G., Morgan-Hughes, J.A. & Harding, A.E. (1992): A molecular genetic study of focal histochemical defects in mitochondrial encephalomyopathies. *Brain* **115**, 343–365.

King, M., Yoga, Y., Davidson, M. & Schon, E.A. (1992): Defects in mitochondrial protein synthesis and respiratory chain activity segregate with the tRNA$^{Leu(UUR)}$ mutation associated with mitochondrial myopathy, encephalopathy, lactic acidosis, and stroke-like episodes. *Mol. Cell Biol.* **12**, 480–490.

Loehr, J.P., Goodman, S.I. & Frerman, F.E. (1990): Glutaric acidemia type II: heterogeneity of clinical and biochemical phenotypes. *Pediatr. Res.* **27**, 311–315.

Mariotti, C., Tiranti, V., Carrara, F., Dallapiccola, B., Di Donato, S. & Zeviani, M. (1994): Defective respiratory capacity and mitochondrial protein synthesis in transformant cybrids harbouring the tRNA$^{Leu(UUR)}$ mutation associated with maternally inherited myopathy and cardiomyopathy. *J. Clin. Invest.* in press.

Moraes, C.T., Ricci, R., Petruzzella, V., Shanske, S., Di Mauro, S., Shon. E. & Bonilla, E. (1992): Molecular analysis of the muscle pathology associated with mitochondrial DNA deletions. *Nature Genet.* **1**, 359–367.

Penn, A.M.W., Lee, J.W.K., Thuilliere, P., Wagner, M., Maclure, K.M., Menard, M.R., Hall, L.D. & Kennaway, N.G. (1992): MELAS syndrome with mitochondrial tRNA$^{Leu(UUR)}$ mutation: correlation of clinical state, nerve conduction, and muscle ^{31}P magnetic resonance spectroscopy during treatment with nicotinamide and riboflavin. *Neurology* **42**, 2147–2152.

Servidei, S., Zeviani, M., Manfredi, G., Ricci, E., Silvestri, G., Bertini, E., Gellera, C., Di Mauro, S., Di Donato, S. & Tonali, P. (1991): Dominantly inherited mitochondrial myopathy with multiple deletions of mitochondrial DNA. *Neurology* **41**, 1053–1059.

Shoffner, J.M., Lott, M.T., Lezza, A.M.S., Seibel, P., Ballinger, S.W. & Wallace, D.C. (1990): Myoclonic epilepsy and ragged-red fiber disease (MERRF), is associated with a mitochondrial tRNA^{lys} mutation. *Cell* **61**, 931–937.

Shoffner, J.M. & Wallace, D.C. (1992): Mitochondrial genetics: principles and practice. *Am. J. Hum. Genet.* **51**, 1179–1186.

Shoubridge, E.A., Karpati, G. & Hastings, K.E.M. (1990): Deletion mutants are functionally dominant over wild-type mitochondrial genomes in skeletal muscle fiber segments in mitochondrial diseases. *Cell* **62**, 43–49.

Suomalainen, A., Kollmann, A.P., Octave, J.N., Soderlund, H. & Sylvanen, A.C. (1993): Quantification of mitochondrial DNA carrying the tRNA^{lys} mutation associated with mitochondrial myopathy, encephalopathy, lactic acidosis, and stroke-like episodes. *Eur. J. Hum. Genet.* **1**, 88–95.

Taroni, F., Verderio, E., Fiorucci, S., Cavadini, P., Finocchiaro, G., Uziel, G., Lamantea, E., Gellera, C. & Di Donato, S. (1992): Molecular characterization of inherited carnitine palmitoyltransferase II deficiency. *Proc. Natl Acad. Sci. USA* **89**, 8429–8433.

Taroni, F., Verderio, E., Dworzak, F., Willems, P.J., Cavadini, P. & Di Donato, S. (1992): Identification of a common mutation in the carnitine palmitoyltransferase II gene in familial recurrent myoglobinuria patients. *Nature Genet.* **4**, 314–320.

Tiranti, V., Barat-Gueride, M., Bijl, J., Di Donato, S. & Zeviani, M. (1991): A full-length cDNA encoding a mitochondrial DNA-specific single-stranded binding protein from *Xenopus laevis*. *Nucl. Acid Res.* **19**, 4291.

Tiranti, V., Rocchi, M., Di Donato, S. & Zeviani, M. (1993): Cloning of the human and the rat cDNAs encoding the mitochondrial single-stranded-DNA binding protein (SSB). *Gene* **126**, 219–225.

Van Tuyle, G.C. & Pavco, P.A. (1985): The rat liver mitochondrial DNA-protein complex: displaced single strands of replicative intermediates are protein coated. *J. Cell. Biol.* **100**, 251–257.

Wu, M. & Tzagaloff, A. (1987): Mitochondrial and cytoplasmic fumarases in *Saccharomyces cerevisiae* are encoded by a single nuclear gene FUM 1. *J. Biol. Chem.* **262,** 12275–12282.

Yamaguchi, S., Orii, T., Maeda, K., Oshima, M. & Hashimoto, T. (1990): A new variant of glutaric aciduria type II: deficiency of β-subunit of electron transfer flavoprotein. *J. Inherit. Metab. Dis.* **13,** 783–786.

Zeviani, M., Moraes, C.T., Di Mauro, S. *et al.* (1988): Deletions of mitochondrial DNA in Kearns–Sayre syndrome. *Neurology* **38,** 1339–1346.

Zeviani, S., Servidei, S., Gellera, C., Bertini, E., Di Mauro, S. & Di Donato, S. (1989): An autosomal dominant disorder with multiple deletions of mitochondrial DNA starting at the D-loop region. *Nature* **339,** 309–311.

Zeviani, M., Bresolin, N., Gellera, C., Bordoni, A., Pannacci, M., Amati, P., Moggio, M., Servidei, S., Scarlato, G. & Di Donato, S. (1990): Nucleus-driven multiple large-scale deletions of the human mitochondrial genome: a new autosomal dominant disease. *Am. J. Hum. Genet.* **47,** 904–914.

Zeviani, M., Gellera, C., Antozzi, C., Rimoldi, M., Morandi, L., Villani, F., Tiranti, V. & Di Donato, S. (1991): Maternally inherited myopathy and cardiomyopathy: association with mutation in mitochondrial DNA tRNA$^{Leu(UUR)}$. *Lancet* **338,** 143–147.

Zeviani, M. and Di Donato, S. (1991): Neurological disorders due to mutations of the mitochondrial genome. *Neuromuscular Disorders* **1,** 165–172.

Zeviani, M., Muntoni, F., Savarese, N., Serra, G., Titranti, V., Carrara, F., Mariotti, C. & Di Donato, S. (1993): A MERRF/MELAS overlap syndrome associated with a new point mutation in the mitochondrial DNA tRNA^{lys} gene. *Eur. J. Hum. Genet.* **1,** 80–87.

Zeviani, M. & Tiranti, V. (1993): Inherited Mendelian defects. In: *Mitochondrial DNA in human pathology*, eds. S. Di Mauro & D.C. Wallace, pp. 85–95. New York: Raven Press.

Chapter 2

Fatty acid oxidation disorders

Graziella Uziel*, Franco Taroni† and Stefano Di Donato†

*Division of Child Neuropsychiatry, †Division of Biochemistry and Genetics, Istituto Nazionale Neurologico Carlo Besta, via Celoria 11, 20133 Milan, Italy

Introduction

Inborn errors of mitochondrial fatty acid oxidation are a group of disorders with a wide spectrum of clinical features, mainly affecting infants and children. Fatty acids are the major source of energy for tissues such as skeletal muscle and myocardium with a high rate of mechanical work. In the liver, fatty acid oxidation gives rise to ketone bodies, an important oxidative substrate for many organs, including the brain, when glucose availability is restricted. In some physiological conditions such as prolonged physical exercise or fasting, fatty acids catabolism is a major biochemical pathway for maintaining fuel homoeostasis. Infants and young children are particularly at risk of having problems with fasting adaptation because basal metabolism is higher than in adults, and brain energy needs are elevated and highly dependent on glucose availability (Pildes *et al.*, 1973), and some of the key enzymes involved in energy production and glucose homoeostasis work at lower rates than in adults (Pagliara *et al.*, 1973).

Fatty acid catabolism

Fatty acid oxidation in mammals is largely localized in the mitochondrial compartment; its main physiological role is ATP production.

Different steps must be accomplished in order to obtain energy from fatty acid catabolism: fats are mobilized from adipose tissue and transported to the cytosolic compartment of the target tissues where they are activated to the corresponding acylCoA esters by an adenosine triphosphate-dependent acylCoA ligase (Osmundsen, 1984). Since the inner mitochondrial membrane is impermeable to long-chain acylCoA esters (length of more than 10 carbon atoms) a specific transport mechanism, which requires carnitine, is needed to transfer long-chain fatty acids across the mitochondrial membranes. This 'carnitine shuttle' involves the enzymes carnitine palmitoyl tranferase (CPT) I and CPT II and acylcarnitine translocase. CPT I is located with tissue-specific isoforms on the inner side of the outer mitochondrial membrane and catalyses the production of acylcarnitine esters. CPT II is located on the inner side of the inner mitochondrial membrane, has no tissue specificity and in the presence of CoA catalyses the formation of acylCoA esters and free carnitine in the matrix (Woeltje *et al.*, 1987). In the matrix fatty acylCoA are eventually oxidized by a repeated cycle of four concerted reactions each catalysed by enzymes which exhibit chain length specificity. According to the length of the carbon chain the first step in β-oxidation is catalysed by three distinct

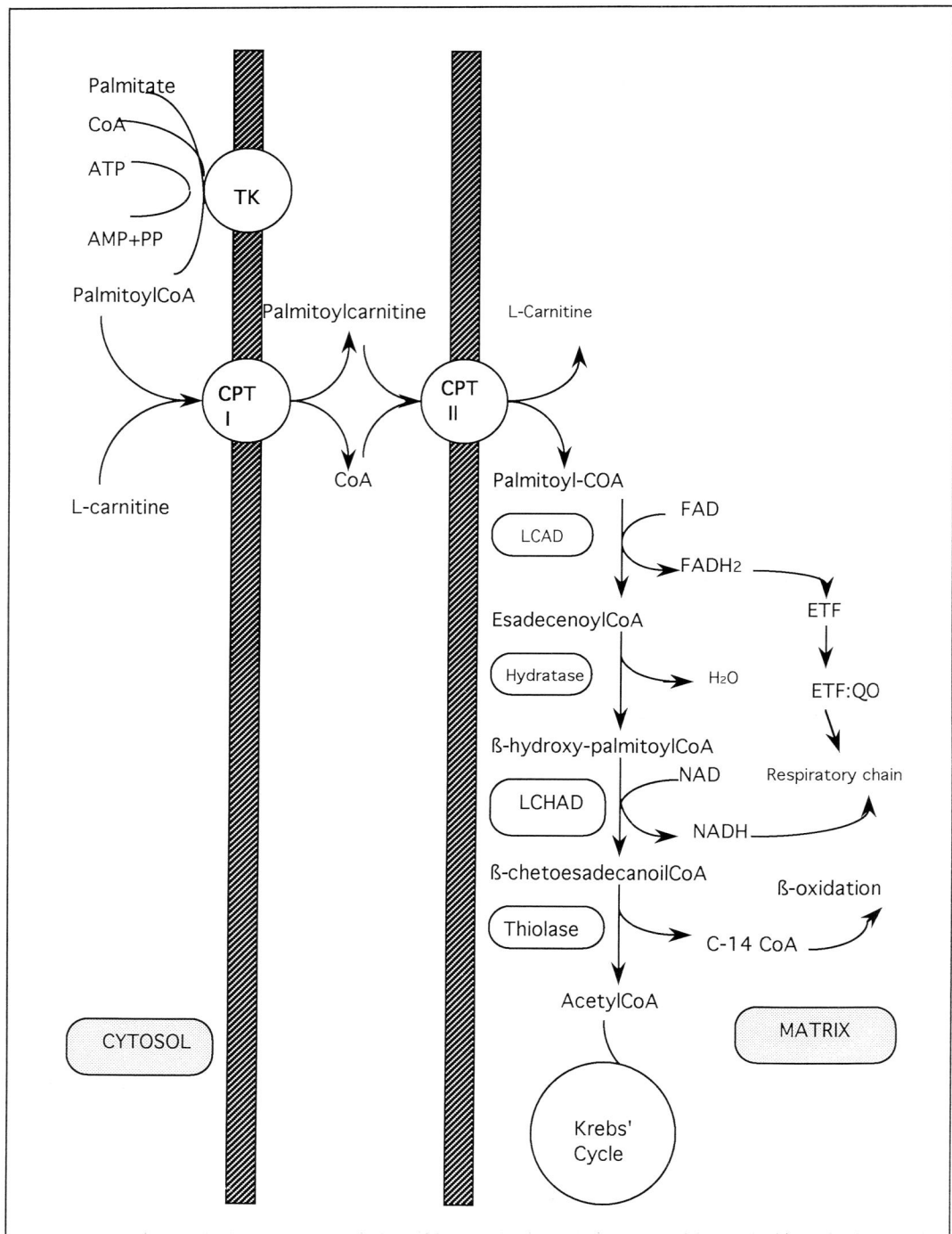

Fig. 1. Mitochondrial fatty acid oxidation pathway.

acylCoA dehydrogenases: long-chain (LCAD), medium chain (MCAD) and short-chain (SCAD) acylCoA dehydrogenases. These enzymes are all homotetramers with a molecular weight varying between 165 and 185 kDa and have as their coenzyme flavine adenine dinucleotide (FAD) (Ikeda et al., 1983). Recently a new acylCoA dehydrogenase has been isolated from liver mitochondrial membranes, and defined as very-long-chain acylCoA dehydrogenase (VLCAD) because of its high activity toward fatty acids with more than 16 carbons (Izai et al., 1992). The other enzymes of the β-oxidation spiral are: enoylCoA hydratase, 3-hydroxyacylCoA dehydrogenase and 3-ketoacylCoA thiolase, three distinct enzymes located in the matrix. In the inner mitochondrial membrane the same reactions are catalysed by the recently discovered trifunctional heterodimeric protein (Uchida et al., 1992).

During fatty acid oxidation FAD and NAD coenzymes become reduced: the corresponding electrons are transferred to the respiratory chain to complete the oxidative pathway yielding ATP. While NADH is oxidized directly by NADH-coenzyme Q reductase, the first complex of the respiratory chain, FADH needs the presence of two proteins to transfer its electrons to coenzyme Q: electron transfer flavoprotein (ETF) and electron transfer flavoprotein coenzyme Q oxidoreductase (ETF-QO). Both these enzymes contain FAD as coenzyme (Hall & Kamin, 1975). An outline of β-oxidation is shown in Fig. 1.

Clinical features

The presenting symptoms of fatty acid β-oxidation disorders are monomorphous and only in a few disorders do the clinical features suggest the specific diagnosis. Accurate metabolic, biochemical, and enzymatic analyses are needed to point out the precise defect. A classification of the β-oxidation disorders based on the different inborn errors of metabolism is proposed in Table 1. The main clinical features are listed in Table 2.

Recurrent episodes of hypoketotic hypoglycaemia, with or without brain involvement, are the most common clinical presentation; sometimes these episodes are triggered by fasting or minor viral infection. Patients can survive the acute metabolic attacks, although severe disorders have been described. Babies with marked defects of either CPT II or ETF and ETF-QO present multiple congenital malformations involving the brain and the kidney, facial dysmorphisms reminiscent of Zellweger's syndrome, and severe hypoglycaemia; death usually occurs in the first weeks of life (Goodman et al., 1983; Hug et al., 1991). Since the myocardium is highly dependent on fatty acid

Table 1. Classification of fatty acid oxidation disorders

A	Transport defect
	Primary carnitine deficiency
	Translocase deficiency
	CPT I deficiency
	CPT II deficiency
B	Deficiency of single enzymes of β-oxidation
	Long-chain acylCoA deydrogenase deficiency
	Medium-chain acylCoA dehydrogenase deficiency
	Short-chain acyl CoA dehydrogenase deficiency
	Very-long-chain acylCoA dehydrogenase deficiency
	Long-chain 3-hydroxyacylCoA dehydrogenase deficiency or combined deficiency
	Short-chain 3-hydroxyacylCoA dehydrogenase deficiency
C	Multiple acylCoA dehydrogenation disorders
	Electron transfer flavoprotein deficiency
	Electron transfer flavoprotein dehydrogenase deficiency
	Riboflavin responsive multiple acylCoA dehydrogenase deficiency

Table 2. Clinical features

Hepatic signs
  Hypoketotic hypoglycaemia
  Reyes'-like syndrome
  Steatosis
  Acute hepatic failure

Muscle signs
  Hypotonia
  Weakness
  Lipid storage myopathy
  Exercise intolerance and muscle pain
  Episodes of rhabdomyolysis with or without myoglobinuria

Cardiac signs
  Hypertrophic and dilatative cardiomyopathy
  Progressive heart failure
  Arrhythmias
  Cardiac arrest

Malformations
  Renal dysplasia
  Polycystic kidney
  Facial dysmorphism
  Brain malformation

catabolism for its energy supply, the heart is one of the target organs in these disorders. Primary carnitine deficiency, CPT II deficiency and long-chain acylCoA dehydrogenase deficiency are associated with progressive cardiomyopathy. Skeletal muscle is also frequently affected and weakness, muscle wasting, pain and sometimes myoglobinuria are manifestations of these diseases, particularly in the forms with later onset. Nervous system involvement is rarer, usually secondary to severe hypoglycaemic status and coma, although in progressive peripheral neuropathy and retinitis pigmentosa have been described long-chain 3-hydroxyacyl-CoA dehydrogenase deficiency.

Primary carnitine deficiency

For many years the term 'carnitine deficiency' has been used to define conditions characterized by metabolic disease, lipid storage in skeletal muscle, with or without associated liver pathology, and, as a common hallmark, reduced levels of carnitine in plasma and tissues. Two forms of carnitine deficiency (CD) were recognized: a muscular form and a systemic form. It has become clear recently that the majority of patients reported as having systemic carnitine deficiency suffered from other disorders, including some genetic defects of β-oxidation. The cause for carnitine deficiency in those diseases is probably the accumulation in mitochondria of metabolites that can easily react with carnitine, leading to reduced availability of free carnitine and increased renal loss of carnitine esters. A number of inherited and acquired disorders such as organic acidurias, respiratory chain defects or valproate therapy can cause, through the mechanisms mentioned above, tissue carnitine depletion. These diseases have been defined as secondary carnitine deficiency (Chalmers *et al.*, 1984).

The first description of a disorder due to true primary carnitine deficiency was reported by Morand *et al.* (1979) in a girl who completely recovered from heart failure after carnitine supplementation. Since then more than 20 patients have been described (Stanley *et al.*, 1991). Primary carnitine deficiency is a genetic disorder inherited as an autosomal recessive trait. The onset is always in infancy or childhood. Progressive dilatative cardiomyopathy, hypoketotic hypoglycaemia and muscular weakness are the main clinical findings. These different clinical phenotypes may coexist in members of the same family or even in the same patient. Chronic cardiomyopathy is usually diagnosed when it becomes symptomatic with persistent cough, dyspnoea, and fatigue. The carnitine content is very low in muscle, heart, liver and plasma. Total and free carnitines in plasma are less than 10 per cent of the normal and carnitine esters are not increased. Morphological study of skeletal muscle biopsy reveals lipid storage myopathy with increased lipid droplets in type I muscle fibres. Urinary organic acids excretion is normal: notably, no dicarboxylic aciduria is present which differs from other disorders of β-oxidation.

The biochemical defect underlying this disease is a carnitine membrane transport defect (Eriksson *et al.*, 1988; Treem *et al.*, 1988). The cellular uptake of carnitine by skeletal muscle and heart depends on the presence of high-affinity receptors which are functionally absent in patients with primary carnitine deficiency. Accordingly almost all tissues, including heart, skeletal muscle, bowel and kidney, have an impaired uptake of carnitine. Tubular carnitine leakage accounts for the low levels of carnitine in the plasma.

Palmitate oxidation by cultured fibroblasts, markedly reduced in the absence of exogenously supplemented carnitine, is almost completely corrected by the presence of 0.1 mM carnitine in the culture medium. Measurement of carnitine uptake by cultured fibroblasts in the presence of carnitine concentrations ranging from 0.05 to 10 µM is diagnostic: in patients' cells uptake is barely detectable. Fibroblasts from obligate heterozygotes show K_m values for carnitine uptake similar to those of controls, while V_{max} values are reduced to approximately 50 per cent of normal, suggesting that parents' cells have about 50 per cent of the normal receptor pool (Garavaglia *et al.*, 1991).

Treatment with high doses of carnitine (2–4 g per day) produces a dramatic clinical response: attacks of hypoglycaemia disappear, heart function and muscle strength improve, and eventually the patients fully recover.

Carnitine palmitoyltransferase deficiency

CPT I deficiency

CPT I deficiency is a rare disease identified in a few patients who presented episodes of severe hypoglycaemia with hypoketonaemia triggered by fasting or intercurrent illness. Hepatomegaly with steatosis has been found on histological examination in nearly all patients. Plasma and tissue carnitine contents as well as the excretion of urinary organic acids are normal. Palmitate oxidation in cultured fibroblasts is low. CPT I deficiency has been demonstrated in the liver (Bougnieres *et al.*, 1981) and fibroblasts (Demaugre *et al.*, 1988) but CPT I activity was normal in skeletal muscle (Tein *et al.*, 1989) suggesting the presence of tissue specific isoforms for CPT I. In order to distinguish CPT I from CPT II activity the enzymatic assays are performed in the presence and absence of malonylCoa, a specific inhibitor of CPT I (McGarry *et al.*, 1978).

CPT II deficiency

Three different clinical phenotypes are associated with CPT II deficiency: a myopathic form with juvenile-adult onset, an infantile form with liver and heart involvement and a lethal neonatal form.

Adult-onset muscular presentation

Since the first description by Di Mauro & Melis Di Mauro (1973) of a young adult with exercise-induced myoglobinuria due to CPT deficiency in muscle, more than 50 patients complaining of muscle pain, rhabdomyolysis, and myoglobinuria after prolonged exercise have been reported (Di Mauro & Papadimitrou, 1986). The disease is inherited as an autosomal recessive trait, but is most frequently seen in young adult males, probably because environmental and hormonal factors influence the expression of the defect. The attacks are triggered by prolonged exercise in fasting conditions, and consist of muscle pain and weakness. Sometimes, the metabolic attacks may cause massive rhabdomyolysis with myoglobinuria which may lead to acute renal failure. Although the disease is more frequent in adults, some infants with CPT II deficiency have been reported; in children rabdomyolytic attacks are more easily induced by fever rather than prolonged exercise (Schiffmann et al., 1992). Following acute episodes serum CK levels tend to be enormously increased up to 100 000 mU/l. Plasma and tissue carnitine and acylcarnitine levels are normal, as is the excretion of urinary organic acids. The morphology of muscle fibres is usually normal; only transient signs of necrosis and mild lipid storage may be present if the biopsy is performed immediately after an acute episode.

Biochemically, CPT activity in patients' muscles ranges from 'not detectable' to 30 per cent of normal and the enzyme defect is present in all tissues that have been tested: leucocytes, fibroblasts (Di Donato et al., 1978; Sacrez et al., 1982) platelets, and liver (Di Donato et al., 1981).

Infantile hepatomuscular phenotype

A less common variant of CPT II deficiency, also reported as a 'hepatic form', has been detected in infants with acute attacks of fasting hypoglycaemia, seizures, coma and, sometimes, sudden death (Demaugre et al., 1988, 1991; Taroni et al., 1992). In one of these patients cardiomyopathy associated with abnormal heartbeat was also present. Arrhythmia, which is rather uncommon in β-oxidation disorders, may be related to the accumulation of long-chain acylcarnitines that could elicit arrhythmias (Corr et al., 1989). Biochemically, data obtained in these children overlap with those found in patients with the 'muscular' form: deficiency of CPT II, with normal CPT I activity, is seen in cultured fibroblasts, leucocytes and skeletal muscle.

Lethal neonatal-early infantile phenotypes

A rare severe infantile form of CPT II deficiency with neonatal manifestations has been reported (Hug et al., 1991). These patients present at birth with severe hypoketotic hypoglycaemia, renal cystic dysplasia, and generalized steatosis, and die in their early days of life. CPT II enzyme activity in patients' cells was either barely detectable or reduced to less than 10 per cent of normal. Prenatal diagnosis in a family with this disease was successfully reached in both an affected and an unaffected pregnancy (Witt, 1991).

Molecular studies of CPT II allow some interesting observations. Subsequent to the cloning of the cDNA encoding CPT II, several different mutations segregating with specific clinical phenotypes have been identified, suggesting that clinical variants were the phenotypic expression of different genotypes (Taroni et al., 1992, 1993).

Carnitine acylcarnitine translocase (CT)

Only one patient with proven CT deficiency has been reported by Stanley et al. (1992) who described a child with poor growth, vomiting, coma and a defect in fatty acid oxidation. At the age of 2 and a half years, he had muscle weakness, cardiomyopathy and fasting hypoglycaemia. Increased excretion of medium-chain dicarboxylic acids was noticed, in the absence of ketonuria. The plasma free carnitine concentration was very low. By contrast, the level of plasma long-chain acylcarnitines was markedly increased; under L-carnitine treatment nearly all plasma carnitines were carnitine esters. Oleate oxidation in patient's cultured fibroblasts was low, and CPT activity normal. The measurement of carnitine-acylcarnitine translocase in the patient's cells showed a reduction of translocase activity to less than 5 per cent of the control value. Translocase activity of the parents was intermediate between that of the patient and that of controls suggesting heterozygosity in both parents.

AcylCoA dehydrogenases deficiency

LCAD deficiency

LCAD deficiency has been identified in infants presenting in the first 6 months of life with hypertrophic cardiomyopathy, failure to thrive and muscle weakness; less frequently, metabolic crises characterized by episodic vomiting, hypoglycaemia and coma started the clinical picture (Hale et al., 1985). A small number of patients with later onset had recurrent episodes of muscle pain, rhabdomyolysis and myoglobinuria. As seen in other disorder of β-oxidation, myopathic signs and symptoms develop in LCAD patients who reach childhood or adult age, while acute metabolic attacks seem to be confined to infancy. Biochemically, total and free carnitine are lowered in patients' plasma, liver and muscle, but long-chain carnitine esters tend to be increased (Hale et al., 1990a). Gas chromatography–mass spectrometry (GC–MS) analysis of the patients' urine showed marked C_6–C_{16} dicarboxylic aciduria. Pathologically, LCAD deficiency is characterized by liver steatosis. In patients' fibroblasts LCAD activity is less than 10 per cent of control values; it is also markedly lowered in leucocyte and liver homogenates (Treem et al., 1991). Avoiding fasting, a low-fat diet and oral administration of medium-chain tryglycerides (MCT) are the current therapeutic tools. Carnitine supplementation is controversial because of the risk of increasing long-chain acylcarnitine which may facilitate heart arrhythmias.

MCAD deficiency

MCAD deficiency is, together with CPT deficiency, the most frequent disease of β-oxidation: but MCAD deficiency seems to be confined to patients of anglosaxon origin. Although the severity of clinical presentation varies, symptoms include fasting intolerance, nausea, vomiting, hypoketotic hypoglycaemia, lethargy and coma (Stanley et al., 1983): in some of the patients the onset may be so acute and unexpected as to lead to sudden infant death (Arens et al., 1993). Investigations in members of families with at least one affected patient, showed, by contrast, MCAD deficiency in asymptomatic subjects. (Roe et al., 1986).

Gas chromatography–mass spectrometry of urine samples collected during the acute phase of the disease reveals increased levels of adipic, suberic and sebacic acids, but during remissions these markers may be normal and specific metabolites such as hexanoylglycine, suberylglycine and octanoylcarnitine must be sought. Their detection is considered pathognomonic of MCAD, but requires sophisticated procedures such as stable isotope dilution or fast atom bombardment mass spectrometry (FAB-MS) (Millington et al., 1984; Rinaldo et al., 1988). Free carnitine is reduced in plasma but medium-chain acyl carnitine esters are increased during intercritical periods. Oxidation of medium-chain fatty acids in cultured cells is impaired, while long- and short-chain substrates are oxidized normally (Duran et al., 1985).

Deficiency of MCAD can be detected in patients' cultured fibroblasts, lymphocytes and liver biopsies (Rhead et al., 1983; Coates et al., 1985). The enzyme activity is between 2 and 10 per cent of normal.

The molecular cloning of a full-length cDNA encoding the human MCAD enzyme (Kelly et al., 1987), the assignment of the gene to the short arm of chromosome 1, band p31, and the knowledge of the genomic structure of the MCAD gene (Matsubara et al., 1986) allowed molecular studies in numerous independent patients. These studies proved that most MCAD patients carry a point mutation at nucleotide 985 of the coding region (Matsubara et al., 1990). This mutation is an A→G transition which changes an highly conserved lysine at position 304 of the mature MCAD subunit into glutamate. The mutation causes impairment of tetramer assembly and instability of the protein.

SCAD deficiency

This disease has been documented in only a few patients (Amendt et al., 1987; Coates et al., 1988). Myopathy is frequently described as the only sign in adult patients, but is invariably associated with vomiting and failure to thrive in infancy. All SCAD-deficient patients excrete in their urine increased amounts of ethylmalonic, methylsuccinic acids and, in some instances, butyrylglycine.

Biochemical data obtained from these patients are somewhat controversial: SCAD activity and the oxidation of short-chain fatty acids was impaired both in muscle and cultured fibroblasts of patients with early onset, while in a patient with the late-onset myopathic form the enzyme deficiency was restricted to skeletal muscle (Turnbull et al., 1984). It is still unclear whether in these patients muscle-specific SCAD deficiency was due to a defect of a tissue specific SCAD isoenzyme, or it was secondary to another enzyme defect.

Very-long-chain acylCoA dehydrogenase deficiency

Very recently two groups of investigators reported two patients with a neonatal severe disorder involving heart and liver, and demonstrated mitochondrial very-long-chain acylCoA dehydrogenase deficiency (Aoyama et al., 1993; Bertrand et al., 1993). Cultured cells from six patients previously diagnosed as having LCAD deficiency were reexamined by immunoblot analysis for VLCAD and in three cell lines no VLCAD band was detectable (Yamaguchi et al., 1993). These results indicate that other patients previously identified as having LCAD deficiency may suffer from VLCAD deficiency.

3-Hydroxy acylCoA dehydrogenase (HAD) deficiency

HAD is the third enzyme of the β-oxidation cycle. Mammalian mitochondria contain two different HAD enzymes (Osumi & Hashimoto, 1980). One acts on long-chain 3-OH acylCoA substrates and is bound to the inner membrane, while the other, which acts on short-chain 3-OH acylCoA substrates, is located in the matrix. A third type of HAD activity is present in peroxisomes as part of the bifunctional protein in the peroxisomal β-oxidation system.

To date, 10 cases of LCHAD deficiency have been reported (Hale et al., 1990b; Przyrembel et al., 1991). Clinical features in these infants include Reye's like episodes, hypoketotic hypoglycaemia, myopathy and/or cardiomyopathy and sudden infant death. Two patients presented with peripheral sensory-motor polyneuropathy, which in one patient was associated with pigmentary retinopathy (Bertini et al., 1992). Significant dicarboxylic aciduria involving 3-hydroxydicarboxylic acids was detected in patients' urine.

Biochemically, all patients had a marked deficiency of the long-chain HAD in cultured fibroblasts, with normal activity of the enzyme that is active on short-chain substrates. The other enzymes of β-oxidation were all normal, except for a partial reduction of 3-ketoacylCoA thiolase observed in three patients. The very existence of long-chain HAD deficiency is now questioned by the discovery that some of these patients suffer from a combined defect of β-oxidation enzymes (see below).

Combined deficiency of β-oxidation enzymes

A young girl suffering from recurrent episodes of muscle weakness with a fatal outcome at the age of 4.5 years due to acute respiratory failure has been reported (Jackson et al., 1992). The activity of long-chain 3-hydroxyacylCoA dehydrogenase was severely decreased in her muscle, heart, liver and fibroblasts; also, long-chain, but not short-chain, 2-enoylCoA hydratase and 3-ketoacylCoA thiolase were markedly low in her muscles, liver and heart, pointing to a combined defect of these enzymes of β-oxidation. The recent discovery of a trifunctional enzyme in human liver mitochondria (Uchida et al., 1992) suggests that this patient, and probably others with long-chain HAD deficiency, suffer from a genetic defect of the mitochondrial trifunctional protein.

Multiple acylCoA dehydrogenation disorder, or glutaric aciduria type II

Glutaric aciduria type II (GA II) is a genetic disorder firstly described by Przyrembel et al. (1976) and characterized clinically by metabolic acidosis, hypoketotic hypoglycaemia and early death. Pathologically, fatty degeneration of several organs occurs, including liver, kidney, heart and skeletal muscle (Frerman & Goodman, 1989). The biochemical hallmark is the excretion in the urine of massive amounts of several metabolites which accumulate as the consequence of a block of the mitochondrial flavin-dependent acylCoA dehydrogenases. Accordingly, the disorder has been named multiple acylCoA dehydrogenase deficiency or glutaric aciduria type II, because glutaric acid is invariably increased in the patients' urine. In most patients, this disease is due to a defect of either ETF or ETF:QO (Frerman & Goodman, 1985). A third type of glutaric aciduria type II has no identified aetiology and is treatable with riboflavin (Gregersen et al., 1982).

ETF and ETF-dehydrogenase deficiencies

ETF is a mitochondrial flavoprotein which transfers electrons from the reduced form of several acylCoA dehydrogenases to the respiratory chain via ETF-QO. ETF consists of an α-subunit and a β-subunit of 32 and 27 kilodaltons, respectively: both subunits are synthesized in the cytosol (Ikeda et al., 1986). The α-subunit is synthesized as a 35 kD precursor and processed to the mature form in mitochondria, but the β-subunit is synthesized in its ultimate size. Each mole of β-ETF binds one mole of FAD and interacts directly with acylCoA dehydrogenase. ETF-QO is a 68 kD protein, partially embedded in the inner mitochondrial membrane, which transfers electrons from ETF to ubiquinone. The protein monomer contains two different redox centres, i.e. a flavin site which interacts with ETF, and a Fe_4S_4 cluster which donates electrons to ubiquinone (Frerman & Goodman, 1989).

At least three groups of patients with glutaric aciduria type II have been identified (Goodman & Frerman, 1984): (a) patients with the neonatal form characterized by hypotonia, hepatomegaly, severe hypoglycaemia and metabolic acidosis, multiple congenital anomalies, typical 'sweaty feet' odour and early death; (b) infants without congenital anomalies, with a similar clinical course to patients with the neonatal form, but with longer survival up to a few months of age; these patients may develop cardiomyopathy; (c) patients with later onset and variable clinical presentation, frequently characterized by vomiting, hypoglycaemia, hepatomegaly and proximal myopathy. Analysis of urinary organic acids is essential for the diagnosis. Infants with the severe MAD form present with metabolic acidosis and urinary excretion of glutaric, ethylmalonic, isovaleric, isobutyric, 2-methyl-butyric, and saturated and unsaturated dicarboxylic acids and sarcosine. In patients with the milder and later onset form organic acidaemia may be variable and inconstant: in these patients analysis should be performed during acute metabolic decompensation. The evaluation of substrate oxidation in cultured fibroblasts is often informative: a decreased rate of oxidation of branched chain amino acids, palmitate, octanoate and butyrate is demonstrated in cultured cells of MAD patients. The carnitine content in plasma, muscle and liver may be low both in the early-onset and late-onset cases (Mandel et al., 1988). Treatment with carnitine and riboflavin, although advisable, is mostly unsuccessful. Dietary management with low fat and low protein intake and careful surveillance avoiding fasting and stress has to be considered.

Riboflavin-responsive glutaric aciduria type II

This disorder has been described both in infants with acute metabolic attacks (Gregersen et al., 1982) and in young adults with progressive weakness and lipid storage myopathy (Carrol et al., 1981). The patients have a urinary pattern of organic acids compatible with GA II. The carnitine content in plasma and tissues is variably reduced. The clinical, morphological, biochemical, and physiological responses to oral riboflavin supplementation are dramatic. In infants, metabolic attacks and hypotonia disappear (Harpey et al., 1983). In myopathic adults, muscle weakness and wasting improve within weeks, and muscle biopsy after-therapy shows the disappearance of lipid droplets (Di Donato et al., 1989). In both groups of patients organic acids in urine also normalize within a few days. Biochemically, the disease is characterized by multiple deficiency of several flavin-dependent acylCoA dehydrogenases. Recent studies in muscle mitochondria isolated from these patients showed that the defect involves the primary dehydrogenases active on acylCoA substrates and is more marked at the level of SCAD and MCAD (Di Donato & Gellera, 1990). In a young girl, oral riboflavin not only was able to normalize the deficient activities of the SCAD and MCAD, but also restored to normal the amount of SCAD antigen in the patient's muscle mitochondria (Di Donato et al., 1989). The pathogenetic mechanism of this disorder is still unknown. Studies performed in cultured fibroblasts showed that riboflavin uptake and FAD synthesis are unaffected in this condition.

References

Amendt, B.A., Greene, C., Sweetman, L., Cloherty, J., Shih, V., Moon, A., Teel, L. & Rhead, W.J. (1988): Short-chain acyl-CoA dehydrogenase deficiency. Clinical and biochemical studies in two patients. *J. Clin. Invest.* **79**, 1303–1309.

Arens, R., Gozal, D., Jain K., Muscati, S., Heuser, E.T., Williams, J.C., Keens T.G. & Davidson Ward, S.L. (1993): Prevalence of medium-chain acyl-coenzyme A dehydrogenase deficiency in the sudden infant death syndrome. *J. Pediatr.* **122**, 715–718.

Aoyama, T., Uchida, Y., Kelley, R.I., Marble, M., Hofman, K., Tonsgard, J.H., Rhead, W.J. & Hashimoto T. (1993): A novel disease with deficiency of mitochondrial very-long-chain acyl-CoA dehydrogenase. *Biochem. Biophys. Res. Commun.* **191**, 1369–1372.

Bertini, E., Dionisi-Vici, C., Garavaglia, B., Burlina, A.B., Sabatelli, M., Rimoldi, M., Bartuli, A., Sabetta, G. & Di Donato, S. (1992): Peripheral sensory-motor neuropathy, pigmentary retinopathy, and fatal cardiomyopathy in long-chain 3-hydroxyacylCoA dehydrogenase deficiency. *Eur. J. Pediatr.* **151**, 121–126.

Bertrand, C., Largilliere, C., Zabot, M.T., Mathieu, M. & Vianey-Seban, C. (1993): Very-long-chain acyl-CoA dehydrogenase deficiency: identification of a new inborn error of mitochondrial fatty acid oxidation in fibroblasts. *Biochim. Biophys. Acta* **1180**, 327–329.

Bougnieres, P.J., Saudubray, J.M., Marsac, C., Bernard, O., Odievere, M. & Girard, J. (1981): Fasting hypoglycemia resulting from hepatic carnitine palmitoyl transferase deficiency. *J. Pediatr.* **98**, 742–746.

Carroll, J.E., Shumate, J.B., Brooke, M.H. & Hagberg, J.M. (1981): Riboflavin-responsive lipid myopathy and carnitine deficiency. *Neurology* **31**, 1557–1559.

Chalmers, R.A., Roe, C.R., Stancey, J.E. & Happel, C.R. (1984): Urinary excretion of L-carnitine and acylcarnitines by patients with disorders of organic acid metabolism: evidence for secondary insufficiency of L-carnitine. *Pediatr. Res.* **18**, 1325–1326.

Coates, P.M., Hale, D.E., Stanley, C.A., Corkey, B.E. & Cortner, J.A. (1985): Genetic deficiency of medium-chain acylcoenzyme A dehydrogenase: studies in cultured skin fibroblasts and peripheral mononuclear leucocytes. *Pediatr. Res.* **19**, 671–676.

Coates, P.M., Hale, D.E., Finocchiaro, G., Tanaka, K. & Winter, S.C. (1988): Genetic deficiency of short-chain acylcoenzyme A dehydrogenase in cultured fibroblasts from a patient with muscle carnitine deficiency and severe skeletal muscle weakness. *J. Clin. Invest.* **81**, 171–175.

Corr, P.B., Creer, M.H., Yamada, K.A., Saffitz, J.E. & Sobel, B.E. (1989): Prophylaxis of early ventricular fibrillation by inhibition of acylcarnitine accumulation. *J. Clin. Invest.* **83**, 927–936.

Demaugre, F., Bonnefont, J.P., Mitchell, G., Nguyen-Hoang, N., Pelet, A., Rimoldi, M., DiDonato, S. & Saudubray, J.M. (1988): Hepatic and muscular presentations of carnitine palmitoyl transferase deficiency: two distinct entities. *Pediatr. Res.* **24**, 308–311.

Demaugre, F., Bonnefont, J.P., Colonna, M., Cepanec, C., Leroux, J.P. & Saudubray, J.M. (1991): Infantile form of carnitine palmitoyltransferase II deficiency with hepatomuscular symptoms and sudden death. Physiopathological approach to carnitine palmitoyltransferase II deficiency. *J. Clin. Invest.* **87**, 859–864.

Di Donato, S., Cornelio, F., Pacini, L., Peluchetti, D., Rimoldi, M. & Spreafico, S. (1978): Muscle carnitine palmitoyltransferase deficiency: a case with enzyme deficiency in cultured fibroblasts. *Ann. Neurol.* **4**, 465–467.

Di Donato, S., Castiglione, A., Rimoldi, M., Cornelio, F., Vendemia, F., Cardace, G. & Bertagnolio, B. (1981): Heterogeneity of carnitine palmitoyltransferase deficiency. *J. Neurol. Sci.* **50**, 207–215.

Di Donato, S., Gellera, C., Peluchetti. D., Uziel, G., Antonelli, A., Lus, G. & Rimoldi, M. (1989): Normalization of short-chain acylcoenzyme A dehydrogenase after riboflavin treatment in a girl with multiple acylcoenzyme A dehydrogenase deficient myopathy. *Ann. Neurol.* **25**, 479–484.

Di Donato, S. & Gellera, C. (1990): Short-chain and medium-chain acylCoA dehydrogenases are lowered in riboflavin-responsive lipid myopathies with multiple acylCoA dehydrogenase deficiency. In: *Fatty acid oxidation: clinical, biochemical and molecular aspects*, eds. K. Tanaka & P.M. Coates, pp. 325–332. New York: Alan R. Liss.

Di Mauro, S. & Melis Di Mauro, P. (1973): Muscle carnitine palmitoyltransferase deficiency and myoglobinuria. *Science* **118**, 929–931.

Di Mauro, S. & Papadimitrou, A. (1986): Carnitine palmitoyltransferase deficiency. In: *Myology*, eds. A.G. Engel & B.Q. Banker, pp. 1697–1708. New York: McGraw-Hill.

Duran, M., Mitchell, G., de Klerk, J.B.C., de Jager, J.P., Hofkamp, M., Bruinvis, L., Ketting, D., Saudubray, J.M. & Wadman, S.K. (1985): Octanoic acidemia and octanoylcarnitine excretion with dicarboxylic aciduria due to defective oxidation of medium-chain fatty acids. *J. Pediatr.* **107**, 397–404.

Eriksson, B.O., Gustafson, B., Lindstedt, S. & Nordin, I. (1988): Hereditary defect in carnitine membrane transport is expressed in skin fibroblasts. *Eur. J. Pediatr.* **147**, 662–666.

Frerman, F.E. & Goodman, S.I. (1985): Deficiency of electron transfer flavoprotein or electron transfer flavoprotein: ubiquinone oxidoreductase in glutaric aciduria type II fibroblasts. *Proc. Natl. Acad. Sci. USA* **82**, 4517–4520.

Frerman, F.E. & Goodman, S.I. (1989): Glutaric aciduria type II and defects of mitochondrial respiratory chain. In: *The metabolic basis of inherited disease*, eds. C.R. Scriver, A.R. Beaudet, W.S. Sly & D. Valle, pp. 915–931. New York: McGraw-Hill.

Garavaglia, B., Uziel, G., Dworzak, F., Carrara, F. & Di Donato, S. (1991): Primary carnitine deficiency: heterozygote and intrafamilial phenotypic variation. *Neurology* **41**, 1691–1693.

Goodman, S.I., Reale, M. & Barlow, S. (1983): Glutaric acidemia type II: a form with deleterious intrauterine effect. *J. Pediatr.* **102**, 411–413.

Goodman, S.I. & Frerman, F.E. (1984): Glutaric acidemia type II (multiple acyl-CoA dehydrogenation deficiency). *J.Inherit. Metab. Dis.* **7 suppl. 1**, 33–37.

Gregersen, N., Wintzensen, H., Kolvraa, S., Christensen, E., Christensen, M.F., Brandt, N.J. & Rasmussen, K. (1982): C_6–C_{10}-Dicarboxylic aciduria: investigation of a patient with riboflavin responsive multiple acyl-CoA dehydrogenase defect. *Pediatr. Res.* **16**, 861–868.

Hale, D.E., Batshaw, M.L., Coates, P.M., Frerman, F.E., Goodman, S.I., Singh, I. & Stanley, C.A. (1985): Long-chain acylCoA dehydrogenase deficiency. An inherited cause of non-ketotic hypoglycemia. *Pediatr. Res.* **19**, 666–671.

Hale, D.E., Stanley, C.A. & Coates, P.M. (1990a): The long-chain acyl-CoA dehydrogenase deficiency. In: *Fatty acid oxidation: clinical, biochemical and molecular aspects*, eds. K. Tanaka & P.M. Coates, pp. 303–312. New York: Alan R. Liss.

Hale, D.E., Thorpe, C., Braat, K., Wright, J.H., Roe, C.R., Coates, P.M., Hashimoto, T. & Glasgow, A.M. (1990b): The L-3-hydroxyacyl-CoA dehydrogenase deficiency. In: *Fatty acid oxidation: clinical, biochemical and molecular aspects*, eds. K. Tanaka & P.M. Coates, pp. 503–510. New York: Alan R. Liss.

Hall, C.L. & Kamin, H. (1975): The purification and some properties of electron transfer flavoprotein and general fatty acyl coenzyme A dehydrogenase from pig liver mitochondria. *J. Biol. Chem.* **250**, 3476–3486.

Harpey, J.P., Charpentier, C., Goodman, S.I., Darbois, Y., Lefebvre, G. & Sebbah, J. (1983): Multiple acyl-CoA dehydrogenase deficiency occurring in pregnancy and caused by a defect in riboflavin metabolism in the mother. *J.Pediatr.* **103**, 394–398.

Hug, G., Bove, K.E. & Soukup, S. (1991): Lethal neonatal multiorgan deficiency of carnitine palmitoyltransferase II. *N. Engl. J. Med.* **325**, 1862–1864.

Ikeda, Y., Dabrowski, C. & Tanaka, K. (1983): Separation and properties of five distinct acylCoA dehydrogenases from rat liver mitochondria. *J. Biol. Chem.* **258**, 1066–1076.

Ikeda, Y., Keese, S.M. & Tanaka, K. (1986): Biosynthesis of electron transfer flavoprotein in a cell-free system and in cultured fibroblasts. Defect in the alpha subunit synthesis is the primary lesion in glutaric aciduria type II. *J. Clin. Invest.* **78**, 997–1002.

Izai, K., Uchida, Y., Orii, T., Yamamoto, S. & Hashimoto, T. (1992): Novel fatty acid β-oxidation enzymes in rat liver mitochondria. I. Purification and properties of very-long-chain acyl-coenzyme A dehydrogenase. *J. Biol. Chem.* **267**, 1027–1003.

Jackson, S., Singh Kler, R., Bartlett, K., Briggs, H., Bindoff, L.A., Pourfarzam, M., Gardner-Medwin, D. & Turnbull, D.M. (1992): Combined enzyme defect of mitochondrial fatty acid oxidation. *J. Clin. Invest.* **90**, 1219–1225.

Kelly, D.P, Kim, J.J., Billadello, J.J., Hainline, B.E., Chu, T.W. & Strauss, A.W. (1987): Nucleotide sequence of medium-chain acyl-CoA dehydrogenase mRNA and its expression in enzyme deficient human tissue. *Proc. Natl. Acad. Sci. USA* **84**, 4068–4072.

Mandel, H., Africk, D., Blitzer, M. & Shapira, E. (1988): The importance of recognizing secondary carnitine deficiency in organic acidaemias: case report in glutaric acidaemia type II. *J. Inherit. Metab. Dis.* **11**, 397–402.

Matsubara, Y., Kraus, J.P., Yang-Feng, T.L., Francke, U., Rosenberg, L.E. & Tanaka, K. (1986): Molecular cloning of cDNAs encoding rat and human medium-chain acyl-CoA dehydrogenase and assignment of the gene to human chromosome 1. *Proc. Natl. Acad. Sci. USA* **83**, 6543–6547.

Matsubara, Y., Narisawa, K., Miyabayashi, S., Tada, K., Coates, P.M., Bachmann, C., Elsas II, L.J., Pollit, R.J., Rhead, W.J. & Roe, C.R. (1990): Identification of a common mutation in patients with medium-chain acyl-CoA dehydrogenase deficiency. *Biochem. Biophys. Res. Commun.* **171**, 498–505.

McGarry, J.D., Leatherman, G.F. & Foster D.W. (1978): Carnitinepalmitoyltransferase I. The site of inhibition of hepatic fatty acid oxidation by malonylCoA. *J. Biol. Chem.* **253**, 4128–4136.

Millington, D.S., Roe, C.R. & Maltby, D.A. (1984): Application of high resolution fast atom bombardment and constant B/E linked scanning to the identification and analysis of acylcarnitine in metabolic disease. *Biomed. Mass Spectrom.* **11**, 236–241.

Morand, P., Despert, F. & Carrier, H.N. (1979): Myopathie lipidique avec cardiomyopathie sévère par deficit generalisé en carnitine. *Arch. Mal. Coeur* **5**, 536–544.

Osmundsen, B.J. (1984): Fatty acid oxidation and its regulation. In: *Fatty acid metabolism and its regulation*, ed. S. Numa, pp. 113–154. New York: Elsevier.

Osumi, T. & Hashimoto, T. (1980): Purification and properties of mitochondrial and peroxisomal 3-hydroxyacylCoA dehydrogenase from rat liver. *Arch. Biochem. Biophys.* **203**, 372–383.

Pagliara, A.S., Karl, I.E., Haymond, M. & Kipnis, D.M. (1973): Hypoglycemia in infancy and childhood. II. *J. Pediatr.* **82**, 558–577.

Pildes, R.J., Patel, D.A. & Nitzam, M. (1973): Glucose disappearance rate in symptomatic neonatal hypoglycemia. *Pediatrics* **52**, 75–82.

Przyrembel, H., Wendel, U., Becker, K., Bremer, H.J., Bruinvis, L., Ketting, D. & Wadman, S.K. (1976): Glutaric aciduria type II: report on a previously undescribed metabolic disorder. *Clin. Chim. Acta* **66**, 227–239.

Rhead, W.J., Amendt, B.A., Fritchman, K.S. & Felts, S. (1983): Dicarboxylic aciduria: deficient $1\text{-}^{14}C$ octanoate oxidation and medium-chain acylCoA dehydrogenase in cultured fibroblasts. *Science* **221**, 73–75.

Rinaldo, P., O'Shea, J.J., Coates, P.M., Hale, D.E., Stanley, C.A. & Tanaka, K. (1988): Medium chain acyl-CoA dehydrogenase deficiency: diagnosis by stable isotope dilution measurement of urinary n-hexanoylglycine and 3-phenylpropionylglycine. *N. Engl. J. Med.* **319**, 1308–1313.

Roe, C.R., Millington, D.S., Maltby, D.A. & Kinnebrew, P. (1986): Recognition of medium-chain acyl-CoA dehydrogenase deficiency in asymptomatic siblings of children dying of sudden infant death or Reye-like syndrome. *J. Pediatr.* **108**, 13–18.

Sacrez, A., Porte, A., Hindengland, C., Bieth, R. & Merian, B. (1982): Myocardiopathie avec surcharge lipidique et deficit en palmityl carnitine transferase (PCT) leucocytaire. *Arch. Mal. Coeur.* **21**, 1371–1379.

Schiffmann, R., Lahat, E. & Schechter, A. (1992): Severe periodic myalgia in infancy due to carnitine palmitoyltransferase deficiency. *Neuromusc. Disord.* **2**, 285–288.

Stanley, C.A., DeLeeuw, S., Coates, P.M., Vianey-Liaud, C., Divry, P., Bonnefont, J.P., Saudubray, J.M., Haymond, M., Trefz, F.K., Breningstall, G.N., Wappner, R.S., Byrd, D.J., Sansarcq, C., Tein, I., Grover, W., Valle, D., Rutledge, S.L. & Treem, W.R. (1991): Chronic cardiomyopathy and weakness or acute coma in children with a defect in carnitine uptake. *Ann. Neurol.* **30**, 709–716.

Stanley, C.A., Hale, D.E., Coates, P.M., Hall, C.L., Corkey, B.E., Yang, W., Kelley, R.I., Gonzales, E.L., Williamson, J.R. & Baker, L. (1983): Medium-chain acyl-CoA dehydrogenase deficiency in children with non-ketotic hypoglycemia and low carnitine levels. *Pediatr. Res.* **17**, 877–883.

Stanley, C.A., Hale, D.E., Berry, G.T., Deleeuw, S., Boxer, J. & Bonnefont J.P. (1992): Brief report: a deficiency of carnitine translocase in the inner mitochondrial membrane. *N. Engl. J. Med.* **327**, 19–23.

Taroni, F., Verderio, E., Fiorucci, S., Cavadini, P., Finocchiaro, G., Uziel, G. & Di Donato, S. (1992): Molecular characterization of inherited carnitine palmitoyltransferase II deficiency. *Proc. Natl. Acad. Sci. USA* **89**, 8429–8433.

Taroni, F., Verderio, E., Dworzak, F., Willems, P.J., Cavadini, P. & DiDonato, S. (1993): Identification of a common mutation in the carnitine palmitoyltransferase II gene in familial recurrent myoglobinuria patients. *Nature Genet* **4**, 314–320.

Tein, I., Demaugre, F., Bonnefont, J.P. & Saudubray, J.M. (1989): Normal muscle CPT_1 and CPT_2 activities in hepatic presentation patients with CPT_1 deficiency in fibroblasts. Tissue specific isoforms of CPT_1? *J. Neurol. Sci.* **29**, 229–245.

Treem, W.R., Stanley, C.A., Finegold, D.N., Hale, D.E. & Coates, P.M. (1988): Primary carnitine deficiency due to a failure of carnitine transport in kidney, muscle, and fibroblasts. *N Engl. J. Med.* **319**, 1331–1336.

Treem, W.R., Stanley, C.A., Hale, D.E., Leopold, H.B. & Hyams, J.S. (1991): Hypoglycemia, hypotonia, and cardiomyopathy: the evolving clinical picture of long-chain acyl-CoA dehydrogenase deficiency. *Pediatrics* **87**, 328–333.

Turnbull, D.M., Bartlett, K., Stevens, D.L., Alberti, K.G.M.M., Gibson G.J., Johnson, M.A., McCulloch, A.J. & Sherratt, H.S.A. (1984): Short-chain acyl-CoA dehydrogenase deficiency associated with a lipid-storage myopathy and secondary carnitine deficiency. *N. Engl. J. Med.* **311**, 1232–1236.

Uchida, I., Izai, K., Orii, T. & Hashimoto, T. (1992): Novel fatty acid beta-oxidation enzymes in rat liver mitochondria. II. Purification and properties of enoyl coenzyme A (CoA) hydratase/3-hydroxyacyl-CoA dehydrogenase/3-ketoacylCoA thiolase trifunctional protein. *J. Biol. Chem.* **267**, 1034–1041.

Witt, D.R. (1991): Carnitine palmitoyltransferase- type 2 deficiency: two new cases and successful prenatal diagnosis. *Am. J. Hum. Genet.* **49**, A 109.

Woeltje, K.F., Kuwajima, M., Foster, D.W. & McGarry, J.D. (1987): Characterization of the mitochondrial carnitine palmitoyltransferase enzyme system. II. Use of detergent and antibodies. *J. Biol. Chem.* **262**, 9822–9827.

Yamaguchi, S., Indo, Y., Coates, P.M., Hashimoto, T. & Tanaka, K. (1993): Identification of very-long-chain acyl-CoA dehydrogenase deficiency in three patients previously diagnosed with long-chain acyl-CoA dehydrogenase deficiency. *Pediatr. Res.* **34**, 111–113.

Chapter 3

Mitochondrial encephalomyopathies

Carlo Antozzi*, Graziella Uziel†, Caterina Mariotti‡, Marco Rimoldi‡, Stefano Di Donato‡ and Massimo Zeviani‡

*Divisions of *Neuromuscular Diseases, †Child Neuropsychiatry, and ‡Biochemistry and Genetics of the Nervous System, Istituto Nazionale Neurologico Carlo Besta, via Celoria 11, 20133 Milan, Italy*

Summary

Mitochondria, the organelles devoted to energy production, are characterized by unique genetic features. They possess their own DNA (mtDNA) encoding several subunits of the respiratory chain, but the majority of mitochondrial proteins as well as factors controlling mtDNA replication, transcription and translation are encoded by nuclear DNA (nDNA). Due to this dual genetic control of mitochondrial functions, defects of both mtDNA and nDNA can be identified as a source of human disorders. Mutations of mtDNA are sporadic or maternally inherited. Large-scale rearrangements of mtDNA (such as deletions, or rarely duplications) have been detected in sporadic progressive external ophthalmoplegia (CPEO) and in the Kearns–Sayre syndrome (KSS). Maternally inherited point mutations of mtDNA have been reported in several syndromes including Leber's hereditary optic neuroretinopathy (LHON), myoclonus epilepsy with ragged-red fibres (MERRF), mitochondrial encephalomyopathy with lactic acidosis and stroke-like episodes (MELAS), maternally inherited myopathy and cardiomyopathy (Mimyca) and in the neuropathy, ataxia and retinitis pigmentosa complex (NARP). However, several disorders, transmitted as Mendelian traits, can be ascribed to nDNA defects. The majority of these syndromes are still largely identified on the basis of their biochemical features (as defects of the respiratory chain complexes). Recently, qualitative and quantitative defects of mtDNA have been described, presenting as autosomal dominant progressive external ophthalmoplegia (associated with multiple deletions of mtDNA) or as severe infantile tissue-specific syndromes (associated with depletion of mtDNA). Clinical, morphological, biochemical and molecular genetic criteria are necessary for a correct diagnosis of mitochondrial encephalomyopathies, a rapidly expanding area of adult and paediatric neurology.

Introduction

Mitochondrial myopathies and encephalomyopathies are relatively rare disorders characterized by significant dysfunction of the respiratory chain and oxidative phosphorylation (Oxphos). Until recently, diagnosis was largely based on the detection of ragged red fibres under the light microscopy examination of the muscle biopsy. Ultrastructural studies demonstrated that the ragged-red transformation of the muscle fibres is caused by an increase in number and size of structurally abnormal subsarcolemmal mitochondria.

Since the study of Holt *et al.* (1988), the interest in mitochondrial diseases has increased remarkably, due to the identification of gene mutations in a small extranuclear genome, the mitochondrial

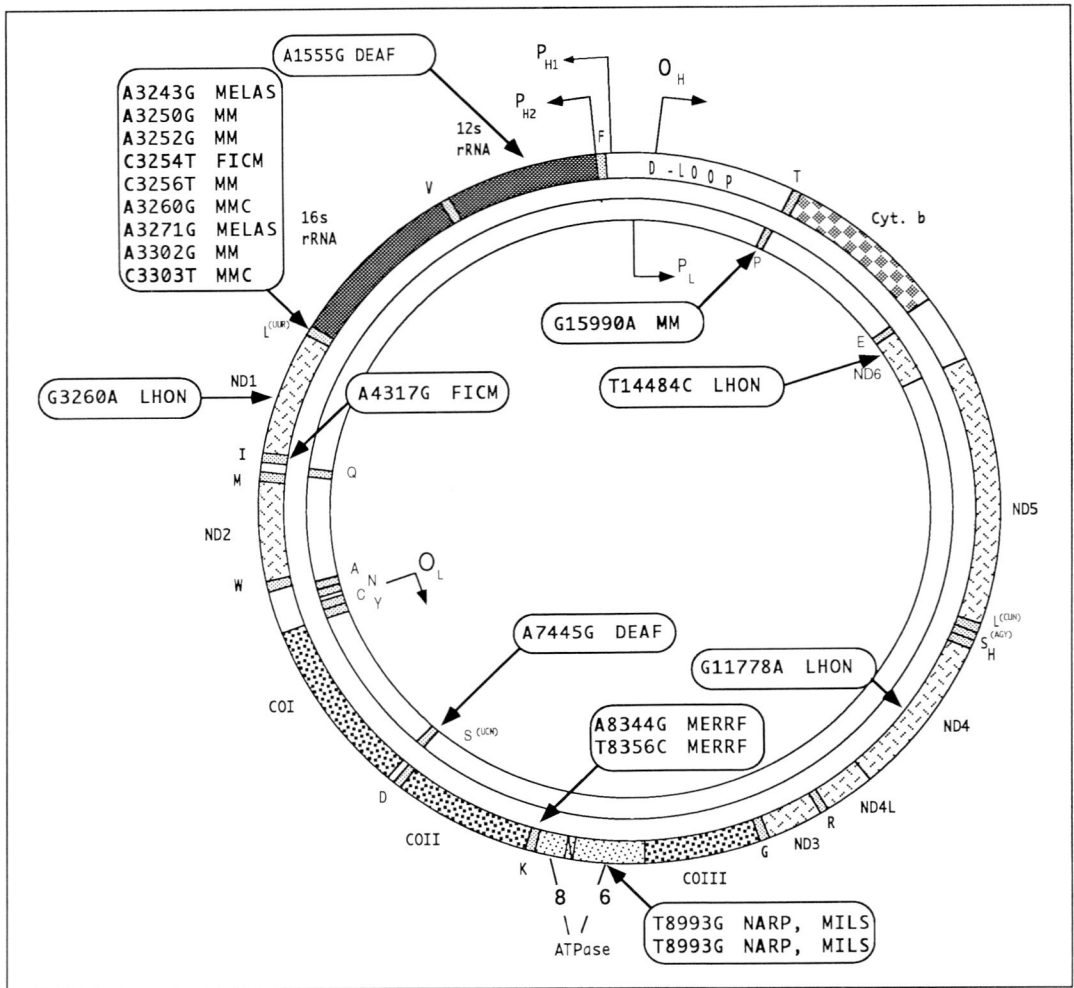

Fig. 1. Map of human mitochondrial genome and localization of the principal point mutations. O_H, origin of heavy strand replication; O_L, origin of light strand replication; cyt. b, cytochrome b; ND 1–6, complex I subunits; CO I–III, cytochrome c oxidase subunits; capital letters, tRNA genes; 12S rRNA and 16S rRNA, mitochondrial ribosomal rRNA; MM, mitochondrial myopathy; FICM, fatal infantile cardiomyopathy; MMC, mitochondrial myopathy and cardiopathy; LHON: Leber's hereditary optic neuropathy; DEAF, deafness; MILS, maternally inherited Leigh syndrome.

DNA (mtDNA), which encodes for some of the protein constituents of the Oxphos enzymes. These studies have provided both relevant pathogenetic insights and new diagnostic clues for many mitochondrial syndromes.

Molecular and genetic features of the mitochondrial genome

Mitochondria possess an autonomous DNA (mtDNA), organized as a small, circular, double-stranded chromosome, 16.5 kb long (Tzagoloff, 1982). Each mitochondrion contains from 2 to 10 mtDNA copies. Compared to nuclear DNA (nDNA), the mtDNA has a very compact gene organization since all coding sequences are contiguous, with no introns. Moreover, since the genetic code of mtDNA is different from the universal code, mitochondrial gene expression relies upon the complementation of numerous nuclear gene products involved in transcription and translation, with mitochondrion-specific transfer RNAs (tRNAs) and ribosomal RNSs (rRNAs). Therefore, the mtDNA, whose sequence has been fully elucidated (Anderson *et al.*, 1981), contains two sets of genes, one encoding mitochondrial proteins (corresponding to the yeast *mit* genes) and one involved in mitochondrial protein synthesis (corresponding to the yeast *syn* genes) (Tzagoloff, 1982). The *mit* genes encode for 13 messenger RNAs (mRNAs) corresponding to as many subunits of the respiratory chain: seven subunits of complex I (NADH-coenzyme Q reductase), apocytochrome *b* of complex III (coenzyme Q-cytochrome *c* reductase), three subunits of complex IV (cytochrome *c* oxidase, COX), and two subunits of complex V (mitochondrial ATPase). The *syn* genes encode for 22 tRNAs and two rRNAs. A map of human mtDNA is shown in Fig. 1.

From a genetic point of view, mtDNA is transmitted according to non-Mendelian, maternal inheritance, since during fertilization mitochondria are contributed only by the oocyte. Thus, affected mothers will transmit the disease to all of their children, but only their daughters will transmit the disease to subsequent generations. Moreover, each cell contains hundreds of mitochondria and each mitochondrion is endowed with several copies of mtDNA; as a consequence, thousands of copies of mtDNA will determine the mitochondrial genotype of each cell. During mitosis mtDNAs are transmitted to the progeny according to a statistical distribution: if cells in the first generation are heteroplasmic (i.e. they contain different forms of mtDNA), the relative proportion of different populations of mtDNAs might shift considerably at each subsequent generation. This phenomenon, called mitotic segregation, increases the variability of the mitochondrial genotypes and contributes to the different degrees of mtDNA heteroplasmy observed in different tissues from the same patient. Finally, a given phenotype will be evident whenever the relative proportion of mutant *vs* wild-type mtDNA will reach a critical value, so as to impair energy metabolism significantly (threshold effect). However, the threshold for phenotypic expression will vary in different tissues, depending on the intrinsic energy demands and the activity of aerobic metabolism.

Clinical considerations

The clinical presentation of mitochondrial disorders is extremely heterogeneous, as it can range from pure myopathies to encephalomyopathies, cardiomyopathies and complex multisystem syndromes. Most commonly, patients with mitochondrial diseases show the involvement of tissues characterized by the highest aerobic demand, such as skeletal muscle, brain and heart, while the liver and kidneys are less frequently affected. Although some mitochondrial syndromes are well established as nosologically defined entities, clinical data are not sufficient to provide a systematic classification of mitochondrial diseases, because overlap syndromes or aspecific phenotypes are frequent. Likewise, identical biochemical and morphological abnormalities, including the ragged-red fibres (RRF), can be found in different clinical presentations. On the other hand, RRF and other hallmarks of mitochondrial abnormalities may be absent in patients with biochemically and/or genetically proven mitochondrial phenotypes, such as Leigh's disease. Because of the rapid pro-

Table 1. Genetic classification of mitochondrial encephalomyopathies

Defects of mitochondrial DNA:
    Deletions, duplications (usually sporadic)
    Point mutations (maternally inherited)

Defects of nuclear DNA (Mendelian inheritance):
    Defects of genes encoding subunits of the respiratory chain
    Defects of mitochondrial protein importation
    Defects of nDNA–mtDNA communication

gress of the molecular genetic studies in this field, the most useful classification is perhaps one that links the clinical, biochemical and morphological features to the molecular abnormalities associated with these disorders (Table 1).

As shown in Table 1, since mitochondrial functions are regulated by a dual genetic control, mitochondrial diseases can be divided into two main groups: defects of mitochondrial DNA and defects of nuclear DNA.

Defects of mitochondrial DNA

Mutations of mtDNA can be classified according to their molecular nature in (a) large-scale rearrangements (such as deletions or duplications) and (b) point mutations (Fig. 1).

(a) Large scale rearrangements of mtDNA are heteroplasmic and are either sporadic or inherited as Mendelian traits (see defects of nuclear DNA). mtDNA deletions are usually associated with marked proliferation of mitochondria in muscle cells, leading to the typical ragged-red appearance under light microscope examination.

We will consider here the phenotypes associated with single deletions of mtDNA.

Kearns–Sayre syndrome (KSS)

The disease is characterized by the 'obligatory' triad: (1) progressive external ophthalmoplegia (PEO), (2) pigmentary retinopathy, and (3) onset before the age of 20. These obligatory features are usually associated with one or more of the following: cerebellar syndrome, heart block, and increased CSF protein content. The prognosis is poor and most patients die within the fourth decade of life, even after receiving a pacemaker.

Sporadic progressive external ophthalmoplegia (PEO)

The disease is defined by the presence of bilateral ptosis and ophthalmoplegia, frequently associated with exercise intolerance and variable degrees of muscle weakness and wasting.

Pearson's syndrome

This rare syndrome is characterized by the association of pancytopaenia and exocrine pancreatic dysfunction (Rotig *et al.*, 1990). It is interesting to observe that an infant who survived into adolescence developed the clinical picture of KSS (McShane *et al.*, 1991). Thus, Pearson's and KSS may represent different clinical expressions of the same molecular defect, presumably due to the tissue distribution and relative amount of deleted mtDNA.

Single large-scale deletions have been found by Southern blot analysis in about 50 per cent of patients with PEO and in almost all patients affected with KSS, but not in other mitochondrial encephalomyopathies (Holt *et al.*, 1988; Zeviani *et al.*, 1988; Moraes *et al.*, 1989). Deleted mtDNA species (mtDNA$^{\Delta+}$) were restricted to muscle tissue in patients affected with sporadic PEO and widely distributed in several tissues in the multisystem KS syndrome; the same type of deletion was found in different tissues in the same patient (Shanske *et al.*, 1990; Zeviani *et al.*, 1990). Moreover, single deletions were heteroplasmic, and the proportion of wild-type (mtDNA^{wt}) *vs* mtDNA$^{\Delta+}$ was correlated with the severity of the clinical picture. The majority of reported mtDNA deletions ranged from 1.3 to 7.6 kb, and have been localized between the end of the D-loop and the origin of the L-strand replication of the mtDNA molecule (see Fig. 1) (Holt *et al.*, 1988; Moraes *et al.*, 1989). The junctional regions of mtDNA$^{\Delta+}$ have been sequenced and shown to be flanked by direct repeats of variable length. The most frequently observed deletion, hence called 'common deletion', 4.9 kb in length, spans for a total of 4.9 kilobases from mtDNA nucleotide position 8470 to 13460, and occurs across two perfect direct repeats of 13 base pairs (Schon *et al.*, 1989). The molecular mechanisms leading to these large-scale rearrangements are still unclear. However, sequence analysis of deleted mtDNAs suggested two possibilities: unequal crossing-over during recombination and slipped mispairing during replication. Crossing-over is thought to be unlikely since available data suggest that recombination does not occur in the mitochondria of mammalian cells. Therefore, a mismatch of mtDNA strands during replication seems to be more likely (Shoffner et al., 1989); the presence of direct repeats as complementary single strands could allow pairing and facilitate recombination.

Both PEO and KSS are sporadic disorders associated with a single deletion of mtDNA in each individual, suggesting the clonal amplification of a single mutational event. Mitotic segregation will further influence the variability in the tissue distribution of mtDNA$^{\Delta+}$, leading to different clinical phenotypes. Even though mtDNA$^{\Delta+}$ is widely distributed in the multisystem KSS, it is not maternally transmitted, possibly because cells containing substantial amounts of mtDNA$^{\Delta+}$ are not viable for gametogenesis.

At the cellular level, mtDNA$^{\Delta+}$ are not able to synthesize functional Oxphos enzymes since several genes encoding tRNAs are encompassed by deletions. Studies performed by *in situ* hybridization of mtDNA in muscle and by mitochondrial translation *in vitro* demonstrated that RRF are rich in mtDNA$^{\Delta+}$ but the levels of mtDNA^{wt} and mRNAs are normal. These findings suggested that RRF are competent for mtDNA transcription but not for translation, the latter being impaired by the reduced availability of tRNAs (Mita et al., 1989; Shoubridge et al., 1990). Moreover, experiments on cybrids obtained by introducing different amounts of mtDNA^{wt} and mtDNA$^{\Delta+}$ into human ρ° cells, i.e. cells permanently deprived of mtDNA, showed that the reduction of mtDNA translation is proportional to the relative amount of mtDNA$^{\Delta+}$ (Hayashi et al., 1991).

Table 2. Biochemical classification of the mitochondrial encephalomyopathies

1. Defects of substrate transport:
    CPT deficiency
    Carnitine deficiency

2. Defects of substrate utilization:
    Pyruvate dehydrogenase deficiency
    Pyruvate carboxylase deficiency
    Defects of fatty acids oxidation

3. Defects of the Krebs' cycle:
    Ketoglutarate dehydrogenase deficiency
    Fumarase deficiency

4. Defects of oxidation–phosphorylation coupling:
    Luft's syndrome

5. Defects of the respiratory chain complexes:
    Complex I deficiency
    Complex II deficiency
    Complex III deficiency
    Complex IV deficiency
    Complex V deficiency
    Combined defects of respiratory chain complexes

(b) Point mutations of mtDNA have been reported in association with several, rather well-defined clinical phenotypes. All of the point mutations of mtDNA are maternally inherited. However, due to the high mutational rate of mtDNA, the pathogenic relevance of a point mutation must be demonstrated. In particular, the following criteria should be fulfilled: (1) high phylogenetic conservation of the mutated nucleotide, (2) presence of heteroplasmy (not obligatory), (3) specific segregation with the disease, and (4) correlation between the degree of mtDNA heteroplasmy and the severity of the clinical and biochemical phenotype. Due to the variable degree of mtDNA heteroplasmy observed in several pedigrees, an extensive clinical assessment is mandatory since both symptomatic patients and asymptomatic maternal relatives can be observed in each candidate's pedigree. With a few exceptions, RRF are observed in patients with mutations involving tRNA genes (*syn⁻* mutations) while they are absent in patients with mutations affecting genes encoding subunits of the mitochondrial respiratory chain (*mit⁻* mutations).

A list of point mutations of mtDNA and associated phenotypes is reported in Fig. 1. We briefly describe here the main clinical features of the syndromes associated with point mutations of mtDNA.

(1) *syn⁻* point mutations:

Myoclonus epilepsy with ragged-red fibres (MERRF) is a severe and progressive neuromuscular disorder characterized by myoclonus or myoclonus epilepsy, muscle weakness and wasting, deafness, cerebellar ataxia, and dementia (Wallace *et al.*, 1988b). The molecular genetic investigation disclosed an A → G transition at nt 8344 in the tRNA^{Lys} gene (Shoffner *et al.*, 1990). A positive correlation was found between mtDNA heteroplasmy and clinical severity, age of onset and defective mtDNA-dependent respiratory chain enzymes (Shoffner *et al.*, 1990).

Genetic heterogeneity occurs also in the MERRF syndrome since the 8344 mutation has not been found in all pedigrees. Indeed, a second mutation in the same tRNA^{Lys}gene at nt 8356 has been recently reported in two families (Silvestri *et al.*, 1992; Zeviani *et al.*, 1993).

Mitochondrial encephalomyopathy, lactic acidosis, and stroke-like episodes (MELAS). Diagnosis of MELAS is based on the following obligatory criteria: (1) stroke-like episodes (with corresponding focal brain lesions confirmed by CT or MRI scan), and (2) lactic acidosis and/or presence of RRF in the muscle biopsy, frequently associated with other signs of central nervous system involvement, including focal or generalized seizures, headache, deafness, recurrent vomiting and dementia (Pavlakis *et al.*, 1984; Ciafaloni *et al.*, 1992). MELAS was first associated with a heteroplasmic A → G transition at nucleotide 3243, involving one of the two tRNA for leucine (Goto *et al.*, 1990). As already observed in MERRF pedigrees, mtDNA heteroplasmy correlated with the severity of the clinical involvement, since levels above 90 per cent of mutant mtDNA were found only in severely compromised patients. A second point mutation involving the same gene but at nucleotide 3271 was reported in some 3243-negative patients (Goto *et al.*, 1991). It must be underlined that the phenotypic expression of the 3243 mutation is quite variable since it has been reported in a few patients with PEO without stroke not associated with mtDNA deletions (Hammans *et al.*, 1991).

Recently, the mtDNA 3243 mutation has been found in two pedigrees affected with maternally transmitted diabetes mellitus and deafness (Reardon *et al.*, 1992; van den Ouweland *et al.*, 1992).

Maternally-inherited myopathy and cardiomyopathy (Mimyca) has been reported in two pedigrees (Zeviani *et al.*, 1991; Sweeney *et al.*, 1993). The clinical features are those of a proximal myopathy with exercise intolerance, increased blood lactate at rest and during exercise, and a reduced cardiac ejection fraction, without clinical signs of central nervous system involvement. The most severely compromised patient had a severe myopathy associated with hypertrophic cardiomyopathy. A heteroplasmic A → G transition was found at nt 3260, affecting the same tRNA gene for leucine involved in the MELAS syndrome. A positive correlation was found between mtDNA heteroplasmy, clinical compromise, oxygen consumption *in vivo* and the activity of the respiratory chain in muscle.

In addition to the tRNA^{Leu} gene mutations associated with MELAS, Mimyca and maternally inherited diabetes and deafness, other point mutations have been identified in the same gene in patients affected with myopathy, or myopathy and cardiomyopathy (Moraes *et al.*, 1993). Therefore, the tRNA^{Leu} gene appears to be a mutational hot-spot in the mitochondrial genome, suggesting the need for extensive molecular genetic studies in patients negative for the A3243G mutation.

(2) *mit* − point mutations:

Leber's hereditary optic neuroretinopathy (LHON) is a maternally inherited disease characterized by juvenile onset and acute or subacute loss of central vision due to bilateral optic atrophy. The disease has a variable penetrance and a characteristic male predominance. The visual defect can be the only clinical feature or, less frequently, it can be associated with cardiac conduction abnormalities, peripheral neuropathy or ataxia. The first point mutation of mtDNA associated with LHON was a homoplasmic G → A transition at nt 11778 in the gene encoding subunit 4 of complex I (ND4). This mutation has been reported in about two-thirds of LHON families (Wallace *et al.*, 1988a). The genetic heterogeneity of the disease has been confirmed by the identification of other point mutations involving genes encoding different subunits of the respiratory chain complexes, including subunits ND1, ND2 and ND5 of complex I, subunit I of COX, and cytochrome *b* (Wallace & Lott, 1993). Some of these mutations probably act as primary mutations, since they are able to determine the LHON phenotype in isolation ('major mutations'), while others may interact synergistically ('minor mutations'). The pathogenic potential of the minor mutations must be rather mild, since some of them have been reported with low frequencies in the general population.

Apart from the pathogenic significance of the mtDNA mutations associated with LHON, several aspects of the disease remain unexplained. For instance, the mutations are usually homoplasmic in all of the maternal relatives of a LHON pedigree, regardless of the clinical status. The lack of genetic differences in the mtDNA of affected and normal individuals implies that other factors, either genetic or epigenetic, contribute to the penetrance and expressivity of the disease. The multifactorial aetiopathogenesis of LHON could also explain other puzzling aspects of this disease, such as the male predominance, the variable penetrance, the reported later onset for females, and the apparently selective involvement of the optic nerve. The hypothesis of LHON as a two-loci – mitochondrial and X-linked – disorder has been proposed to explain male predominance (Vilkki *et al.*, 1991), but it has not been confirmed by further linkage studies.

Neuropathy, ataxia and retinitis pigmentosa complex (NARP) is a rare maternally inherited syndrome characterized by the association of retinitis pigmentosa, ataxia, seizures, proximal neurogenic muscle weakness, sensory neuropathy and dementia. Ragged-red fibres have not been found in the muscle biopsy. The disease has been associated with a heteroplasmic point mutation at nt 8993 involving subunit 6 of mitochondrial ATPase. A positive correlation was found between the degree of heteroplasmy and the clinical compromise, which becomes evident for levels of mutant mtDNA above 80 per cent (Holt *et al.*, 1990). Further investigation in another family demonstrated that when mutant mtDNA is more than 95 per cent of total mtDNA, the mutation is associated with a severe infantile encephalopathy with neuropathological lesions in the basal ganglia and brainstem typical of Leigh's syndrome (Tatuch *et al.*, 1992; Santorelli *et al.*, 1993). Moreover, patients with NARP and Leigh's syndrome were observed in the same pedigree. An important consequence of this observation is that the NARP mutation should be investigated in patients affected with Leigh's syndrome, especially in those with no cytochrome *c* oxidase or pyruvate dehydrogenase deficiency (see below).

Molecular pathogenesis of the *syn* − mutations

Data from studies on muscle tissue demonstrated that, in the presence of the most common *syn*$^-$ mutations, the overall mitochondrial protein synthesis is markedly impaired *in vitro*. Point mutations involving tRNA genes are thought to be responsible for a reduced availability of functional tRNAs and hence reduced translation of mtDNA. Cybrids containing either the MERRF or the MELAS mutations (Chomyn *et al.*, 1991; Yoneda *et al.*, 1992) showed that above a given threshold of mutant mtDNA, mitochondrial protein synthesis and the respiratory activity are reduced, confirming the correlation between the mitochondrial genotype and the clinical and biochemical phenotypes. However, the pathogenetic linkage between the molecular defect and the clinical expression is still missing. It is surprising that mutations that involve the same biochemical pathway (i.e. Oxphos) are associated with strikingly different clinical phenotypes. For instance, MELAS and Mimyca are different disorders associated with mutations involving the same tRNA gene. Moreover, the A3243G mutation can cause phenotypes as different as MELAS, PEO or isolated diabetes mellitus. We already mentioned the case of LHON, in which the same mutation can cause blindness in one individual and be completely silent in another. Epigenetic factors, different nuclear backgrounds, or the association with other, still unknown, mutations of mtDNA have been invoked to explain the variable expressivity of the mutations. An additional explanation could be the existence of cryptic functions in different regions of the mtDNA molecule, whose impairment could produce specific effects and therefore have different consequences at the phenotypic level. For instance, the A3243G mutation affects the binding site of mtTERM, a nuclear protein involved in the control of transcription of the rRNA genes (Hess et al., 1991). Therefore, it is possible that the mutation can affect ribosomal function, in addition to causing abnormality of the tRNALeu. Further studies are necessary to determine as to whether this double molecular effect can influence the specific clinical expression of the A3243G mutation.

Defects of nuclear DNA

Defects of genes encoding subunits of the mitochondrial respiratory chain

As already mentioned, most of the protein subunits of the mitochondrial respiratory chain complexes are encoded by nDNA. The possibility of a respiratory chain deficiency caused by a defect of a nuclear gene was suggested by the clinical observation of familial cases with Mendelian inheritance, and by the biochemical finding of severe isolated enzyme defects. However, no molecular defects have been identified to date, and the current classification is based on biochemical findings only (Table 2).

Table 3. Clinical features associated with defects of the respiratory chain

Complex I:	– Fatal infantile syndrome
	– Myopathy (childhood or adult onset)
	– Encephalomyopathy (childhood or adult onset)
Complex II:	– Infantile encephalomyopathy
	– Infantile myopathy
Complex III:	– Myopathy
	– Encephalomyopathy (from birth to adult onset)
	– Histiocytoid cardiomyopathy of infancy
Complex IV:	– Fatal infantile myopathy
	– Benign infantile myopathy
	– Subacute necrotizing encephalopathy (Leigh's Syndrome)
Complex V:	– Myopathy (congenital)
	– Encephalomyopathy

The clinical features of the respiratory chain defects are extremely heterogeneous (Table 3). Several cases have been reported in the literature, with neonatal, infantile, juvenile or adult onset (Di Mauro & Moraes, 1993). We will focus here on the main clinical pictures of paediatric interest.

Fatal infantile multisystem disorders or severe encephalomyopathic syndromes are frequently associated with defects of respiratory complex I or complex III. The clinical features are usually those of severe psychomotor delay, generalized hypotonia, lactic acidosis and signs of cardiorespiratory failure. Patients with onset in childhood usually have various combinations of signs of central and peripheral nervous system involvement such as dementia, ataxia, seizures, hearing loss, pigmentary retinopathy, movement disorders and polyneuropathy.

Defects of complex IV (cytochrome c oxidase, COX) need particular attention. Two main clinical forms, myopathic and encephalomyopathic, have been identified.

The *myopathic* form is characterized by severe muscle weakness, leading to ventilatory insufficiency, and lactic acidosis. The disease must be thoroughly investigated since the fatal form, causing death before 1 year of age, must be differentiated from the benign form, which is initially indistinguishable, but that later undergoes a spontaneous and progressive improvement up to remission by the age of 3 years.

The *encephalomyopathic* form (Leigh's syndrome or subacute necrotizing encephalopathy) is characterized by a severe and predominant involvement of the central nervous system (Van Coster *et al.*, 1991). Affected children are usually normal up to 1 year of age, when they present psychomotor delay, recurrent vomiting, ophthalmoplegia, cerebellar and pyramidal signs, dystonia, seizures, and respiratory abnormalities. Lactic acid is increased in both plasma and cerebrospinal fluid. MRI of the brain is particularly important in the diagnosis of this severe fatal encephalomyopathy. The disease is associated with focal and symmetrical lesions in the brainstem, thalamus and posterior columns of the spinal cord. Biochemically, a defect of complex IV was found in the majority of patients; defects of the pyruvate dehydrogenase complex or respiratory complex I are less frequent. As already mentioned, the NARP point mutation at nt 8993 has been recently reported in children affected with Leigh's syndrome without COX or pyruvate dehydrogenase deficiency.

Defects of mitochondrial protein importation

The majority of mitochondrial peptides are synthesized in the cytoplasm as larger precursors containing a leader peptide. After addressing the protein to mitochondria by interaction with specific receptors, the leader peptide is cleaved before the mature protein is assembled in its final intramitochondrial compartment. A defect of protein importation caused by abnormalities of the leader peptide was first described by Ledley *et al.* (1990). They reported a variant of methylmalonic acidaemia caused by a nonsense mutation in the leader sequence of the enzyme methylmalonyl CoA-mutase that, as a consequence, could not be imported into mitochondria. Another example of impaired translocation was proposed by Schapira *et al.* (1990) in a patient affected with a congenital myopathy. Morphological studies revealed the complete absence of the histochemical stain for succinate dehydrogenase (complex II) in muscle. Biochemical studies demonstrated a specific defect of two iron-sulfur proteins, one belonging to succinate dehydrogenase and the other, the Riske protein, to complex III. Since the Riske protein was detected in the cytosol and in the muscle homogenate but was absent in isolated mitochondria, the authors suggested that, in this patient, the primary defect propably involved mitochondrial protein importation.

Defects of nuclear DNA – mitochondrial DNA communication

Several housekeeping functions of mtDNA, such as replication, transcription and translation, rely upon enzymes encoded by nuclear genes. Two human disorders, transmitted by Mendelian inheritance, have been recently identified and considered as examples of impaired cross-talk between the mitochondrial and the nuclear genomes.

Autosomal dominant chronic progressive external ophthalmoplegia (AD-CPEO) was first reported by Zeviani *et al.*, (1989, 1990) in several Italian families. The clinical features of the disease are that of adult-onset CPEO associated with proximal muscle weakness and wasting, and, in several cases, ataxia, vestibular areflexia, cataracts, and sensory-motor peripheral neuropathy. Ragged-red fibres, partially COX-depleted fibres and neurogenic changes were found in muscle biopsy specimens, and reduced activities of mtDNA-encoded enzymes were measured in the muscles. Southern blot analysis demonstrated the presence of multiple deletions of mtDNA. Most deletions spanned the mtDNA molecule between the end of the D-loop and the gene for COX I, but spared the origins of both H-strand and L-strand replication. The autosomal dominant transmission observed in several families pointed to a mutation in a nuclear gene, whose abnormal product might interact, presumably during replication, with mtDNA, causing the accumulation of deleted molecules.

Depletion of mtDNA has been recently reported as the first disorder associated with a quantitative alteration of mtDNA (Moraes *et al.*, 1991; Tritschler *et al.*, 1992). The clinical manifestations of reported cases fall into three main groups. The first was affected by a fatal infantile hepatopathy causing liver failure and death by the age of 9 months, or by a congenital severe myopathy with ragged-red fibres causing respiratory insufficiency and death by age 11 months; in some of these (the second group) patients muscle involvement was associated with a DeToni–Fanconi syndrome. The third group had a later onset, usually at about 1 year of age, with a progressive proximal myopathy and death due to respiratory failure by 3 years of age. Southern blot analysis revealed a severe depletion of mtDNA in affected tissues. Inheritance of the disease was autosomal recessive, suggesting a mutation in a nuclear gene involved in mtDNA replication. Molecular genetic analysis of mtDNA is particularly important in these patients since the clinical manifestations may be indistinguishable from those of isolated COX deficiency reported above.

Diagnostic considerations

The diagnosis of mtDNA disorders relies on clinical, morphological, biochemical and molecular genetic data.

Detailed clinical observation is important in addressing the subsequent diagnostic protocol. Particular attention must be paid to patients with well-defined maternally inherited syndromes, in which the investigation of the whole pedigree is mandatory to identify asymptomatic maternal relatives carrying a given point mutation of mtDNA. The general concept of tissue vulnerability is helpful in suspecting a mitochondrial disorder in patients with atypical presentations: the association of symptoms and signs suggesting the involvement of apparently unrelated tissues may lead to the correct diagnosis.

Examination of the muscle morphology is necessary in the majority of candidate patients, even though the absence of ragged-red fibres or other morphological signs does not exclude the diagnosis. Moreover, the availability of muscle tissue is particularly important for biochemical studies and for molecular genetic analysis, particularly in patients with maternally inherited phenotypes, since the percentage of detectable mutant mtDNA is significantly higher in muscle than in other tissues, such as peripheral blood lymphocytes.

Recent advances in molecular genetic analysis of mtDNA have provided powerful diagnostic tools. Indeed, mtDNA analysis is positive in more than 50 per cent of patients with morphologically and/or biochemically proven mitochondrial phenotypes. Due to the heterogeneity and variable clinical presentation of mitochondrial encephalomyopathies, mtDNA analysis may be of considerable help in the differential diagnosis of several identified and still unidentified syndromes.

References

Anderson, S., Bankier, A.T., Barrel, B.G., de Bruijn, M.H.L., Coulson, A.R., Drouin, J., Eperon, I.C., Nierlich, D.P., Roe, B.A., Sanger, F., Schreier, P.H., Smith, A.J.H., Staden, R. & Young, I.G. (1981): Sequence and organization of the human mitochondrial genome. *Nature* **290**, 457–465.

Chomyn, A., Meola, G., Bresolin, N., Lai, S.T., Scarlato, G. & Attardi, G. (1991): *In vitro* genetic transfer of protein synthesis and respiration defects to mitochondrial DNA-less cells with myopathy- patient mitochondria. *Mol. Cell. Biol.* **11**, 2236–2244.

Ciafaloni, E., Ricci, E., Shanske, S., Moraes, C.T., Silvestri, G., Hirano, M., Angelini, C., Donati, A., Garcia, C., Martinuzzi, A., Mosewich, R., Servidei, S., Zammarchi, E., Bonilla, E., De Vivo, D.C., Rowland, L.P., Schon, E.A. & DiMauro, S. (1992): MELAS: clinical features, biochemistry and molecular genetics. *Ann. Neurol.* **31,** 391–398.

Di Mauro, S. & Moraes, C.T. (1993): Mitochondrial encephalomyopathies. *Arch. Neurol.* **40,** 1197–1208.

Goto, Y., Nonaka, I., & Horai, S. (1990): A mutation in the tRNA$^{Leu(UUR)}$ gene associated with the MELAS subgroup of mitochondrial encephalomyopathies. *Nature* 348–653.

Goto, Y., Nonaka, I. & Horai, S. (1991): A new mtDNA mutation associated with mitochondrial myopathy, encephalopathy, lactic acidosis and stroke-like episodes (MELAS). *Biochim. Biophys. Acta* **1097,** 238–240.

Hammans, S.R., Sweeney, M.G., Brockington, M., Morgan Hughes, J.A. & Harding, A.E. (1991): Mitochondrial encephalopathies: molecular genetic diagnosis from blood samples. *Lancet* **337,** 1311–1313.

Hayashi, J.I., Ohta, S., Kikuchi, A., Takemitsu, M., Goto, Y.I. & Nonaka, I. (1991): Introduction of disease-related mitochondrial DNA deletions into HeLa cells lacking mitochondrial DNA results in mitochondrial dysfunction. *Proc. Natl. Acad. Sci. USA* **88,** 10614–10618.

Hess, J.F., Parisi, M.A., Bennet, J.L. & Clayton, D.A. (1991): Impairment of mitochondrial transcription termination by a point mutation associated with the MELAS subgroup of mitochondrial encephalomyopathies. *Nature* **351,** 236–239.

Holt, I.J., Harding, A.E. & Morgan Hughes, J.A. (1988): Deletions of muscle mitochondrial DNA in patients with mitochondrial myopathies. *Nature* **331,** 717–719.

Holt, I.J., Harding, A.E., Petty, R.H.K. & Morgan Hughes, J.A. (1990): A new mitochondrial disease associated with mitochondrial DNA heteroplasmy. *Am. J. Hum. Genet.* **46,** 428–433.

Ledley, F.D., Janse, R., Nham, S.U., Fenton, W.A. & Rosenberg, L.E. (1990): Mutation eliminating mitochondrial leader sequence of methylmalonyl-CoA mutase causes mut^{o}methylmalonic acidemia. *Proc. Natl. Acad. Sci. USA* **87,** 3147–3150.

McShane, M.A., Hammans, S.R., Sweeney, M., Holt, I.J., Beattie, T.J., Brett, E.M. & Harding, A.E. (1991): Pearson syndrome and mitochondrial encephalomyopathy in a patient with a deletion of mtDNA. *Am. J. Hum. Genet.* **48,** 39–42.

Mita, S., Schmidt, B., Schon, E.A., Di Mauro, S. & Bonilla, E. (1989): Detection of deleted mitochondrial genomes in cytochdrome *c* oxidase-deficient muscle fibers of a patient with Kearns–Sayre syndrome. *Proc. Natl. Acad. Sci. USA* **86,** 9509–9513.

Moraes, C.T., Di Mauro, S., Zeviani, M., Lombes, A., Shanske, S., Miranda, A.F., Nakase, H., Bonilla, E., Werneck, L.C., Servidei, S., Nonaka, I., Koga, Y., Spiro, A.J., Brownell, K.W., Schmidt, B., Schotland, D.L., Zupanc, M., De Vivo, D.C., Schon, E. & Rowland, L.P. (1989): Mitochondrial DNA deletions in progressive external ophthalmoplegia and Kearns–Sayre syndrome. *N. Engl. J. Med.* **320,** 1293–1299.

Moraes, C.T., Shanske, S., Tritschler, H-J., Aprille, J.R., Andreetta F., Bonilla, E., Schon, E.A. & Di Mauro, S. (1991): mtDNA depletion with variable tissue expression: a novel genetic abnormality in mitochondrial diseases. *Am. J. Hum. Genet.* **48,** 492–501.

Moraes, C.T., Ciacci, F., Bonilla, E., Jansen, C., Hirano, M., Rao, N., Lovelace, R.E., Rowland, L.P., Schon, E.A. & Di Mauro, S. (1993): Two novel pathogenic mitochondrial DNA mutations affecting organelle number and protein synthesis. Is the tRNA$^{Leu(UUR)}$ gene an etiologic hot spot? *J. Clin. Invest.* **92,** 2906–2915.

Pavlakis, S.G., Phillips, P.C., Di Mauro, S., DeVivo D.C. & Rowland, L.P. (1984): Mitochondrial myopathy, encephalomyopathy, lactic acidosis and stroke-like episodes: a distinctive clinical syndrome. *Ann. Neurol.* **16,** 481–488.

Reardon, W., Ross, R.J.M., Sweeney, M.G., Luxon, L.M., Pembrey, M.E., Harding, A.E. & Trembath, R.C. (1992): Diabetes mellitus associated with a pathogenic point mutation in mitochondrial DNA. *Lancet* **340,** 1376–1379.

Rotig, A., Cormier, V., Blache, S., Bonnefont, J-P., Ledeist, F., Romero, N., Schmitz, J., Rustin, P., Fischer, A., Saudubray, J-M. & Munnich A. (1990): Person's marrow–pancreas syndrome. A multisystem mitochondrial disorder of infancy. *J. Clin. Invest.* **86,** 1601–1608.

Santorelli, F.M., Shanske, S., Macaya, A., De Vivo, D.C. & Di Mauro, S. (1993): The mutation at nt 8993 of mitochondrial DNA is a common cause of Leigh's syndrome. *Ann. Neurol.* **34,** 827–834.

Schapira, A.H.V., Cooper, J.M., Morgan Hughes, J.A., Landon, D.N. & Clark, J.B. (1990): Mitochondrial myopathy with a defect of mitochondrial protein transport. *N. Engl. J. Med.* **323,** 37–42.

Schon, E., Rizzuto, R., Moraes, C.T., Nakase, H., Zeviani, M. & Di Mauro, S. (1989): A direct repeat is a hot spot for large-scale deletions of human mitochondrial DNA. *Science* **244,** 346–349.

Shanske, S., Moraes, C.T., Lombes, A., Miranda, A.F., Bonilla, E., Lewis, P., Whelan, M.A., Ellsworth, C.A. & Di Mauro, S. (1990): Widespread tissue distribution of mitochondrial DNA deletions in Kearns–Sayre syndrome. *Neurology* **40,** 24–28.

Shoffner, J.M., Lott, M.T., Voljavec, A.S. Soueidan, S.A., Costigan, D.A. & Wallace, D.C. (1989): Spontaneous Kearns–Sayre/chronic external ophthalmoplegia plus syndrome associated with a mitochondrial DNA deletion: a slip replication model and metabolic therapy. *Proc. Natl. Acad. Sci. USA* **86**, 7952–7856.

Shoffner, J.M., Lott, M.T., Lezza, A.M.S., Seibel, P., Ballinger, S.W. & Wallace, D.C. (1990): Myoclonic epilepsy and ragged-red fibers disease (MERRF) is associated with a mitochondrial DNA tRNA^{Lys} mutation. *Cell* **61**, 931–937.

Shoubridge, E.A., Karpati, G. & Hastings, K.E.M. (1990): Deletion mutants are functionally dominant over wild-type mitochondrial genomes in skeletal muscle fiber segments in mitochondrial diseases. *Cell* **62**, 43–49.

Silvestri, G., Moraes, C.T., Shanske, S., Oh, S.J. & DiMauro, S. (1992): A new mtDNA mutation in the tRNA^{Lys} gene associated with myoclonic epilepsy and ragged-red fibers (MERRF). *Am. J. Hum. Genet.* **51**, 1213–1217.

Sweeney, M.G., Brockington, M.J., Morgan-Hughes, J.A. & Harding, A.E. (1993): Mitochondrial DNA transfer mutation Leu(UUR) A $\rightarrow$ G 3260: a second family with myopathy and cardiomyopathy. *Q.J. Med.* **86**, 435–438.

Tatuch, Y., Christodoulou, J., Feigenbaum, A., Clarke, J.T.R., Wherret, J., Smith C., Rudd, N., Petrova-Benedict, P. & Robinson, B.H. (1992): Heteroplasmic mtDNA mutation (T $\rightarrow$ G) at 8993 can cause Leigh disease when the percentage of abnormal mtDNA is high. *Am. J. Hum. Genet.* **50**, 852–858.

Tritschler, H-J., Andreetta, F., Moraes, C.T., Bonilla, E., Arnaudo, E., Danon, M.J., Glass, S., Zelaya, B.M., Vamos, E., Telerman-Toppet, N., Shanske, S., Kadenbach, B., Di Mauro, S. & Schon, E.A. (1992): Mitochondrial myopathy of childhood with depletion of mitochondrial DNA. *Neurology* **42**, 209–217.

Tzagoloff, A. (1982): *Mitochondria*. ed. P. Siekievitz. New York, London: Plenum Press.

Van Coster, R., Lombes, A., De Vivo, D.C., Chi, L.T., Dodson, W.E., Rothman, S., Orrechio, E.J., Grover, W., Bery, G.T., Schwartz, J.F., Habib, A. & Di Mauro, S. (1991): Cytochrome *c* oxidase-associated Leigh syndrome: phenotypic features and pathogenetic speculations. *J. Neurol. Sci.* **104**, 97–111.

Van den Ouweland, J.M.W., Lemkes, H.H.P.J., Ruitenbeek, W., Sandkuijl, L.A., de Vijlder M.F., Struyvenberg, P.A.A., van de Kamp, J.J.P. & Maassen, J.A. (1992): Mutation in mitochondrial tRNA$^{Leu(UUR)}$ gene in a large pedigree with maternally transmitted type II diabetes mellitus and deafness. *Nature Genet* **1**, 368–371.

Vilkki, J., Ott, J., Savountas, M.L., Aula, P. & Nikoskelainen, E.K. (1991): Optic atrophy in Leber hereditary optic neuroretinopathy is probably determined by an X-chromosomal gene linked to DXS7. *Am. J. Hum. Genet.* **48**, 486–491.

Wallace, D.C., Singh, G., Lott, M.T., Hodge, J.E., Schur, T.G., Lezza, A.M.S. Elsas, II, L.J. & Nikoskelainen, E.K. (1988a): Mitochondrial DNA mutation associated with Leber's hereditary optic neuropathy. *Science* **242**, 1427–1430.

Wallace, D.C., Zeng, X., Lott, M.T., Shoffner, J.M., Hodge, J.A., Kelley, R.I., Epstein, C.M. & Hopkins, L.C. (1988b): Familial mitochondrial encephalomyopathy (MERRF): genetic, pathophysiological and biochemical characterization of a mitochondrial DNA disease. *Cell* **55**, 601–610.

Wallace, D.C. & Lott M.T. (1993): Maternally inherited diseases. In: *Mitochondrial DNA in human pathology*, eds. S. Di Mauro & D.C. Wallace, pp. 63–83. New York: Raven Press.

Yoneda, M., Chomyn, A., Martinuzzi, A., Hurko, O. & Attardi, G. (1992): Marked replicative advantage of human mtDNA carrying a point mutation that causes the MELAS encephalomyopathy. *Proc. Natl. Acad. Sci. USA* **89**, 11164–11168.

Zeviani, M., Moraes, T., Di Mauro, S., Nakase, H., Bonilla, E., Schon, E.A. & Rowland, L.P. (1988): Deletions of mitochondrial DNA in Kearn–Sayre syndrome. *Neurology* **38**, 1339–1346.

Zeviani, M., Servidei, S., Gellera, C., Bertini, E., Di Mauro, S. & Di Donato, S. (1989): An autosomal dominant disorder with multiple deletions of mitochondrial DNA starting at the D-loop region. *Nature* **339**, 309–311.

Zeviani, M., Bresolin, N., Gellera, C., Bordoni, A., Pannacci, M., Amati, P., Moggio, M., Servidei, S., Scarlato, G. & Di Donato, S. (1990): Nucleus-driven multiple large-scale deletions of the human mitochondrial genome: a new autosomal dominant disease. *Am. J. Hum. Genet.* **47**, 904–914.

Zeviani, M., Gellera, C., Pannacci, M., Uziel, G., Prelle, A., Servidei, S. & Di Donato, S. (1990): Tissue distribution and transmission of mitochondrial DNA deletions in mitochondrial myopathies. *Ann. Neurol.* **28**, 94–97.

Zeviani, M., Gellera, C., Antozzi, C., Rimoldi, M., Morandi, L., Villani, F., Tiranti, V. & Di Donato, S. (1991): Maternally inherited myopathy and cardiomyopathy: association with mutation in mitochondrial DNA tRNA$^{Leu(UUR)}$. *Lancet* **338**, 143–147.

Zeviani, M. & Antozzi, C. (1992): Defects of mitochondrial DNA. *Brain Pathol.* **2**, 121–132.

Zeviani, M., Muntoni, F., Savarese, N., Serra, G., Tiranti, V., Carrara, F., Mariotti, C. & Di Donato, S. (1993): A MERRF/MELAS overlap syndrome associated with a new point mutation in the mitochondrial DNA tRNA^{Lys} gene. *Eur. J. Hum. Genet.* **1**, 80–87.

Chapter 4

Lactic acidaemia: clinical diagnosis, treatment, and prognosis

Darryl C. De Vivo and Christine K. Wade

Departments of Neurology and Pediatrics, Division of Pediatric Neurology, Program in Physical Therapy, Columbia Presbyterian Medical Center, New York, NY 10032, USA

Summary

Lactic acidaemia signifies a primary or secondary disturbance of pyruvate metabolism. Genetically determined abnormalities of pyruvate metabolism include enzyme defects of gluconeogenesis, pyruvate dehydrogenase, Krebs cycle, respiratory chain, or more remote defects involving organic acid and fatty acid metabolism. Associated metabolic abnormalities facilitate the identification of the underlying biochemical defect causing lactic acidaemia. Hypoglycaemia suggests a gluconeogenic defect, or a more remote abnormality affecting fatty acid oxidation. Relative resistance to hypoglycaemia suggests pyruvate dehydrogenase deficiency. Normal lactate:pyruvate ratios occur with pyruvate dehydrogenase deficiency, and may be associated with gluconeogenic defects, Krebs cycle defects, respiratory chain defects, and several organic acidurias. Increased ratios of lactate:pyruvate and β-hydroxybutyrate: acetoacetate signify a defect involving the respiratory chain. Elevated lactate:pyruvate ratios and lowered β-hydroxybutyrate:acetoacetate ratios suggest pyruvate carboxylase deficiency.

Cerebrospinal fluid lactate values may be informative. Primary disorders affecting cerebral metabolism are distinguished by elevated cerebrospinal fluid lactate values, usually higher than blood lactate values. On occasion, only the CSF lactate will be elevated, a condition referred to as cerebral lactic acidosis.

The genetic patterns of inheritance associated with the lactic acidaemias include autosomal recessive, X-linked, and maternal inheritance. Pyruvate dehydrogenase deficiency may be transmitted as an X-linked or autosomal recessive trait. Defects of gluconeogenesis and the Krebs cycle are transmitted as autosomal recessive traits. Respiratory chain defects may be transmitted as autosomal recessive, autosomal dominant, or maternal traits. Maternal inheritance signifies a mutation of mitochondrial DNA.

Treatment options are limited in most cases of lactic acidaemia. Continuous intragastric feedings are useful in the hypoglycaemic syndromes, and may be helpful in the other disorders of energy metabolism. Cofactor supplementation may be helpful in selected instances, most notably biotinidase deficiency. Supplementation with thiamine, lipoic acid, riboflavin, coenzyme Q_{10}, folic acid, and L-carnitine have been tried, but double-blind placebo-controlled studies will be necessary to evaluate the efficacy of these supplements. Sodium bicarbonate has been used traditionally to correct the metabolic acidosis. This agent has no effect on the lactic acidaemia, and may paradoxically lower the cerebral pH. Sodium dichloroacetate, an experimental agent, specifically lowers the lactate concentrations, and may be specifically useful in treating cerebral lactic acidosis.

Prognosis is determined by the underlying mechanism causing the lactic acidaemia. In general, those biochemical conditions that directly involve the central nervous system have a more guarded prognosis. The family must be counselled regarding the genetic implications, and the availability of prenatal diagnosis.

Introduction

Lactic acidaemia is the laboratory signature of many conditions that interfere with the metabolism of pyruvate. Pyruvate and lactate are linked together by a pyridine nucleotide-dependent reaction catalysed by the enzyme, lactate dehydrogenase:

$$\text{Pyruvate} + \text{NADH} + \text{H}^+ \leftrightarrow \text{Lactate} + \text{NAD}^+$$

Under normal metabolic conditions, this equilibrium is maintained by the mass action of the reactants, and the blood lactate value ranges from 1–2 mmol/l. The ratio of lactate to pyruvate is also tightly maintained in the range of 10–15. Ratios exceeding 20 are abnormal, and increasingly signify a disturbance of the cellular oxidation–reduction state.

Pyruvate has several metabolic fates. This substrate is mainly synthesized by the glycolytic metabolism of glucose in the cytosolic compartment of the cell. A few tissues have no oxidative capability, and pyruvate is converted to lactate. Erythrocytes are a good example. Other tissues may have a high glycolytic rate, and oxidative metabolism is suppressed, the so-called Crabtree effect. Again, lactate is synthesized. The other tissues are metabolically able to oxidize pyruvate aerobically to carbon dioxide and water, and only small amounts of lactate are produced in these tissues.

Lactate production from these various mechanisms has been quantified under physiological conditions (Kreisberg *et al.*, 1970) as shown in Table 1.

Table 1. Lactate production by body tissues (data shown as per cent of total)

Tissue	Per cent total:
Erythrocytes	25
Skin	25
Brain	15
Skeletal muscle (white)	14
Intestinal mucosa	7
Renal medulla	13

About 65 per cent of the lactate produced by these body tissues is removed by the liver for gluconeogenesis. The remaining 35 per cent is removed by extrahepatic tissues such as red muscle and kidney cortex for oxidation to carbon dioxide and water.

The resting blood lactate values will be altered by vigorous physical activity, and blood values as high as 22 mmol/l have been documented in athletes subjected to exhausting exercise (Hermansen *et al.*, 1975). Under such circumstances, the lactic acidaemia returns slowly over 6–8 h to normal resting values. These physiological observations underscore the difficulty of interpreting exercise-provoked lactate elevations in unconditioned subjects, and patients with suspected enzyme defects in intermediary metabolism.

Normally, the lactate values differ in various body fluids such as arterial blood, venous blood, and cerebrospinal fluid. The values are lowest in the arterial blood, intermediate in the venous blood, and slightly higher in the cerebrospinal fluid. Artifacts of sampling also may confuse the observations. Skin has a high content of lactic acid reflecting the fact that this tissue is mainly anaerobic. Application of a tourniquet may compromise oxygen supply to a limb and contribute to venous congestion of the tissue. These factors may cause the venous lactate to rise and disturb the lactate: pyruvate ratio. The cerebrospinal fluid lactate concentrations are more durable, but these values may also change with episodes of cerebral hypoxia and ischaemia. It is impossible to predict, in a given case, the rate at which the lactate value will return to normal. Interpretations of laboratory data under such conditions should be viewed cautiously. In our experience, these artefacts have been interpreted incorrectly on occasion, and patients have been investigated for a genetically-deter-

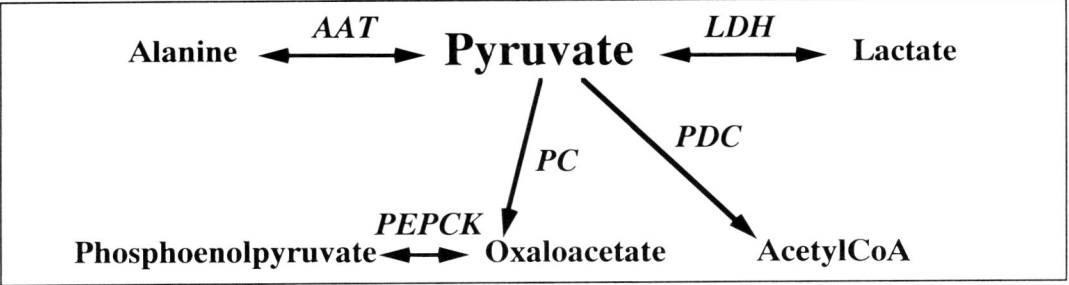

Fig. 1. The primary metabolic fates of pyruvate.

mined metabolic disease causing lactic acidaemia when an environmental stress is the more likely possibility. These caveats usually relate to elevated venous lactate values, in particular.

Elevations of the cerebrospinal fluid lactate values in the absence of systemic lactic acidaemia are particularly meaningful, and suggest that a primary disturbance of cerebral energy metabolism exists. In a study of 34 subjects, we obtained a mean cerebrospinal fluid lactate value of 1.63 mmol/l. Brown and colleagues have introduced the term 'cerebral lactic acidosis' to describe the situation when the biochemical defect is limited primarily or exclusively to the brain (Brown et al., 1988). Tissue-specific disturbances in mitochondrial metabolism are instructive examples.

Conversely, lactic acidaemia may exist in the absence of elevated cerebrospinal fluid lactate values. Having dismissed the artifactual possibilities mentioned earlier, this finding suggests that the enzyme defect involves non-neural tissues with sparing of the brain. Examples include gluconeogenic defects such as von Gierke's disease and fructose 1,6-bisphosphatase deficiency. This finding indicates that lactate diffuses across the blood–brain–barrier very slowly, and also supports the finding that lactate is a poor substrate for cerebral oxidative metabolism (Pardridge, 1983).

Metabolic fates of pyruvate

Pyruvate can be converted to several metabolites including oxaloacetate, acetyl-CoA, lactate, alanine, and phosphoenolpyruvate. These metabolic conversions are catalysed respectively by pyruvate carboxylase, the pyruvate dehydrogenase complex, lactate dehydrogenase, alanine aminotransferase, and phosphoenolpyruvate carboxykinase. These metabolic interrelationships are shown in Fig. 1.

Lactate and alanine are in equilibrium with pyruvate, and the steady-state concentrations of the metabolites are determined by the relative concentrations of the reactants, and by the hydrogen ion pressure in the case of lactate.

The conversion of pyruvate to acetyl-CoA is an irreversible step, and is dependent upon the mitochondrial availability of coenzyme A. This step also is modulated by the mitochondrial oxidation–reduction potential, the ratio of acetyl-CoA to coenzyme A, the phosphorylation potential, and other regional microchemical and hormonal influences. The conversion of pyruvate to oxaloacetate is influenced by the mitochondrial acetyl-CoA concentration as an allosteric effector. These modulating influences of the pyruvate dehydrogenase complex and pyruvate carboxylase can be perturbed by cellular factors related to various disease states. Therefore, lactic acidaemia can arise from more distant biochemical defects that directly affect tissue concentrations of coenzyme A, acyl-CoA pools, phosphorylation states, etc. Examples of such deficiencies include the organic acidurias, and fatty acid oxidation defects.

Pathological states affecting pyruvate metabolism

Many biochemical conditions can affect the tissue concentrations of pyruvate and lactate. The

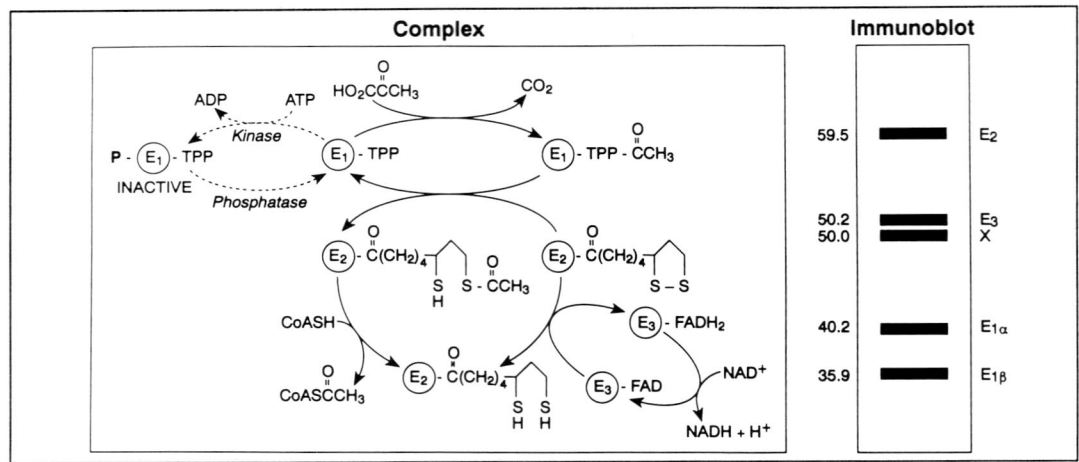

Fig. 2. The pyruvate dehydrogenase complex is composed of three catalytic steps (E_1, E_2, and E_3) and two regulatory steps (the kinase and the phosphatase). The principal subunits of the catalytic steps and the anchoring protein X are shown in the schematic immunoblot.

primary disorders directly affect the metabolism of pyruvate. The secondary disorders indirectly affect pyruvate metabolism. Lactic acidaemia has been reviewed recently by several authors (Robinson, 1989; De Vivo, 1994; Di Mauro & De Vivo, 1994), either specifically or in the context of mitochondrial diseases. The most common primary disorder of pyruvate metabolism is pyruvate dehydrogenase deficiency.

Pyruvate dehydrogenase deficiency

The net reaction of pyruvate conversion to acetyl-CoA is shown below:

$$\text{Pyruvate} + \text{CoASH} + \text{NAD}^+ \rightarrow \text{acetyl–CoA} + \text{NADH} + \text{H}^+ + \text{CO}_2$$

This reaction is catalysed by a multi-enzyme complex, pyruvate dehydrogenase complex (PDC), located in the mitochondria. The components of PDC are shown in Fig. 2. PDC is composed of five enzyme reactions, and at least nine different proteins. Four genes have been cloned. Two genes, one located on the X-chromosome and the other on chromosome 4, encode the E_1 alpha subunit. This subunit is pivotal in the catalytic activity of the enzyme complex, and is the site for phosphorylation. Mutations of the E_1 alpha subunit gene on the X-chromosome affect the catalytic efficiency of the complex directly, or indirectly by altering the phosphorylation–dephosphorylation regulation sequence. Mutations affecting the phospho E_1-phosphatase have a similar effect.

The gene for the E_1 beta subunit is located on chromosome 3; and the gene for the E_3 alpha subunit is located on chromosome 7.

A molecular defect involving the E_1 alpha subunit has emerged as the most common cause for PDC deficiency (Robinson et al., 1987; Brown et al., 1989; Dahl et al., 1992; Fujii et al., 1994). Robinson and colleagues (1987) grouped 54 cases of E_1 deficiency into four categories as determined by age at clinical presentation and death. Thirteen patients died before the age of 6 months, 12 died between the ages of 7 and 36 months, and 23 were alive at the time of publication with evidence of chronic psychomotor retardation, and six had a more benign recurrent syndrome manifested primarily by ataxia. The intensity of lactic acidaemia correlated roughly with the clinical grouping, but the residual enzyme activity in cultured skin fibroblasts correlated less well. The most severely affected infants presenting in the neonatal period had the lowest residual enzyme activity.

Our review of approximately 100 cases in the medical literature produced similar observations. We subdivided the patients into three categories: neonatal, infantile/early childhood, and benign (De Vivo & Van Coster, 1990).

The neonatal group presented with hypotonia, convulsions, episodic apnoea, poor suck, dysmorphic features, lethargy, low birth weight, failure to thrive, and coma. There was a male predominance. These patients usually died before age 8 months, and the neuropathology showed destructive lesions of the subcortical white matter, basal ganglia, and brainstem. Dismyelination, optic atrophy, hydrocephalus, agenesis of the corpus callosum, ectopic olivary nuclei, reactive gliosis, spongy degeneration of the neuropil, neuronal loss, and vascular proliferation represented associated pathological findings.

Patients in the infantile/early childhood group demonstrated psychomotor retardation, hypotonia, convulsions, episodic apnoea, pyramidal tract signs, ataxia, dysmorphic features, lethargy, deceleration of head growth with acquired microcephaly, optic atrophy and ophthalmoplegia, ptosis, dysphagia, peripheral neuropathy, deceleration in somatic growth, cranial nerve palsies, and extrapyramidal signs. Eighty-three percent of patients coming to autopsy (21 cases) had the neuropathological findings of Leigh's syndrome.

Seven male children had a more benign phenotype with episodic symptomatology. The clinical findings included post-exercise fatigue, fluctuating ataxia, transient paraparesis, and thiamine responsiveness. These boys demonstrated normal mental and motor development between episodes of metabolic decompensation.

A small number of patients have been reported with other biochemical defects involving the pyruvate dehydrogenase complex. One patient, a 3½-year-old girl, had an E_2 defect (Robinson et al., 1990). Clinical findings included psychomotor retardation, acquired microcephaly, moderate lactic acidosis and associated hyperammonaemia. Four patients have also been described with abnormalities of protein X (Robinson et al., 1990; Marsac et al., 1993). The first patient was symptomatic in infancy with hypotonia, poor head control, and subsequent psychomotor retardation. The parents were first cousins. The second patient was asymptomatic until the age of 3 years, when he developed an unstable gait. The CT scan demonstrated bilateral basal ganglia lucencies. The third and fourth cases were brothers of a consanguineous marriage. Protein X is important in the organization and function of the pyruvate dehydrogenase complex, and participates in the shuttling of electrons and acetyl groups between the E_2 and E_3 components.

Several patients have been described with defects of the E_3 component (Robinson et al., 1977, 1981; Munnich et al., 1982; Yoshida et al., 1990). The urinary organic acid profile is distinctive in these cases because the E_3 component is shared by pyruvate dehydrogenase, alpha-ketoglutarate dehydrogenase, and the alpha ketoacid dehydrogenase. As a result, these patients demonstrate elevated lactate, pyruvate, alanine, alpha-ketoglutarate, and branched-chain alpha-ketoacids.

Mutations affecting the pyruvate dehydrogenase complex may be transmitted genetically as autosomal recessive traits, or X-linked traits. Defects involving the E_2 and the E_3 components are likely to be transmitted as autosomal recessive traits, whereas defects involving the E_1 alpha subunit gene are transmitted as X-linked traits. The region of the E_1 alpha subunit gene on the X-chromosome is highly conserved. To date, 23 mutations of the E_1 alpha subunit gene have been described (Fujii et al., 1994). There is remarkable allelic heterogeneity in this group of mutations with point mutations, micro-deletions, and insertions. Eighteen of the mutations are unique, with a clustering of mutations at the C-terminus of the gene involving exons 10 and 11. Most mutations appear to be sporadic, and the clinical expression of the mutation and the phenotype is influenced by the non-random pattern of X-chromosome inactivation (Brown & Brown, 1993).

Defects of gluconeogenesis

Pyruvate, and other gluconeogenic substrates, are converted to glucose principally in the liver. The

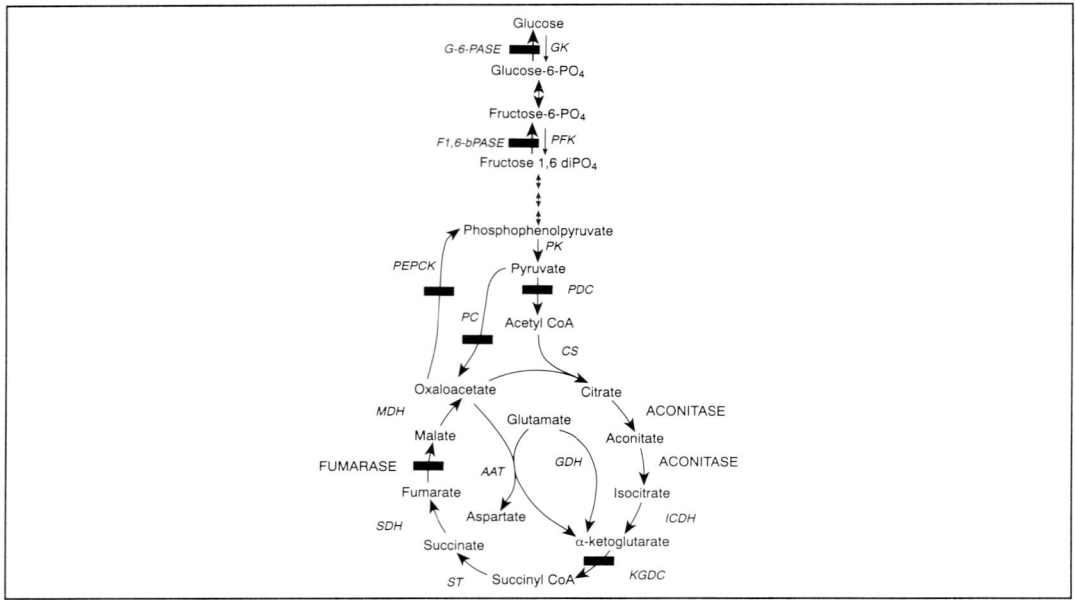

Fig. 3. Schematic overview of gluconeogenesis and the Krebs cycle showing the major blocks associated with lactic acidaemia.

four key steps in this pathway include glucose 6-phosphatase, fructose 1,6-bisphosphatase, phosphoenolpyruvate carboxykinase, and pyruvate carboxylase (Fig. 3).

An enzyme deficiency of the gluconeogenic pathway causes fasting hypoglycaemia and lactic acidaemia. The hypoglycaemia may be least severe in pyruvate carboxylase deficiency because some gluconeogenic precursors may enter the pathway beyond the site of the enzymatic block. The brain is not dependent on the gluconeogenic pathway directly. Therefore, neurological symptoms largely result from fasting hypoglycaemia. Pyruvate carboxylase is also essential in replenishing oxaloacetate to maintain optimal Krebs cycle activity. This anapleurotic function of pyruvate carboxylase is essential for brain metabolism.

Pyruvate carboxylase deficiency

Pyruvate carboxylase, one of the four known biotin-containing proteins found in mammalian tissues, catalyses the conversion of pyruvate to oxaloacetate as shown below:

$$\text{Pyruvate} + \text{ATP} + \text{HCO}_3^- \rightarrow \text{oxaloacetate} + \text{ADP}^- + P_i$$

Pyruvate carboxylase deficiency has been described in 35 patients, and usually has two distinct clinical presentations. These phenotypes are determined by the presence or absence of any residual enzyme activity (Robinson *et al.*, 1984).

The North American phenotype is associated with the presence of immunoreactive enzyme protein and residual catalytic activity (De Vivo *et al.*, 1977; Atkin *et al.*, 1979b). These infants present with severe psychomotor delay, and death occurs in infancy or early childhood. The metabolic findings include lactic acidosis, ketosis, an increased lactate: pyruvate ratio, and a decreased β-hydroxybutyrate:acetoacetate ratio.

The French phenotype is more severe, and associated with decreased or absent cross-reacting material and negligible catalytic activity (Saudubray *et al.*, 1976; Wong *et al.*, 1986). The tissue oxaloacetate concentrations are depleted, and aspartic acid concentrations are markedly decreased.

These deficiencies interfere with the conversion of citrulline to argininosuccinate in the urea cycle. As a result, the metabolic features include the findings in the North American phenotype, in addition to hyperammonaemia, citrullinaemia, and hyperlysinaemia. Impaired Krebs cycle activity is the most devastating consequence of pyruvate carboxylase deficiency leading to cellular energy failure.

One patient has been described with a benign variant of pyruvate carboxylase deficiency (Van Coster et al., 1991). This girl was repeatedly hospitalized for vomiting and dehydration. Her growth and development were normal interictally. The molecular basis for this benign variant remains obscure.

There appears to be only one form of pyruvate carboxylase in human tissues. Prenatal and postnatal diagnoses, therefore, are possible by enzyme assay in cultured fibroblasts, amniocytes, or lymphocytes. It is presumed that all cases result from mutations of the gene located on chromosome 11q. Pyruvate carboxylase deficiency is transmitted as an autosomal recessive trait, and heterozygotes can be identified by residual enzyme activity in cultured skin fibroblasts or lymphocytes (Atkin, 1979).

Phosphoenolpyruvate carboxykinase deficiency

This enzyme defect is extremely rare, and little clinical information is available (Robinson, 1989). Phosphoenolpyruvate carboxykinase is equally distributed between a cytosolic isoform and a mitochondrial isoform. The cytosolic form is responsive to fasting and various hormonal stimuli. Both isoforms have similar molecular weights but differ in their kinetic and immunochemical properties. Hypoglycaemia is severe and intractable in this condition. The two children with mitochondrial phosphoenolpyruvate carboxykinase deficiency had hypoglycaemia, lactic acidaemia, failure to thrive, hypotonia, and hepatomegaly. The first patient died at age 6 months, and the second patient had survived to the age of 10 years. The older patient had muscular weakness and hypotonia, suggesting primary involvement of the skeletal musculature. The reported cases of cytosolic phosphoenolpyruvate carboxykinase deficiency are more problematic since this isoform is influenced by induction and repression. Nevertheless, a small number of patients have been reported with a deficiency of the cytosolic isoform.

Fructose 1,6-bisphosphatase deficiency

This condition was first described by Baker & Winegrad (1970). An autosomal recessive disorder, it is more prevalent in females. Neonatal hypoglycaemia is the common presenting sign associated with metabolic acidosis, irritability or coma, apnoeic spells, dyspnoea, tachycardia, hypotonicity, and moderate hepatomegaly. Lactate, alanine, uric acid, and ketone bodies are elevated in the blood and urine, and the initial manifestations are similar to those of glucose 6-phosphatase deficiency. The enzyme is deficient in liver, kidney, jejunum, and leucocytes, and is normal in muscles. When properly managed, these patients do well and have a normal life expectancy.

Glucose 6-phosphatase deficiency

This enzyme defect is otherwise known as glycogenosis type I, or Von Gierke's disease. The enzyme deficiency causes hypoglycaemia, lactic acidaemia, hyperuricaemia, and hyperlipidaemia. These metabolic disturbances reflect an accumulation of intracellular glucose 6-phosphate. Glucose 6-phosphatase deficiency type Ib results from a defective translocation system moving glucose 6-phosphate into the microsomal compartment for conversion to glucose by glucose 6-phosphatase. Clinically, patients with the type Ia form are similar to the patients with the type Ib form. However, the glucose 6-phosphatase activity is normal in the type Ib form. These patients also have hepatomegaly, bleeding diathesis and neutropoenia. Recent studies suggest that lactate may be used by the brain as an alternative cerebral fuel when hypoglycaemia is associated with lactic acidaemia. A higher than expected incidence of cognitive impairment and seizures is seen in patients with glucose

6-phosphatase deficiency. Presumably, the neurological symptoms result from chronic or recurrent hypoglycaemia. Frequent daytime meals and nocturnal intragastric feeding minimize the neurological complications and improve the clinical and metabolic abnormalities in this condition.

Defects of the Krebs cycle

During the past few years, examples of partial enzyme defects involving the Krebs cycle have been reported, including deficiencies of fumarase, alpha-ketoglutarate dehydrogenase, combined defects of succinate dehydrogenase and aconitase, and dihydrolipoyl dehydrogenase (E_3 component). The latter defect was discussed previously in relationship to pyruvate dehydrogenase deficiency. The combined defect of succinate dehydrogenase and fumarase is limited to a single patient with a muscle-specific syndrome of exercise intolerance, muscle fatigue and weakness, and myoglobinuria (Haller et al., 1991). This patient did not have evidence of lactic acidaemia. The two deficiencies relevant to a discussion of lactic acidaemia are fumarase deficiency and alpha-ketoglutarate dehydrogenase deficiency (Fig. 3).

Fumarase deficiency

The fumarate hydratase gene is located on the long arm of chromosome 1. This gene encodes six electrophoretically different fumarase isoforms, four located in the mitochondria, and two located in the cytoplasm (Petrova-Benedict et al., 1987).

Seven patients with fumarase deficiency have been described since 1986 (Zinn et al., 1986; Petrova-Benedict et al., 1987; Walker et al., 1989; Gellera et al., 1990; Elpeleg et al., 1992; Remes et al., 1992). Two phenotypes have emerged, both presenting in infancy. Three patients had a fatal infantile encephalopathy with hypotonia, deceleration of head growth, and psychomotor deterioration. Death occurred between 6 and 8 months. Fumaric aciduria was the characteristic metabolic signature, and lactic acidaemia was more variable, with normal values reported on occasion. Lactic acidaemia was marked particularly during metabolic crises.

The second phenotype involved a more slowly progressive course. One patient had hypotonia, microcephaly and delayed development, and was the product of a consanguineous marriage. A second patient had congenital hypotonia and was later considered to have cerebral palsy with psychomotor retardation and hypotonia. Two brothers had intrauterine cerebral ventriculomegaly and polyhydramnios. Infantile spasms became evident after birth.

This phenotypic heterogeneity is similar to the clinical features seen with PDC deficiency including the presence of brain malformations.

Alpha-ketoglutarate dehydrogenase deficiency

Alpha-ketoglutarate dehydrogenase catalyses the oxidative decarboxylation of alpha-ketoglutarate to succinyl CoA as shown in the equation below:

$$\text{Alpha-ketoglutarate} + \text{CoASH} + \text{NAD}^+ \rightarrow \text{succinyl CoA} + \text{CO}_2 + \text{NADH} + \text{H}^+$$

Deficiencies of the alpha-ketoglutarate dehydrogenase complex have been described in isolation (Kohlschuetter et al., 1982; Bonnefont et al., 1992), or combined with deficiencies of the pyruvate dehydrogenase complex and the branched chain alpha-ketoacid dehydrogenase complex.

Kohlschuetter et al. (1982) reported a brother and sister with slowly progressive neurodegenerative disease after normal development during the first year of life. The initial clinical features were dominated by extrapyramidal symptoms. Pyramidal tract findings became evident later. Ultimately, the siblings were severely disabled with motor dysfunction and less severe cognitive disturbances. The parents were consanguineous, suggesting an autosomal recessive pattern of inheritance.

Bonnefont et al. (1992) reported three brothers, also born to a consanguineous couple. Unlike the first report, these siblings were symptomatic in the newborn period with hypotonia, metabolic acidosis, and lactic acidaemia. Generalized seizures and pyramidal tract dysfunction were present

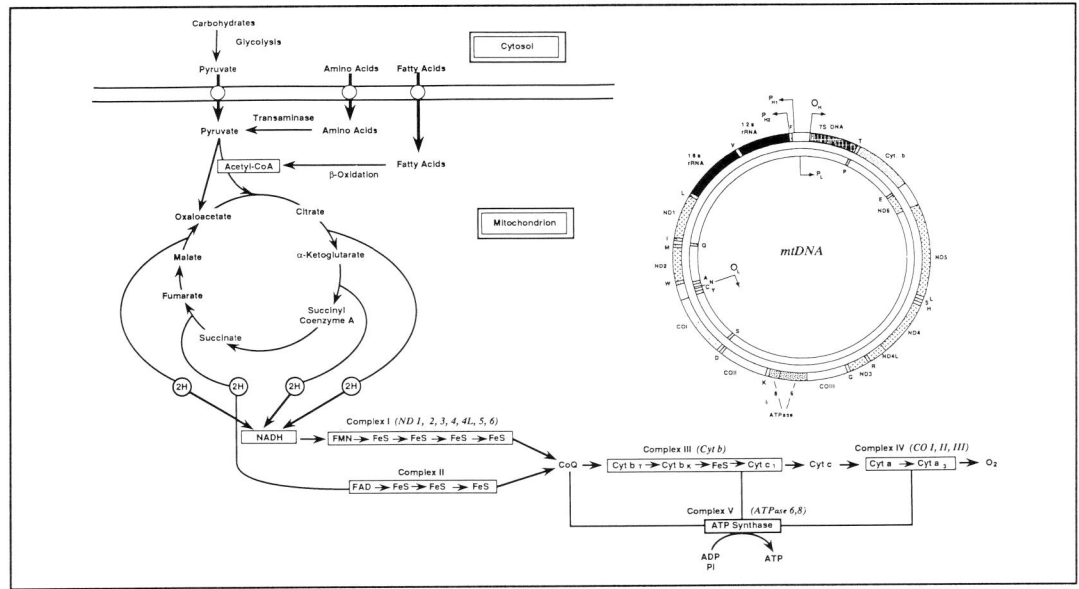

Fig. 4. Scheme of intermediary metabolism showing pyruvate metabolism, the Krebs cycle, and the respiratory chain. The respiratory chain is genetically controlled by the nuclear genome and the mitochondrial genome (upper right).

early, and extrapyramidal signs developed later in infancy. The blood lactate concentrations and the lactate:pyruvate ratios were elevated. Blood ketone concentrations were mildly increased, but the β-hydroxybutyrate:acetoacetate ratio was low. An E_3 defect was ruled out, but the primary enzyme defect was not determined.

Defects of the respiratory chain

Much attention has been focused on defects of the respiratory chain because of the extraordinary scientific advances that have been made in this area over the past several years. This subject is discussed elsewhere in these proceedings, and will be reviewed only briefly in this chapter. Several reviews have also been published recently on mitochondrial diseases with particular emphasis on defects of oxidative phosphorylation (Wallace, 1992; De Vivo, 1993; Di Mauro & De Vivo, 1994). The respiratory chain is uniquely influenced by the mitochondrial and nuclear genomes (Fig. 4).

Thirteen subunits are encoded by the mitochondrial DNA: seven in complex I, one in complex III, three in complex IV, and two in complex V. Unlike nuclear DNA mutations, mitochondrial DNA mutations are transmitted exclusively through the maternal lineage, variably expressed in both male and female progeny. This pattern of vertical transmission through successive generations is unmistakable when recognized. All the subunits in complex II, and the remaining subunit in complexes I, III, IV and V are encoded by nuclear genes. Genetically determined diseases of these subunits are transmitted mainly as autosomal recessive traits. A new group of mitochondrial diseases has also been recognized – defects of intergenomic signalling. These conditions result from nuclear mutations, and affect the stability or replication of the mitochondrial genomes. Examples include the dominantly inherited multiple mitochondrial DNA mutation syndrome, and the recessively inherited mitochondrial DNA depletion syndrome.

In general, genetic defects of complexes I–V present either as myopathies or as generalized disturbances predominantly affecting muscle and brain. Lactic acidaemia is particularly striking in the infantile syndromes, and less striking in the older patients. Because these defects affect the reoxidation of NADH or $FADH_2$, the lactate:pyruvate ratio is elevated. Similarly, the intramitochondrial oxidation–reduction potential is affected, with an elevation of the β-hydroxybutyrate/acetoacetate ratio.

The diagnosis of respiratory chain defects requires several laboratory techniques. Polarographic studies can document differential impairment of oxidizable substrates by isolated intact mitochondria. Defective respiration of NAD-dependent substrates like pyruvate and malate, and normal respiration of FAD-dependent substrates like succinate, strongly suggest a complex I defect, for example. Direct enzyme assays of the respiratory chain complexes can complement these polarographic studies. Molecular strategies, also, are helpful in defining a point mutation or large-scale rearrangement of the mitochondrial DNA. The skeletal muscle biopsy has particular value in this group of disorders that cause lactic acidaemia. Ragged-red fibres are the histological signature of a genetic disease that affects the mitochondrial DNA. The presence of ragged-red fibres signifies a disturbance in intramitochondrial protein synthesis. This disturbance, almost invariably, indicates the presence of a point mutation in a mitochondrial gene coding for one or more transfer RNAs. Mitochondrial DNA deletions and mitochondrial DNA depletion are associated with ragged-red fibres, for the same reason.

Remote defects affecting pyruvate metabolism

Lactic acidaemia has been described as an associated finding in various organic acidurias and defects of fatty acid oxidation. Of particular note is the elevation of lactate in the recently described trifunctional enzyme defect (Jackson *et al.*, 1992) involving the mitochondrial oxidation of long-chain fatty acids. This association indicates the need to evaluate the urinary organic acid profile in all patients presenting with lactic acidaemia. Diagnostic possibilities include fatty acid oxidation defects, biotinidase and multiple carboxylase deficiencies, propionic acidaemia, methylmalonic acidaemia, and other organic acidurias. The mechanisms underlying the associated lactic acidaemia are manifold, and include alterations of the oxidation–reduction potential, sequestration of free coenzyme A, and accumulation of potentially toxic acyl-CoA derivatives. Secondary carnitine deficiency may also exacerbate these microchemical environmental perturbations.

Treatment options

The treatment of lactic acidaemia depends in part upon the underlying enzyme defect. Pyruvate dehydrogenase has a cofactor requirement for thiamine and lipoic acid. On rare occasions, these cofactors will improve the catalytic efficiency of the complex and improve the lactic acidaemia. In theory, a ketogenic diet may be helpful in the chronic management of patients with pyruvate dehydrogenase deficiency. Ketone bodies are metabolized in extrahepatic tissues producing acetyl-CoA. There are no control studies to document the benefit of this dietary regimen. Some patients with an intermittent ataxia secondary to pyruvate dehydrogenase deficiency have benefited from acetazolamide therapy. Gluconeogenic defects, specifically fructose 1,6-bisphosphatase deficiency and glucose 6-phosphatase deficiency, are managed by frequent daily and continuous nocturnal feedings to prevent hypoglycaemia and brain damage. This approach is effective in the management of patients with these two gluconeogenic defects, and the prognosis is good to excellent, depending upon the age at diagnosis and the compliance with treatment.

Pyruvate carboxylase deficiency has no effective treatment. Aspartic acid supplementation will increase the tissue concentrations of oxaloacetate, and will benefit intermediary metabolism in non-neural tissues. Unfortunately, aspartic acid provides no benefit for the neurological consequences of this enzyme deficiency.

There are no specific treatments available for the partial defects involving the Krebs cycle. Management of defects involving the respiratory chain is equally difficult. A single patient with complex III deficiency benefited from high doses of vitamins K and C (Argov *et al.*, 1986). This vitamin replacement therapy has been ineffective in other patients with respiratory chain defects. Combinations of coenzyme Q10, L-carnitine, and high dose folic acid have been attempted in patients with mitochondrial DNA mutations and deletions, but the benefits are modest and controversial (De Vivo, 1993).

Dietary therapy has been tried in various organic acidurias and fatty acid oxidation defects with anecdotal success. Biotin supplementation is of remarkable benefit in patients with biotinidase deficiency and milder forms of holocarboxylase synthetase deficiency.

The management of the metabolic acidosis associated with lactic acidaemia is more controversial. Sodium bicarbonate has been the recommended mode of treatment for over 50 years (Arieff, 1991). The fundamental rationale is the administration of a base to correct the metabolic acidosis. Recent studies indicate that this approach may have subtle and chronic disadvantages. These include venous hypercapnia causing decreased tissue pH, a paradoxical decrease in the cerebrospinal fluid pH, aggravation of the tissue hypoxia and circulatory collapse, hypernatremia, and no direct effect on the lactic acidaemia. In adult studies, sodium bicarbonate is no longer recommended routinely for the management of cardiopulmonary arrest.

The only possible alternative to sodium bicarbonate is an experimental agent, sodium dichloroacetate (Stacpoole *et al.*, 1988, 1992). Recent clinical studies and anecdotal reports suggest possible benefit from this agent. Sodium dichloroacetate inhibits the pyruvate dehydrogenase-specific kinase, thereby fully activating the pyruvate dehydrogenase complex (Stacpoole, 1989). This action facilitates the conversion of pyruvate to acetyl-CoA. The potential advantages of sodium dichloroacetate in treating lactic acidaemia are several. There is no effect of dichloroacetate on blood pCO_2, and presumably no adverse effects on intracellular pH. Similarly, there is no adverse effect on the cerebrospinal fluid pH. Dichloroacetate crosses the blood–brain barrier and acts on brain pyruvate dehydrogenase (Miller *et al.*, 1990). As a result, this agent effectively lowers both blood and brain tissue lactate values. Evidence suggests that dichloroacetate improves cardiovascular function, and there have been no reported adverse effects associated with the acute administration of this agent (Ludvik *et al.*, 1991). Theoretical disadvantages include the possibility of cataract formation, and peripheral neuropathy. At the moment, there is only limited experience with long-term administration of this agent. Clinical trials are needed to determine whether sodium dichloroacetate effectively lowers lactic acidaemia chronically, and whether normal blood and tissue lactate concentrations improve the general health of the patient with these diverse enzymatic conditions.

Prognosis

The prognosis of patients with lactic acidaemia is determined by the underlying biochemical defect. Patients with treatable conditions such as biotinidase deficiency, and gluconeogenic defects such as fructose 1,6-bisphosphatase deficiency and glucose 6-phosphatase deficiency do reasonably well with appropriate management. Patients with pyruvate dehydrogenase deficiency, pyruvate carboxylase deficiency, defects of the Krebs cycle and the respiratory chain do less well. In the absence of effective treatment, accurate clinical diagnosis, prenatal diagnosis, and genetic counselling are of major importance.

Acknowledgement

The authors thank Ms. Alice H. Marti for her secretarial assistance. Parts of this work were supported by the Colleen Giblin Foundation for Pediatric Neurology Research, and a grant from the Muscular Dystrophy Association.

References

Argov, Z., Bank, W.J., Maris, J. *et al.* (1986): Treatment of mitochondrial myopathy due to complex III deficiency with vitamins K_3 and C: a ^{31}P-NMR follow-up study. *Ann. Neurol.* **19**, 598–602.

Arieff, A.I. (1991): Indications for use of bicarbonate in patients with metabolic acidosis. *Br. J. Anaesth.* **67**, 165–177.

Atkin, B.M. (1979): Carrier detection of pyruvate carboxylase deficiency in fibroblasts and lymphocytes. *Pediatr. Res.* **13**, 1101–1104.

Atkin, B.M., Buist, N.R., Utter, M.F., Leiter, A.B. & Banker, B.Q. (1979): Pyruvate carboxylase deficiency and lactic acidosis in a retarded child without Leigh's disease. *Pediatr. Res.* **13**, 109–116.

Baker, L. & Winegrad, A.I. (1970): Fasting hypoglycaemia and metabolic acidosis associated with deficiency of hepatic fructose-1,6-diphosphatase activity. *Lancet* **ii**, 13–16.

Bonnefont, J.P., Chretien, D., Rustin, P. et al. (1992): Alpha-ketoglutarate dehydrogenase deficiency presenting as congenital lactic acidosis. *J. Pediatr.* **121**, 255–258.

Brown, G.K., Haan, E.A., Kirby, D.M. et al. (1988): 'Cerebral' lactic acidosis: defects in pyruvate metabolism with profound brain damage and minimal systemic acidosis. *Eur. J. Pediatr.* **147**, 10–14.

Brown, G.K., Brown, R.M., Scholem, R.D., Kirby, D.M. & Dahl, H.-H.M. (1989): The clinical and biochemical spectrum of human pyruvate dehydrogenase complex deficiency. *Ann. N.Y. Acad. Sci.* **573**, 360–368.

Brown, R.M. & Brown, G.K. (1993): X chromosome inactivation and the diagnosis of X linked disease in females. *J. Med. Genet.* **30**, 177–184.

Dahl, H-H.M., Brown, G.K., Brown, R.M. et al. (1992): Mutations and polymorphisms in the pyruvate dehydrogenase E_1 alpha gene. *Human Mutation* **1**, 97–102.

De Vivo, D.C. (1993): The expanding clinical spectrum of mitochondrial diseases. *Brain Dev.* **15**, 1–21.

De Vivo, D.C. (1994): Intermediary metabolism; In: *Mitochondrial disorders in neurology*, eds. A.H.V. Shapira & S. Di Mauro. pp. 130–144. London: Butterworth-Heinemann.

De Vivo, D.C., Haymond, M.W., Leckie, M.P., Bussman, Y.L., McDougal, D.B., Jr. & Pagliara, A.S. (1977): The clinical and biochemical implications of pyruvate carboxylase deficiency. *J. Clin. Endocrinol. Metab.* **45**, 1281–1296.

De Vivo, D.C. & Van Coster, R.N. (1990): Leigh syndrome: clinical and biochemical correlates; In: *Modern perspectives of child neurology*, eds. Y. Fukuyama, S. Kamoshita, C. Ohtsuka et al., pp. 27–40. Tokyo: The Japanese Society of Child Neurology.

Di Mauro, S. & Moraes, C.T. (1993): Mitochondrial encephalomyopathies. *Arch. Neurol.* **50**, 1197–1208.

Di Mauro, S. & De Vivo, D.C. (1994): Diseases of carbohydrate, fatty acid, and mitochondrial metabolism; In: *Basic neurochemistry: molecular, cellular, and medical aspects*, eds. G.J. Siegel et. al., pp. 723–748. New York: Raven Press.

Elpeleg, O.N., Amir, N. & Christensen, E. (1992): Variability of clinical presentation in fumarate hydratase deficiency. *J. Pediatr.* **121**, 752–754.

Fujii, T., van Coster, R.N., Old, S.E. et al. (1994): Pyruvate dehydrogenase deficiency: molecular basis for intrafamilial heterogeneity. *Ann. Neurol.* **36**, 83–89.

Gellera, C., Uziel, G., Rimoldi, M. et al. (1990): Fumarase deficiency is an autosomal recessive encephalopathy affecting both the mitochondrial and the cytosolic enzymes. *Neurology* **40**, 495–499.

Haller, R.G., Henriksson, K.G., Jorfeldt, L. et al. (1991): Deficiency of skeletal muscle succinate dehydrogenase and aconitase. Pathophysiology of exercise in a novel human muscle oxidative defect. *J. Clin. Invest.* **88**, 1197–1206.

Hermansen, L., Machlum, S., Pruett, E.D., Vagi, O., Waldum, H. & Wesselaas, T. (1975): Lactate removal at rest and during exercise. In: *Metabolic adaptations to prolonged physical exercise*, eds. H. Howald & J.R. Poortman, p. 101. Basel: Birkhauser.

Jackson, S., Kler, R.S., Bartlett, K. et al. (1992): Combined enzyme defect of mitochondrial fatty acid oxidation. *J. Clin. Invest.* **90**, 1219–1225.

Kohlschuetter, A., Behbehani, A.W., Langenbeck, U. et al. (1982): A familial progressive neurodegenerative disease with 2-oxoglutaric aciduria. *Eur. J. Pediatr.* **138**, 32–37.

Kreisberg, R.A., Pennington, L.F. & Boshell, B.R. (1970): Lactate turnover and gluconeogenesis in normal and obese humans. *Diabetes* **19**, 53.

Ludvik, B., Peer, G., Berzlanovich, A., Stifter, S. & Graf, H.: (1991): Effects of dichloroacetate and bicarbonate on haemodynamic parameters in healthy volunteers. *Clin. Sci.* **80**, 47–51.

Marsac, C., Stansbie, D., Bonne, G. et al. (1993): Defect in the lipoyl-bearing protein X subunit of the pyruvate dehydrogenase complex in two patients with encephalomyelopathy. *J. Pediatr.* **123**, 915–920.

Miller, A.L., Hatch, J.P. & Prihoda, T.J. (1990): Dichloroacetate increases glucose use and decreases lactate in developing rat brain. *Metabol. Brain Dis.* **5**, 195–204.

Munnich, A., Saudubray, J.M., Taylor, J. *et al.* (1982): Congenital lactic acidosis, alpha-ketoglutaric aciduria and variant form of maple syrup urine disease due to a single enzyme defect: dihydrolipoyl dehydrogenase deficiency. *Acta Paediatr. Scand.* **71**, 167–171.

Pardridge, W.M. (1983): Brain metabolism: a perspective from the blood–brain barrier. *Physiol. Rev.* **63**, 1481–1535.

Petrova-Benedict, R., Robinson, B.H., Stacey, T.E., Mistry, J. & Chalmers, R.A. (1987): Deficient fumarase activity in an infant with fumaric acidemia and its distribution between the different forms of the enzyme seen on isoelectric focusing. *Am. J. Hum-Genet.* **40**, 257–266.

Remes, A.M., Rantala, H., Kalervo Hiltunen, J., Leisti, J. & Ruokonen, A. (1992): Fumarase deficiency: two siblings with enlarged cerebral ventricles and polyhydramnios in utero. *Pediatrics* **89**, 730–734.

Robinson, B.H. (1989): Lactic acidemia. In: *The metabolic basis of inherited diseases*, eds. C.R. Scriver, A.L. Brandet, W.S. Sly *et al.* pp. 869–888. New York: McGraw Hill.

Robinson, B.H., Taylor, J. & Sherwood, W.G. (1977): Deficiency of dihydrolipoyl dehydrogenase (a component of pyruvate and alpha-ketoglutarate dehydrogenase complexes): a cause of congenital chronic lactic acidosis in infancy. *Pediatr. Res.* **11**, 1198–1202.

Robinson, B.H., Taylor, J., Kahler, S.G. & Kirkman, H.N. (1981): Lactic acidemia, neurological deterioration and carbohydrate dependence in a girl with dihydrolipoyl dehydrogenase deficiency. *Eur. J. Pediatr.* **136**, 35–39.

Robinson, B.H., Oei, J., Sherwood, W.G. *et al.* (1984): The molecular basis for the two different clinical presentations of classical pyruvate carboxylase deficiency. *Am. J. Hum. Genet.* **36**, 283–294.

Robinson, B.H., MacMillan, H., Petrova-Benedict, R. & Sherwood, W.G. (1987): Variable clinical presentation in patients with defective E1 component of pyruvate dehydrogenase complex. *J. Pediatr.* **111**, 525–533.

Robinson, B.H., MacKay, N., Petrova-Benedict, R., Ozalp, I., Coskun, T. & Stacpoole, P.W. (1990): Defects in the E2 lipoyl transacetylase and the X-lipoyl containing component of the pyruvate dehydrogenase complex in patients with lactic acidemia. *J. Clin. Invest.* **85**, 1821–1824.

Saudubray, J.M., Marsac, C., Cathelineau, C.L., Besson Leaud, M. & Leroux, J.P. (1976): Neonatal congenital lactic acidosis with pyruvate carboxylase deficiency in two siblings. *Acta Paediatr. Scand.* **65**, 717–724.

Stacpoole, P.W. (1989): The pharmacology of dichloroacetate. *Metabolism* **38**, 1124–1144.

Stacpoole, P.W., Lorenz, A.C., Thomas, R.G. & Harman, E.M. (1988): Dichloroacetate in the treatment of lactic acidosis. *Ann. Intern. Med.* **108**, 58–63.

Stacpoole, P.W., Wright, E.C., Baumgartner, T.G. *et al.* (1992): A controlled clinical trial of dichloroacetate for treatment of lactic acidosis in adults. *N. Engl. J. Med.* **327**, 1564–1569.

Van Coster, R.N., Fernhoff, P.M. & De Vivo, D.C. (1991): Pyruvate carboxylase deficiency: a benign variant with normal development. *Pediatr. Res.* **30**, 1–4.

Walker, V., Mills, G.A., Hall, M.A., Millward-Sadler, G.H., English, N.R. & Chalmers, R.A. (1989): A fourth case of fumarase deficiency. *J. Inherit. Metab. Dis.* **12**, 331–332.

Wallace, D.C. (1992): Diseases of the mitochondrial DNA. *Annu. Rev. Biochem.* **61**, 1175–1212.

Wong, L.T., Davidson, A.G., Applegarth, D.A. *et al.* (1986): Biochemical and histologic pathology in an infant with cross-reacting material (negative) pyruvate carboxylase deficiency. *Pediatr. Res.* **20**, 274–279.

Yoshida, I., Sweetman, L., Kulovich, S., Nyhan, W.L. & Robinson, B.H. (1990): Effect of lipoic acid in a patient with defective activity of pyruvate dehydrogenase, 2-oxoglutarate dehydrogenase, and branched-chain keto acid dehydrogenase. *Pediatr. Res.* **27**, 75–79.

Zinn, A.B., Kerr, D. & Hoppel, C.L. (1986): Fumarase deficiency: a new cause of mitochondrial encephalomyopathy. *N. Engl. J. Med.* **315**, 469–475.

Chapter 5

Hyperphenylalaninaemia: therapy and follow-up

Enrica Riva, Isabella Basile, Diego Luotti and Giacomo Biasucci

Clinica Pediatrica, Università degli Studi di Milano, Ospedale 'San Paolo', via A. di Rudinì 8, 20142 Milan, Italy

Summary

The term 'hyperphenylalaninaemia' includes different clinical phenotypes, characterized by plasma phenylalanine (phe) levels above 2 mg/dl. They are mostly due to various degrees of deficiency of phenylalanine hydroxylase, which lead to a progressive and severe mental retardation. Therapy is currently based on a phe restricted diet to be continued for life. This comprises foods very poor in whole animal proteins such as vegetables and fruits, special phenylanine lacking amino acid mixtures and proper lipidic and glucidic supplementations. The strict dietetary control, maintained by periodic clinical, nutritional and neurophysiological controls, makes the macronutrient intake closer to the recommended dietary allowances, but at the risk of inadequate intake of some specific components contained only in whole animal foods. Polyunsaturated very-long-chain fatty acids, carnitine, taurine and selenium are lower in treated hyperphenylalaninaemic children in comparison with healthy ones. A new challenge for the adequacy of the dietary intervention is represented by the management of maternal phenylketonuria, for the possible consequences on the developing tissues of the growing organism. The nutritional approach to the treatment of hyperphenylalaninaemic children may not only help to avoid consequences secondary to the dietary deficiencies (in particular those affecting the central nervous system), but may also represent a unique opportunity for better knowledge of the effects and consequences of specific nutrient deficiencies or supplementation, or both, on the metabolic status and body development.

Clinical phenotypes

The term hyperphenylalaninaemia (HPA) refers to various clinical phenotypes, characterized by the inherited deficiency of hepatic phenylalanine (phe) hydroxylase, and of tetrahydrobiopterin (BH4), which is its natural cofactor (Koch & Wenz, 1987).
The consequent HPA (plasma phe levels above 2 mg/dl) characterizes the biochemical picture of the various clinical phenotypes, which are therefore defined as hyperphenylalaninaemic syndromes, whose overall frequency is 1:10 000 live births.
The following forms are currently known:
– Classical phenylketonuria (PKU or HPA type I) which is characterized by a residual enzymatic activity below 1 per cent of the norm, plasma phe levels above 20 mg/dl on a free diet and remarkable urinary excretion of phenyl-ketones. Classical PKU, first described by Fölling (1934), is clinically characterized by a mandatory, severe and progressive mental retardation, on which Jervis (1939) based his definition of 'phenylpyruvic oligophrenia'. About 65 per cent of untreated PKU subjects show an IQ score below 20, while 96 per cent have an IQ of below 50.

The clinical picture, which usually occurs during the second semester of life, also includes microcephaly, muscle hypertone, hyperreflexia, autism, speech disturbances and non-specific electroencephalographic abnormalities. Furthermore, the inhibitory effect on tyrosinase activity of HPA, leading to melanine deficiency, seems to be responsible for the peculiar phenotype 'blonde hair – pale blue eyes' occurring in 62 per cent of PKU subjects as well as the eczema which is present in 34 per cent.

– HPA type II (or mild PKU) with reduced dietary phe tolerance, which is characterized by a residual enzymatic activity ranging between 1 and 3 per cent of the norm, with plasma phe levels between 10 and 20 mg/dl on a free diet. In this form mental retardation does not always occur.

– HPA type III with normal tolerance to dietary phe, residual enzymatic activity above 3 per cent and plasma phe levels below 10 mg/dl on a free diet. This form is accompanied by normal psychomotor development.

– BH4 deficiencies (Valsasina *et al.*, 1989), once called 'atypical PKU' because of the severe neurological damage occurring despite normal phe hydroxylase activity, was then defined as 'malignant PKU' owning to the remarkable psychomotor retardation not responding to dietary treatment. Tetrahydrobiopterin deficiencies are in turn subdivided into four forms according to the different enzymatic defect in the cofactor biosynthesis and regeneration, whose global frequency is 1–3 per cent of all HPAs: the most frequent is pyruvoyltetrahydropterin-synthase deficiency, the rarest guanosine-triphosphate cyclohydrolase deficiency, then dihydropteridine reductase deficiency and, lastly, carbinolimine-dehydratase deficiency (primapterinuria).

Hyperphenylalaninaemia is the common biochemical feature in all BH4 defects. The clinical picture may occur during the first weeks of life even though it generally appears at about 3 months. Major findings are hypotonia of the trunk and hypertone of the limbs, poor head control, convulsions, hyperreflexia, microcephaly, mental retardation, hypersalivation due to swallowing difficulties, and severe psychomotor retardation that progressively leads to death within the third year of life.

Thanks to the occurrence of the biochemical abnormalities, the diagnosis is feasible within the first few days of life, by neonatal screening programmes (Guthrie & Susi, 1963).

This diagnostic approach is made by a semi-quantitative method, requiring to be confirmed by a quantitative assay (ion-exchange chromatography) which enables the definition of the various forms of HPA and by further and more sophisticated investigations which aim to screen for BH4 deficiencies. The final diagnosis should be achieved within 6 weeks, in order to start early and appropriate therapy immediately, thus preventing the development of neurological damage.

Pathogenesis of the neurological damage

Different hypotheses have been proposed to explain the structural (myelin impairments), cytological (impairment of the proteic and proteolipidic components, inhibited oligodendrocyte migration, decreased intracellular protein synthesis) and biochemical (decreased neurotransmitter synthesis) alterations underlying the severe neurological damage in untreated HPA subjects.

The increased plasma phe levels secondary to the enzyme deficiency not only lead to an increased excretion of secondary toxic metabolites, but have also a negative effect on tyrosine and its metabolite synthesis. These events have been and still are indicated as the possible causes of the neurological damage (Michals *et al.*, 1988); however clinical and experimental data show that the tissue concentrations of the toxic metabolites mentioned are not usually high enough to explain the neuropathological modifications observed in HPA subjects (Kaufman, 1989).

The hypothesis that HPA may be directly involved in the pathogenesis of the damage now appears to be more reliable.

Hyperphenylalaninaemia could in fact inhibit the transport of the other large neutral amino acids (tyrosine, leucine, isoleucine, valine, tryptophan, methionine) through the blood–brain barrier (Pardridge & Choi, 1986). The consequent deficiency of tyrosine and its functional metabolites should therefore represent only one aspect of a more complicated alteration. This includes decreased availability of those amino acids involved in neurotransmitter synthesis and of those essential amino acids utilized for cellular synthesis and energy production.

Hommes et al. (1982) demonstrated that high phe levels can inhibit the specific ATP sulphorilases within the nervous tissue. This in turn increases the myelin turnover due to alkaline protein degradation not being balanced by a simultaneous increase of *de novo* synthesis. This theory could well integrate the amino acid competition hypothesis, resulting in a more reliable and proven explanation (Hommes & Moss, 1992) of the structural cerebral damage caused by HPA.

Anyway, it is clear that whatever the underlying pathogenetic mechanism could be, the toxic effect of HPA acts chronically, possibly for life. With respect to the neurological damage in BH4 deficiencies it is very likely to be due to a defective neurotransmitter synthesis, caused by the role of BH4 as the cofactor of tyrosine and tryptophan hydroxylases. Furthermore, very low cerebral concentration of folates have been observed in dihydropteridine reductase deficiencies.

On the basis of these pathogenetic mechanisms, therapy must be based on the administration of the neurotransmitter precursors that are lacking (L-dopa and 5OH-tryptophan), plus chemically synthesized BH4 and folinic acid in selected cases (Irons et al., 1987).

Therapy

The first therapeutical goal should necessarily be to safeguard the cerebral structure and the psychomotor development. 'Safe' plasma phe levels should therefore be restored as early as possible (within 6 weeks of birth), since the growth and maturation rate of the nervous tissue (and therefore its potential for damage) reaches its highest peak during the first years of life.

Since 1954, when Bickel et al. first introduced it, the therapy of HPA is based on a phe-restricted and controlled diet. The dietary regimen, assessed according to the patient's age, phe plasma level and tolerance, is aimed to maintain plasma phe level within the so-called 'safe' range (2–6 mg/dl).

Normal plasma phe values should be achieved by also taking into consideration the patient's calorie and protein needs; furthermore, since phe is an essential amino acid, amounts sufficient to guarantee normal protein synthesis should be included in the dietary regimen, thus preventing the occurrence of impaired psychomotor development and growth secondary to phe lacking diets. The daily phe need (250–550 mg) should be therefore met.

This is obtained by feeding nursing children adequate amounts of breast milk or infant formulas during the first trimester of life, then using hypoproteic natural foods such as vegetables and fruit (whose phe content is minimal). Their intake should be assessed by means of the so called 'ponderal equivalents' table, which enables us to know the exact amount of a given product corresponding to a known phe content (Depondt et al., 1983; Giovannini et al., 1985). The use of this method leads to a better therapeutic compliance and metabolic control, reduces the chance of psychological consequences on the child secondary to a 'different' dietary regimen and makes any dietary variation easier. Since the restriction of phe intake is necessarily linked to a global reduction of natural protein intake (especially of animal origin), the daily protein need is met by administering appropriate amino acid mixtures lacking phe. The diet should then include vegetable oil (olive, sunflower, corn oil) to meet the daily lipid requirements and carbohydrates to satisfy the global calorie need.

The effectiveness of the therapy in terms of metabolic control should then be strictly monitored by frequently assessing plasma phe levels; a periodic clinical examination, as well as the evaluation of nutritional and anthropometric parameters and psychomotor development, represent the best tools for follow-up of the therapy.

Data from previous studies demonstrate an inverse correlation between the IQ score and the age of diet introduction (Smith & Wolff, 1974; Koch et al., 1984).

Only by starting therapy very early can we guarantee a normal psychomotor development, since this becomes progressively less sensitive to the effects of diet; in fact after 4 years of age, the efficacy of diet is only confined to the control of neurological symptoms and behavioural disturbances (Holtzman et al., 1986). However, even early treated and well-controlled HPA patients have shown slight impairments of motor abilities, language, learning and mathematical calculations (Koch et al., 1984), besides a higher frequency of slight behavioural disturbances (Smith et al., 1988). The psychological consequences secondary to the diagnosis and the chronic diet therapy have been claimed to explain the symptoms.

Furthermore in HPA treated early presenting with good metabolic control (mean plasma phe below 6 mg/dl) some modifications of the periventricular white matter have been observed by cerebral MRI (Bick et al., 1989). We could then assume that the pathogenetic mechanisms are always working even in the presence of plasma phe levels just above the physiological range. In particular, it seems that plasma phe fluctuations during the first months of life may contribute to the occurrence of these minimal damages.

New therapeutical tools to be combined with the diet have therefore been studied. Branched-chain (Berry et al., 1990) and/or aromatic (Lou, 1985) amino acid supplementation has been proposed in order to overcome the competitive effect of HPA on their transport through the blood–brain barrier. Clinical and experimental trials showed this supplementation is able to reduce phe concentrations within the central nervous system, meanwhile increasing the neurotransmitter synthesis and improving psychometric abilities. However, it is current opinion that this supplementation should be confined to patients who show a poor dietary compliance, as in restarting diet after previous interruption. Besides the necessity of an even more accurate metabolic control and of specific supplementations useful to improve the efficacy of the dietary intervention, the optimal duration of the diet remains to be fully defined.

The following data should be considered:

(1) biochemical: the chronicity of the pathogenetic mechanisms underlying the acute functional (decreased availability of substrates for the neurotransmitter synthesis) and structural chronic damage (increased myelin turnover);

(2) experimental: increased myelin turnover is induced by HPA even beyond the age of the highest rate of myelin synthesis;

(3) clinical: the negative effects of the interruption of the diet on the modulation of cerebral functions (Smith et al., 1990).

According to these data, we can conclude that the proposal of a life-long therapy appears to be fully justified.

Diet-therapy in maternal phenylketonuria

Once ensured of a good *quoad valetudinem* prognosis, the second 'end-point' of the diet therapy is to prevent the severe embryofoetopathy observed in untreated HPA women.

At the time of conception, maternal plasma phe levels above 20 mg/dl are correlated with a very high risk of embryofetopathy, resulting in mental retardation (92 per cent of the offspring), microcephaly (72 per cent), intrauterine growth retardation (40 per cent), congenital heart defects (12 per cent) and other minor malformations.

The frequency of these abnormalities is significantly related to maternal plasma phe levels during pregnancy and to the age of starting diet, with a remarkable reduction as a good metabolic control is achieved before conception (Lenke & Levy, 1980; Drogari et al., 1987).

However, it is not yet possible to define a safe phe threshold which should not present a risk for fetal abnormalities, even though some recent data from a multicentric American study (Matalon *et al.*, 1991) indicate it may correspond to 6 mg/dl plasma phe.

The maternal PKU derived embryofetopathy should be induced by the same pathogenetic mechanisms as hypothesized for untreated HPA subjects. Experimental studies demonstrated that the maternal placenta does not protect the fetus from the negative effects of maternal HPA; on the contrary, fetal plasma phe levels seem to be 1.48-fold higher than the corresponding maternal value (Hanley *et al.*, 1987), thus suggesting a direct involvement of HPA in the pathogenesis of fetal abnormalities.

Since the toxic effects start immediately after conception, it is mandatory to restore normal maternal plasma phe levels by that time. This is of course easier if the woman has not discontinued the diet, but could anyway be obtained by restarting dietary treatment before conception, if HPA women have been appropriately educated as they entered the fertile age. Anyway it is clear that the best way to prevent maternal PKU embryofetopathy is to keep patients on the diet for life, or at least throughout their fertile age.

The dietary regimen during pregnancy should be updated to take account not only of the tolerance of the subject, but also of the increasing daily requirements linked to the *de novo* protein synthesis of the growing fetus.

However, we need to point out that the efficacy of the diet, even when it starts before conception, is still controversial (Lipson *et al.*, 1984; Lenke & Levy, 1980). This has encouraged research into new therapeutic approaches and new pathogenetic explanations. Branched-chain amino acid supplementation was effective in improving the prognosis for offspring in experimental studies (Vorhees & Berry, 1989), according to the blood–brain barrier competition theory. The 'by exclusion-diet', as the diet for HPA subjects may be called, could itself be responsible for secondary nutritional deficiencies with potential negative effects on tissue synthesis (Giovannini *et al.*, 1989). This is the basic theory for pursuing the third 'end point' of the therapy, which is to monitor the correct balance between all the dietary nutritional components.

Diet-therapy: nutritional consequences and possible variations

With increasing knowledge in the metabolic field, we have been able to redefine the nutritional follow-up so as to not add deficiencies resulting from the limitations imposed by the diet to the potential biochemical damage already present.

Dietary treatment by exclusion means that patients are at risk of being deficient in those dietary factors found electively in products of animal origin. Those dietary components have been referred to as 'conditioned essentiality': they are present and can be synthesized only minimally in animals, but most of them come from exogenous intake. Thus, in situations of increased demand, relative deficiency may occur. Trace elements, taurine, carnitine and lipid (cholesterol and very-long-chain polyunsaturated (VLCP) fatty acids) are currently the molecules most investigated for this, and towards which we have directed our research efforts for the improvement of the dietary treatment of HPA.

Pregnancy is the extreme situation in which a deficiency in nutrients of 'conditioned essentiality' is most likely to occur (Acosta & Stepnick-Gropper, 1986). From the point of view of dietary management, the problem of maternal PKU is two-fold: it is necessary to keep a strictly controlled phe level, and on the other hand to ensure the bioavailability of the nutrients not provided by this semisynthetic regimen, as the demand of the mother–fetus unit is greater.

Minerals and trace elements

The function of trace elements in paediatric nutrition, and the need to supplement formulas with them for semisynthetic diets, form the basis for the first nutritional observation of possible deficiencies caused by the dietary therapy. Interactions between the individual trace elements during absorption can also lower their circulating levels. With the preparations available today, however, no deficiency in the minerals and trace elements most directly involved in the growth is observable. Supplemented formulas have been decidedly helpful in the restoring normal plasma levels of iron, ferritin, zinc and copper (Longhi et al., 1987). The high manganese content of vegetables helps maintain normal circulating levels (Rottoli et al., 1986). By contrast, persistently low blood levels of selenium occur in subjects treated for HPA. The emphasis recently laid on selenium as an antioxidant makes it particularly necessary to revise its intake levels in nursing children fed with special products to supplement semisynthetic diets.

Taurine and carnitine

Taurine plays an important functional role in stabilizing the nerve membranes of the retina and the central nervous system and in regulating the signals between nerve cells (Sturman, 1988). Its intake in people who have a non-supplemented semisynthetic diet mostly comprising vegetable products is minimal, as the low plasma levels show (Agostoni et al., 1990). A similar situation has been observed for carnitine, needed for the oxidation of fatty acids and the production of ketone bodies, which are the main sources of energy for the nursing babies' nerve cells. Treated HPA children aged between 1 and 5 years have low plasma levels of total, free and esterified carnitine (Schulpis et al., 1990). Although no clinical symptoms attributed to a deficiency of taurine and carnitine in HPA subjects have yet been described, in the absence of negative effects supplementing formulas during the period of exclusive breast or bottle feeding may be advisable to complete a diet of itself poor in natural growth factors.

Cholesterol and lipoprotein metabolism

Total cholesterol levels are lower in treated HPA subjects than in controls. The levels of high-density lipoproteins and triglycerides are not different (Galluzzo et al., 1985) nor do they even show a better pattern in HPA (Schulpis & Scarpalezou, 1989).

The diet for HPA subjects is in fact less atherogenic, not so much for the almost-nil cholesterol intake as for the favourable intralipid ratios (high intake of unsaturated fats and low intake of saturated fats).

On the other hand, a cholesterol deficiency in the diet does not appear to have negative consequences on neurological development, since in humans most of the cholesterol is of endogenous origin from the first stages of fetal life (Lin et al., 1977).

Fatty acids

Although regarding the lipoprotein profile, the diet for HPA subjects is to be considered a 'eulipid' model, the levels of VLCP fatty acids appear to be deficient.

As a consequence of the low dietary intake, treated HPAs show low plasma levels of both the n-6 series (e.g. arachidonic acid) and the n-3 series (e.g. eicosapentaenoic acid (EPA) and docosahexaenoic acid (DHA)). The main deficiencies seem to be in arachidonic acid and DHA, which are lower than in controls (Galli et al., 1991). In the absence of foods containing all the VLCP fatty acids, the relative deficiency can be explained both by the characteristics of the diet and by reduced elongation and desaturation.

Substances derived from arachidonic acid mediate immunoallergic responses, regulate cardiovascular parameters and are fundamental to the development of the nerve cell membranes.

A dietary deficiency of arachidonic acid and the consequent limited synthesis of immunoallergic response mediators, together with the low antigen load from complete animal proteins, could thus explain some findings in HPA subjects who showed an overall reduction of allergic symptoms compared to controls, despite higher plasma levels of IgE (Riva et al., 1989) and a lower level of humoral immune stimulation reflected in lower IgG, IgA and IgM levels all at paediatric ages

(Giovannini et al., 1988). Furthermore, the dietary deficiency of n-6 polyunsaturated derivatives seems to reflect negatively on atopic expression (Melnik et al., 1992).

However, although it still cannot be affirmed whether chronically supplementing treated HPA subjects with VLCP fatty acids is worthwhile, the latest studies on breast milk (Clandinin et al., 1989) suggest that supplementing the formulas for HPA subjects is appropriate in the first year of life, since the central nervous system is most vulnerable to dietary deficiencies in this period (Dobbing, 1968).

Furthermore, the conditional intake of VLCP fatty acids can have negative effects on the development of foetal tissues in the third trimester of pregnancy (Neuringer & Connor, 1986), as they selectively accumulate in the fetal membranes, especially in the central nervous system. VLCP n-3 fatty acids were observed to be associated with neurological and electrophysiological parameters of development, while n-6 fatty acids seem to be fundamental to normal growth (Carlson et al., 1990; Uauy et al., 1990; Koletzko & Braun, 1991).

In the first case of maternal PKU that we treated, supplementation of VLCP fatty acids was carried out with equal parts of fish oil and blackcurrant oil (0.3–0.4 per cent of daily caloric requirement) in the fifth month of pregnancy; besides a strict low phe diet, the girl was also supplemented with carnitine and a mixture of vitamins, minerals and trace elements. Third trimester check-ups showed circulating VLCP fatty acids at the same level as in control women on a free diet and the baby, born at term, presented with a perfectly normal clinical picture showing an adequate psychomotor development (Giovannini et al., 1991). In conclusion, almost 40 years after being introduced, the low phenylalanine diet still remains the only effective therapeutic tool for HPA children.

However, growing accuracy in the diagnosis and the deeper knowledge of the pathogenesis of neurological damage allow us to suggest the following indications:

(1) dietary treatment has to be life-long, in order to prevent the toxic effects of pathogenetic mechanisms always working and the need to reintroduce the diet in HPA women during pregnancy.

(2) pathogenetic hypotheses indicate that, besides a phe restricted diet, other possible therapeutical approaches, as supplementation with amino acids modulating the negative biochemical effects of HPA or with those compounds which, although lacking in semisynthetic diets, are fundamental for the growth and the integrity of the central nervous system, are possible.

On the basis of these considerations, the follow-up of HPA subjects will demand an even greater commitment from paediatric nutritionists. The original 'dietary therapy', in fact, is gradually becoming 'nutritional therapy', which is not confined to the elaboration of low-phe alimentary regimens, but contributes to a better prognosis for HPAs by applying the latest knowledge of the biochemistry and physiology of nutrition.

References

Acosta, P.B. & Stepnick-Gropper, S. (1986): Problems related to diet management of maternal phenylketonuria. *J. Inherit. Metab. Dis.* **9 (suppl 2)**, 183–201.

Agostoni, C., Riva, E. & Valsasina, R. (1990): Plasma and urine levels of taurine in PKU children and in normal control population. In: *Abstract book: 5th International Congress of Inborn Errors of Metabolism.* Asilomar, CA.

Berry, H.K., Brunner, R.L., Hunt, M.M. & White, P.P. (1990): Valine, isoleucine, and leucine. A new treatment for phenylketonuria. *Am. J. Dis. Child.* 539–543.

Bick, U., Fahrendorf, G. & Ludolph, A. (1989): MR imaging of the brain in patients with hyperphenylalaninemia. In: *Book of abstracts*, SSIEM 27th Annual Symposium, p. 23.

Bickel, H., Gerrard, J. & Hickmans, E.M. (1954): The influence of phenylalanine intake on the chemistry and behaviour of a phenylketonuric child. *Acta Paediatr.* **43**, 64–77.

Carlson, S.E., Cooke, R.J. & Rhodes, P.G. (1990): n-3 supplementation of the very small premature infant: accumulation and function. In: *Book of abstracts*, 3rd Joint Meeting ESPGAN/NASPGN, Amsterdam, pp. 43–44.

Clandinin, M.T., Chappell, J.E. & Van Aerde, J.E.E. (1989): Requirements of newborn infants for long-chain polyunsaturated fatty acids. *Acta Paediatr. Scand.* **351 (suppl.)**, 63–71.

Depondt, E., Ogier, H. & Munnich, A. (1983): Régime contrôlé en phénylalanine. Le système de parts pondérales. *Arch. Fr. Pediatr.* **40**, 251–256.

Dobbing, J. (1968): Vulnerable periods in developing brain. In: *Applied neurochemistry*, eds. A.N. Davison & J. Dobbing, pp. 287–316. Oxford: Blackwell.

Drogari, E., Smith, I. & Beasley, M. (1987): Timing of strict diet in relation to fetal damage in maternal phenylketonuria. *Lancet* **ii**, 927–930.

Fölling, A. (1934): Über Ausscheidung von Phenylbrenztraubensäure in der Harm als Stoffwechselanomalie in Verbidung mit Imbezillität. *Z. Physiol. Chem.* **227**, 169–176.

Galli, C., Agostoni, C. & Mosconi, C. (1991) Reduced plasma C-20 and C-22 polyunsaturated fatty acids in PKU children under dietary intervention. *J. Pediatr.* **4**, 562–567.

Galluzzo, C., Ortisi, M.T. & Castelli, L. (1985): Plasma lipid concentrations in 42 treated phenylketonuric children. *J. Inherit. Metab. Dis.* **8(suppl.)**, 129.

Giovannini, M., Longhi, R. & Riva, E. (1985): Protocollo per la dietoterapia delle iperfenilalaninemie. *Riv. Ital. Pediatr. (I.J.P.)* **11**, 434–439.

Giovannini, M., Agostoni, C. & Galluzzo, C. (1988): Low serum concentrations of immunoglobulin G, A and M in children on low antigenic charge diets. *Acta Paediatr. Scand.* **77**, 306–307.

Giovannini, M., Agostoni, C., Valsasina, R., Cesa Bianchi, A. & Riva, E. (1989): Intake of linoleic and linolenic acids in phenylketonuric children. In: *Health effects of fish and fish oils*, ed. K. Chandra, pp. 468–477. St. John's, Newfoundland: ARTS Biomedical.

Giovannini, M., Riva, E. & Biasucci, G. (1991): Nutritional and metabolic management in maternal PKU. In: *Abstract Book*, 29th SSIEM Annual Meeting, London.

Guthrie, R. & Susi, A. (1963): A simple phenylalanine method for detecting phenylketonuria in large populations of newborn infants. *Pediatrics* **32**, 338–341.

Hanley, W.B., Clarke, J.T.R. & Schoonkeyt, W. (1987): Maternal phenylketonuria (PKU) – a review. *Clin. Biochem.* **20**, 149–154.

Holtzman, N., Dronmal, R. & Van Doornick, W. (1986): Effect of age at loss of dietary control on intellectual performance and behaviour of children with phenylketonuria. *N. Engl. J. Med.* **14**, 593–595.

Hommes, F.A., Eller, A.G. & Taylor, E.H. (1982): Turnover of the fast components of myelin and myelin proteins in experimental hyperphenylalaninemia. Relevance to termination of dietary treatment in human PKU. *J. Inherit. Metab. Dis.* **5**, 21–25.

Hommes, F.A. & Moss, L. (1992): Myelin turnover in hyperphenylalaninemia. A re-evaluation with the HPH-5 mouse. *J. Inherit. Metab. Dis.* **15**, 243–251.

Irons, M., Levy, H.L. & O'Flynn, M.E. (1987): Folinic acid therapy on the treatment of dihydropteridine reductase deficiency. *J. Pediatr.* **110**, 61–64.

Jervis, G.A. (1939): The genetics of phenylpiruvic oligophrenia. *J. Ment. Sci.* **85**, 719–762.

Kaufman, S. (1989): An evaluation of the possible neurotoxicity of metabolites of phenylalanine. *J. Pediatr.* **114**, 895–900.

Koch, R., Azen, C., Friedman, E.G. & Williamson, M.L. (1984): Paired comparisons between early-treated PKU children and their matched sibling controls on intelligence and school achievement test results at eight years of age. *J. Inherit. Metab. Dis.* **7**, 86–91.

Koch, R. & Wenz, E. (1987): Phenylketonuria. *Ann. Rev. Nutr.* **7**, 117–135.

Koletzko, B. & Braun, M. (1991): Arachidonic acid and early human growth: is there a relation? *Ann. Nutr. Metab.* **35**, 128–131.

Lenke, R. & Levy, H. (1980): Maternal phenylketonuria and hyperphenylalaninemia. *N. Engl. J. Med.* **303**, 1202–1208.

Lin, D.S., Pitkin, R.M. & Connor, W.E. (1977): Placental transfer of cholesterol into human fetus. *Am. J. Obstetr. Gynecol.* **128**, 735–739.

Lipson, A., Beuhler, B., Bartley, J., Walsh, D., Yu, J., O'Halloran, M. & Webster, W. (1984): Maternal hyperphenylalaninemia fetal effects. *J. Pediatr.* **104**, 216–220.

Longhi, R., Rottoli, A. & Vittorelli, A. (1987): Trace elements nutriture in hyperphenylalaninemic patients. Long term follow up study. *Eur. J. Pediatr.* **146 (suppl.),** a32–37.

Lou, H.C. (1985): Large doses of tryptophan and tyrosine as potential therapeutic alternative to dietary phenylalanine restriction in phenylketonuria. *Lancet* **ii,** 150–151.

Matalon, R., Michals, K. & Azen, C. (1991): Maternal PKU collaborative study: the effect of nutrient intake on pregnancy outcome. *J. Inherit. Metab. Dis.* **14,** 371–374.

Melnik, B., Tschung, T. & Plewig, G. (1992): Is atopy caused by defects of omega6 fatty acid and prostaglandin E metabolism? In: *Recent advances in infant feeding,* eds. B. Koletzko, A. Okken, G. Rey, B. Salle & J.P. Van Biervliet. Stuttgart, New York: Springer Verlag-Thieme.

Michals, K., Lopus, M. & Matalon, R. (1988): Phenylalanine metabolites as indicators of dietary compliance in children with phenylketonuria. *Biochem. Med. Metabol. Biol.* **39,** 18–23.

Neuringer, M. & Connor, W. (1986): n-3 fatty acids in the brain and retina: evidence for their essentiality. *Nutr. Rev.* **44,** 285–294.

Pardridge, W.M. & Choi, T.D. (1986): Neutral amino acid transport at the blood–brain barrier. *Fed. Proc.* **45,** 2073–2078.

Riva, E., Fiocchi, A. & Valsasina, R. (1989): Immunologic findings in classical phenylketonuria. *Abstract Book*: SIMS Annual Meeting, Grenelefe, n. 35.

Rottoli, A., Riva, E. & Lista, G. (1986): Plasma chromium and manganese levels in treated PKU patients. *J. Inherit. Metab. Dis.* **9,** 215.

Schulpis, K.H. & Scarpalezou, A. (1989): Triglycerides, cholesterol, HDL, LDL and VLDL cholesterol in serum of phenylketonuric children under dietary control. *Chin. Pediatr.* **28,** 466–469.

Schulpis, K., Namopoulos, C. & Scarpalezou, A. (1990): Serum carnitine level in phenylketonuric children under dietary control in Greece. *Acta Paediatr. Scand.* **79,** 930–934.

Smith, I. & Wolff, O.H. (1974): Natural history of phenylketonuria and influence of early treatment. *Lancet* **ii,** 540–543.

Smith, I., Beasley, M.G., Wolff, O.H. & Ades, A.E. (1988): Behavior disturbance in 8-year-old children with early treated phenylketonuria. *J. Pediatr.* **112,** 403–408.

Smith, I., Beasley, M.G. & Ades, A.E. (1990): Intelligence and quality of dietary treatment in phenylketonuria. *Arch. Dis. Child.* **65,** 472–478.

Sturman, A. (1988): Taurine in development. *J. Nutr.* **118,** 1169–1176.

Uauy, R., Birch, D. & Birch, E. (1990): Effect of omega-3 fatty acids on retinal function of very low birth weight neonates. *Pediatr. Res.* **28,** 485–492.

Valsasina, R., Riva, E. & Biasucci, G. (1989): Study on pteridines metabolism in children affected by hyperphenylalaninemia and phenylketonuria. *Pteridines* **1,** 129–132.

Vorhees, C.V. & Berry, H.K. (1989): Branched chain amino acids improve complex maze learning in rat offspring prenatally exposed to hyperphenylalaninemia: implications for maternal phenylketonuria. *Pediatr. Res.* **25,** 568–572.

Chapter 6

Genotype/phenotype correlation in phenylketonuria

Irma Dianzani*, Luisa de Sanctis*, Sergio Giannattasio†, Carla Alliaudi*, Maria Sartore*, Carlo Dionisi Vici‡, Alberto Burlina§, Massimo Burroni¶, Francesco Papadia**, Gianfranco Sebastio††, Vito Guzzetta††, Ersilia Marra†, Clara Camaschella* and Alberto Ponzone*

*Clinica Pediatrica and Clinica Medica, Università di Torino; †CNR-Centro di Studio sui Mitocondri e Metabolismo Energetico, Bari; ‡Ospedale Bambino Gesù, Roma; §Dipartimento di Pediatria, Università di Padova; ¶Servizio Autonomo di Neuropsichiatria Infantile, Fano; **Divisione di Malattie Metaboliche e Genetiche, Ospedale Pediatrico Giovanni XXIII, Bari; ††Cattedra di Pediatria, II Facoltà di Medicina, Università di Napoli, Italy

Summary

The deficiency of the hepatic enzyme phenylalanine hydroxylase results in hyperphenylalaninaemia of variable severity. The clinical heterogeneity is due to the different residual activity of the mutated enzymes, which depends on the type of DNA change responsible for the defect. Recent studies showed a correlation between the enzymatic activity predicted by *in vitro* expression of the mutated genes and several clinical parameters, such as pretreatment phenylalanine level, phenylalanine tolerance, and the serum phenylalanine level measured after a standardized protein load. Thus, it is well ascertained that several mutations have severe effects on the phenotype, whereas others are associated with a milder variant of the disease. The genotype/phenotype association is apparent particularly in patients homozygous for a mutation or in patients compound heterozygous for two severe or mild mutations. On the other hand, it is difficult to predict the outcome of a compound heterozygous for a mild and a severe mutation. Additional, factors, so far unknown, probably influence the phenotype.

Introduction

Several inherited disorders are characterized by high phenylalanine levels in plasma and urine. They are all caused by disturbance of the hydroxylating system which converts phenylalanine to tyrosine (Scriver *et al.*, 1989). The reaction is catalysed by the enzyme phenylalanine hydroxylase (PAH) whose deficiency, phenylketonuria (PKU), is responsible for more than 97 per cent of hyperphenylalaninaemias (HPA). In this disease the neurological damage caused by persistent HPA may be prevented by the early introduction of a phenylalanine (phe) restricted diet.

The hydroxylating system may also be blocked by a defect of the cofactor tetrahydrobiopterin (BH4). BH4 defects include both defects in biopterin synthesis and in BH4 recycling. Pyruvoyl tetrahydropterin synthase (PTPS) and guanosine triphosphate (GTP) cyclohydrolase deficiencies cause inhibition of the synthetic pathway, whereas in dihydropteridine reductase (DHPR) deficiency the oxidized cofactor is not hydroxylated to the active form.

A transient hyperphenylalaninaemia has been reported in patients with a defect of carbinolamine dehydratase, a further enzyme involved in BH4 recycling (Citron et al., 1993).

Severe neurological symptoms unresponsive to a phenylalanine restricted diet are associated with BH4 deficiency. They are caused by a defective synthesis of the neurotransmitters derived from tyrosine and tryptophan, since the three hydroxylases for aromatic amino acids require BH4 as a cofactor. Thus, the patients require a specific treatment with the precursors of the deficient neurotransmitters.

All the five enzymes whose defects are well-known causes of inherited hyperphenylalaninaemia have been recently cloned and a number of the underlying molecular defects have been identified (Scriver et al., 1989; Howells et al., 1990; Thöny et al., 1992; Togari et al., 1992; Ashida et al.,1993; Blau et al., 1993; Citron et al., 1993; Dianzani et al., 1993a; Scriver, 1994; Smooker et al.,1993).

A novel approach to diagnosis, treatment, prognosis and also prevention of the disease has been implemented by these studies. Prenatal diagnosis and carrier detection are easily performed by tracing the inheritance of the causal mutations in characterized families. On the other hand, several polymorphic markers within the gene (RFLPs, VNTR, STR) (Goltsov et al., 1992, 1993) can be used to identify the mutated uncharacterized alleles by comparison with an affected sibling. At least in PKU, the identification of genotype/phenotype correlation may allow an early, optimal treatment, based on the type of mutation, to be devised (Okano et al., 1991).

Molecular basis for PAH deficiency

The human PAH gene was cloned in 1985 and mapped on the long arm of chromosome 12 (Kwok et al., 1985; DiLella et al., 1986). Analysis of RFLPs at the PAH locus showed a remarkable heterogeneity. Two haplotypes were shown to be frequent in north European PKU patients (haplotypes 2 and 3). The subsequent characterization of these alleles led to the identification of the first two causal mutations in 1987: a base substitution at the splice site of intron 12, associated with haplotype 3, and a mis-sense mutation at codon 408, associated with haplotype 2 (Dilelle et al., 1987; Marvit et al., 1987). The contemporary introduction of PCR technology (Saiki, 1987) and the development of rapid methods for mutation detection (reviewed in Dianzani et al., 1994a) sped up the search for causal mutations. So far more than 100 PKU mutations have been reported (Scriver, 1994). Most of the mutations lie within the 3' portion of the gene and a very high number of mutations have been found in exon 7. The clustering of mutations in this area has been ascribed to the great functional importance of the encoded region of the protein. The putative pterin binding site has been located in the region corresponding to exons 7 and 8 (Jennings et al., 1991), a putative phenylalanine allosteric binding site in the region encoded by exon 6 (Schuster-Gibbs & Benkovic, 1991).

Most of the DNA changes are point mutations: only two large deletions have been reported so far: one includes exons 1 and 2 (Sullivan et al., 1985), the other exon 3 (Avigad et al., 1990). Most mutations lead to amino acid substitution, but also nonsense and splice mutations have been reported. Two of the most common mutations in Caucasians affect a splice site (IVS X-546 and IVS XII-1).

Geographic distribution of PKU mutations

A distinct geographical pattern has been observed in the distribution of PKU mutations. Although PKU is observed both in Asia and Europe, the responsible mutations are completely different, showing that the disease has expanded after racial divergence (Eisensmith et al., 1992).

Two mutations are frequent in northern Europe, IVS XII-1 and R408W: a North to South gradient is shown by the former, but an East to West gradient by the latter. A third mutation, IVS X-546, is frequent in Mediterranean populations, but very rare in northern Europe (Eisensmith et al., 1992).

Interesting data on the migration of ancient populations may be inferred by these studies. Actually, the distribution of these mutations corresponds to three main clines observed by analysing the distribution of non-DNA polymorphisms. These gradients of genetic differentiation could be associated with four main events: (a) the spread of Neolithic farmers from the Near East to all Europe; (b) the admixture of Uralic-speaking people with Northern Europeans; (c) the migrations of speakers of Indo-European languages from the Eurasian steppes (region of the Don river); (d) the effect of Greek colonization (Piazza, 1993). The distribution of IVS X-546 corresponds to pattern (a), that of IVS XII-1 to pattern (b) and that of R408W to pattern (c). Thus the origin of each mutation may be inferred and the corresponding geographical distribution can be explained by the effect of genetic drift and the following admixtures with other populations (Piazza et al., 1993).

Conspicuous difference in the distribution of mutations have also been identified at microgeographical levels. In Italy, we have observed a very different distribution of several PKU mutations in northern and southern regions (Dianzani et al., 1994b). It is noteworthy that a distinct North to South gradient was observed in a genetic map of Italy constructed by using non-DNA polymorphisms (Piazza et al., 1988). The colonization of prehistoric Italy by different small populations was invoked to explain these differences (Piazza et al., 1988), and may account also for the extreme heterogeneity of PKU mutations within the Italian population's differences (Dianzani et al., 1992; and in preparation).

Early studies focused on the analysis of RFLP haplotypes associated with Italian PKU alleles allowed the prediction of many different PKU mutations in Italy (Dianzani et al., 1990). A different distribution of haplotypes in Italy was also observed as compared to PKU alleles from northern Europe. To identify the mutations causing PKU in Italy we have amplified and screened the 13 PAH exons from 20 PKU patients, whose origins are scattered throughout Italy. We employed the chemical cleavage of mismatch (CCM) method to screen couples of exons sufficiently close to be analysed within a single PCR and CCM reaction (exons 7–8, 9–10, 10–11) (Dianzani et al., 1990, 1993b). We directly sequenced exons interspaced by large introns. The frequency of each identified

Table 1. Distribution of PKU mutations in the Italian population; frequencies were estimated by the analysis of 186 unrelated Italian PKU alleles (see text)

Mutations	Frequency (%)
IVS X-546	13.7
L48S	8.6
R261Q	5.4
R158Q	5.4
R261X	4.3
R252W	3.2
delT55	2.7
P281L	2.2
IVS VII-1	2.2
IVS XII-1	2.2
A259V	1.6
R408W	1.1
A403V	1.0
S231P	0.5
S359X	0.5
Undefined	45.4
Total	100.0

mutation was determined by ASO analysis (reviewed in Dianzani et al., 1994a) or restriction digestion (Eiken et al., 1991) within a panel of 186 Italian PKU alleles. This approach allowed us to characterize 54.6 per cent of the Italian PKU alleles. Five new mutations (S67P, S231P, IVS VII-1, S359X, A403V) and ten known mutations (L48S, delT55, R158Q, R252W, R261Q, R261X, P281L, IVS X-546, IVS XII-1, R408W) have been identified, as well as several polymorphisms. Most mutations are represented with a low frequency (Table 1). By analogy with a recent study of the inhabitants of Sicily (Guldberg et al., 1993), we believe that the remaining 46.4 per cent of uncharacterized alleles include rare or private mutations.

In conclusion, the extreme heterogeneity of PKU mutations in Italy precludes the introduction of programmes for carrier detection at a population level and thus prevention by family counselling. In fact, to be effective in terms of costs/benefits a carrier screening programme should be done in populations where at least 95 per cent of mutations are characterized and where the number of mutations is not too great. In families who request prenatal diagnosis the discovery of the mutations might be done by methods able to screen for multiple mutations, such as reverse dot blot (reviewed in Dianzani et al., 1994a) including the 15 mutations which occur more frequently. The utilization of polymorphic markers is probably preferable to detecting mutations for rare or uncharacterized DNA changes.

From genotype to phenotype

Early studies found a correlation between clinical presentation and RFLP haplotypes (Güttler et al., 1987). Haplotypes 2 and 3 were found to be associated with a severe PKU, whereas haplotypes 1 and 4 showed variable phenotypes. This suggested that the heterogeneity observed at clinical level (different tolerance to phenylalanine) and at biochemical level (residual enzyme activity) were accounted for by variable DNA defects. This hypothesis was confirmed by a study of Okano et al., (1991) identifying an association between specific mutations and PKU phenotypes. The enzymatic activity predicted by in vitro expression of the mutated genes correlated with pretreatment phe levels, phe tolerance, and serum phe levels measured after a standardized protein load.

Some mutations, like IVS XII-1, R408W, R243X, and P281L, were associated with a severe phenotype and no enzyme activity was observed when the mutated enzymes were expressed in a COS system ('null' mutations). The absence of immunoreactivity demonstrated lack of the protein. On the other hand, two other mutations, R261Q and Y414C, were generally able to confer a mild PKU, even in compound heterozygosity with a 'severe' mutation. The mutated enzymes showed respectively 30 and 50 per cent of normal activity in the in vitro system. A further mutation, R158Q, was associated with 10 per cent of normal activity, but conferred a severe phenotype in the homozygous state.

The authors proposed a simple calculation to predict the residual enzyme activity in cases of compound heterozygosity (Okano et al., 1991). The predicted value was calculated by averaging the relative levels of PAH activity associated with each mutant enzyme in vitro. Thus a subject compound heterozygote for R408W (0 per cent of normal level) and Y414C (50 per cent) should have a residual activity of 25 per cent of normal level.

This study suggested that early identification of the causal mutations after birth could help towards the choice of the most correct diet for each molecular entity and could be of use even in predicting prognosis.

However, some discrepancies were soon found. A certain overlap was shown between the three cases main phenotypes, identified by phe tolerance (classic, mild, benign). In particular, classification of the cases with a predicted activity around 15 per cent, which represent the boundary between classic and mild phenotypes, was difficult. The same combinations of DNA changes seemed to cause either a mild or a classic phenotype. To account for the overlap a third phenotype was introduced by Güttler et al. (1993a): 'moderate' PKU.

A variable association with phenotype has been observed for R261Q which when homozygous may be associated both with a benign and with a mild PKU. In heterozygosity this mutation is generally associated with a less severe phenotype, but even classic PKU has been reported (Okano et al., 1991; Kleiman et al., 1993).

We evaluated the phenotype/genotype association in the 34 completely characterized patients from our series. To define the clinical phenotype better we considered three clinical parameters: plasma phe levels at diagnosis, plasma phe normalization time after introduction of a phenylalanine-free diet and phe tolerance (expressed as mg of phe ingested per day able to keep the plasma phe levels between 2 and 6 mg/dl) (Table 2). The analysis of the Italian patients showed a certain overlap between the mild and classic phenotypes for some of the parameters mentioned above. We described this overlapping group of patients as having 'moderate' PKU (Guttler et al., 1993a). None of the completely characterized patients showed a benign type. Tables 3 and 4 report the data we obtained by analysing the Italian PKU population.

Table 2. Clinical classification of PKU phenotypes. Seven patients showed intermediate data for some of these parameters and were assigned to 'moderate' PKU.

	Classic	Mild
Pre-treatment phe	> 25 mg %	15–25 mg %
Plasma phe normalization time	> 4 days	< 4 days
Phe tolerance	< 300 mg/day	300–700 mg/day
Patients (n)	20	7

Most of the patients were compound homozygotes for different mutations. Only eleven homozygotes were included in our series, because of the extreme heterogeneity of the Italian PKU population. A tentative clinical classification of PKU mutations is reported in Table 5. We decided to use the following parameters: the amount of residual activity *in vitro* (if data available), the phenotype shown by patients who were homozygous for each mutation, and the phenotype shown when in compound heterozygosity with a severe or a mild mutation. Thus a mutation is severe when a residual activity lower than 15 per cent is shown in *in vitro* expression experiments, or when it confers a severe phenotype both when homozygous or heterozygous with another severe mutation. A mutation is mild when a residual activity higher than 15 per cent is shown in *in vitro* expression experiments, or when it confers a mild phenotype both when homozygous or when heterozygous with another mild mutation. The association of a mild with a severe mutation can result in all possible phenotypes, i.e. mild, moderate or classic.

Thus severe mutations are R261X, IVS X-546, R252W, and P281L, who confer a classic phenotype when homozygous in our series (Table 3). These mutations confer a severe phenotype in compound heterozygosity with other mutations classified as severe by data from the literature, such as IVS

Table 3. Genotype/phenotype association in 11 completely characterized PKU patients homozygous for different PKU mutations; only one patient was identified for each combination, unless indicated in parentheses

Genotype	Phenotype
IVS X-546: IVS X-546	Classic (3)
R261 X: R261 X	Classic (3)
P281 L: P281 L	Classic (2)
R158 Q: R158 Q	Classic
R252 W: R252 W	Classic
R261 Q: R261 Q	Mild

Table 4. Genotype/phenotype association in 23 completely characterized PKU patients compound heterozygous for different PKU mutations; only one patient was identified for each combination, unless indicated in parentheses

Genotype	Phenotype
IVS X-546: IVS VII-1	Classic
IVS X-546: P281L	Classic
IVS X-546: delT55	Classic
IVS X-546: R261Q	Classic
IVS XII-1: P281L	Classic
R252W: L48S	Classic
R408W: L48S	Classic
S231P: R261Q	Classic
S359X: del T55	Classic
L48S: IVS X-546	Moderate; mild (2)
L48S: IVS VII-1	Moderate
L48S: R158Q	Moderate
R158Q: R261Q	Moderate (2)
R158Q: IVS XII-1	Moderate
R261Q: delT55	Moderate
R261Q: L48S	Mild
L48S: delT55	Mild
L48S: S67P	Mild
A403V: P281L	Mild
A403V: R261X	Mild

XII-1 (Okano *et al.*, 1991), delT55 (Konecki & Lichter-Konecki, 1991), and R408W (Okano *et al.*, 1991). A mild phenotype was shown by the single patient homozygote for R261Q.

This tentative classification allowed us to classify as mild the new mutations R403V and S67P, because the first confers a mild phenotype in association with severe mutations, such as P281L and R261X, and the second confers a mild PKU when associated with another mild mutation, such as L48S.

IVS VII-1 and S359X are probably severe mutations since a disruption of the protein is expected by the nature of these defects. In our limited series they give a classic phenotype when associated with a severe mutation, such as IVS X-546 and delT55, respectively. A further new mutation, S231P was shown to have no residual activity when expressed *in vitro* (Dianzanial *et al.*, 1995).

It is interesting to note that mutation R158Q, which gives a severe phenotype when homozygous (Table 3 and Okano *et al.*, 1991), gives an intermediate phenotype when in compound heterozygosity with a severe mutation, such as IVS XII-1 or with a mild mutation such as R261Q (in two patients) or L48S (in one patient). A residual activity of 10 per cent shown by the mutated enzyme in expression experiments might explain this peculiar pattern (Okano *et al.*, 1991).

Similar to other series (Okano *et al.*, 1991; Rey *et al.*, 1992; Kleiman *et al.*, 1993; Konecki *et al.*,

Table 5. Phenotypic classification of PKU mutations

Mutation	Severe	Mild
Activity in expression system	< 15 %	> 15 %
Phenotype in homozygosity	Classic	Mild
Phenotype in compound heterozygosity with a severe mutation	Classic	Mild/moderate/classic
Phenotype in compound heterozygosity with a mild mutation	Mild/moderate/classic	Mild

1993; Svensson *et al.*, 1993), mild mutations such as L48S or R261Q can give either a classic or a mild or an intermediate phenotype when in compound heterozygosity with a severe mutation.

The causes for this variability are unknown. It is obvious that other factors may influence the phenotype. Negative interaction between different mutant subunits might occur in the mature polymeric protein. This might be the case for mutations associated with some residual activity. In addition, the hydroxylating system might be modulated by modifier genes. Finally, it is important to note that expression analyses are usually performed in a monkey kidney cell system or in an *E. coli* system, which are certainly different from the human liver enviroment *in vivo*.

The importance of other unidentified factors *in vivo* is shown also by the impossibility of consistently predicting the degree of mental retardation in untreated PKU subjects. This was clearly observed in several studies (Güttler *et al.*, 1993b; Ramus *et al.*, 1993). In one, 55 untreated patients were genotyped and the degree of mental retardation (ii) was evaluated (Ramus *et al.*, 1993). Even if some of the intellectual phenotypes of patients correlated with the predicted activity of the responsible mutations, major differences in intellectual phenotypes were found in patients with the same genotype, both among unrelated patients and within families. Interestingly, a few untreated cases homozygous for a so-called 'severe' mutation were associated with a normal mental development. Moreover, there was no correlation between serum phe levels and IQ. This shows that other factors (diet, inheritance, intellectual stimulation) clearly influence the final outcome.

Finally, the association of mutations with specific phenotypes accounts for the different clinical presentation of PKU among populations. The frequency of severe mutations, such as R408W and IVS XII-1, in northern Europe is the cause of the greater severity of PKU in these nations as compared to Mediterranean populations (Rey *et al.*, 1992), where mild mutations are more often represented (L48S, R261Q).

References

Ashida, A., Hatakeyama, K. & Kagamiyama, H. (1993): cDNA cloning, expression in *Escherichia coli* and purification of human 6-pyruvoyl-tetrahydropterin synthase. *Biochem. Biophys. Res. Commun.* **195**, 1386–1393.

Avigad, S., Cohen, B.E., Bauer, S., Schwartz, G., Frydman, M., Woo, S.L.C., Niny, Y. & Shiloh, Y. (1990): A single origin of phenylketonuria in Yemenite Jews. *Nature* **334**, 168–170.

Blau, N., Heizmann, C.W., Spert, W., Korenke, G.C., Hoffmann, G.F., Smooker, P.M. & Cotton, R.G.H. (1993): Atypical (mild) forms of dihydropteridine reductase deficiency. Neurochemical evaluation and mutation detection. *Ped. Res.* **32**, 726–730.

Citron, B.A., Kaufman, S., Milstien, S., Naylor, E.W., Greene, C.L. & Davis, M.D. (1993): Mutation in the 4a-carbinolamine dehydratase gene leads to mild hyperphenylalaninemia with defective cofactor metabolism. *Am. J. Hum. Genet.* **53**, 768–774.

Dianzani, I., Devoto, M., Camaschella, C., Saglio, G., Ferrero, G.B., Cerone, R., Romano, C., Romeo, G., Giovannini, M., Riva, E., Angeneydt, F., Trefz, F.K., Okano, Y. & Woo, S.L.C. (1990): Haplotype distribution and molecular defects at the phenylalanine hydroxylase locus in Italy. *Hum. Genet.* **86**, 69–72.

Dianzani, I., Forrest, S.M., Camaschella, C., Saglio, G., Ponzone, A. & Cotton, R.G.H. (1991): Screening for PKU mutations in the phenylalanine hydroxylase gene from Italian patients with phenylketonuria using the chemical cleavage method: a new splice mutation. *Am. J. Hum. Genet.* **48**, 631–635.

Dianzani, I., de Sanctis, L., Ferrero, G.B., Alliaudi, C., Ponzone, A. & Camaschella, C. (1992): Molecular analysis of phenylketonuria in Italy. *Am. J. Hum. Genet.* **51(suppl)**, A349.

Dianzani, I., Howells, D.W., Ponzone, A., Saleeba, J.A., Smooker, P.M. & Cotton, R.G.H. (1993a): Two new mutations in the dihydropteridine reductase gene in patients with tetrahydrobiopterin deficiency. *J. Med. Genet.* **30**, 465–469.

Dianzani, I., Camaschella, C., Saglio, G., Ferrero, G.B., Ramus, S., Ponzone, A. & Cotton, R.G.H. (1993b): Molecular analysis of contiguous exons of phenylalanine hydroxylase: identification of a novel PKU mutation. *J. Med. Genet.* **30**, 228–231.

Dianzani, I., Camaschella, C., Ponzone, A. & Cotton, R.G.H. (1994a): Dilemmas and progress in mutation detection. *Trends Genet.* **9**, 403–405.

Dianzani, I., Giannattasio, S., de Sanctis, L., Marra, E., Ponzone, A., Camaschella, C., & Piazza, A. (1994): Genetic history of phenylketonuria mutations in Italy. *Am. J. Hum. Genet.* **55**, 851–853.

Dianzani, I., Knappskog, P.M., de Sanctis, L., Riva, E., Ponzone, A., Apold, J., & Camascella, C. (1995): Novel missense mutation in the phenylanine hydroxylase gene leading to complete loss of enzymatic activity. *Hum. Mut.* (in press).

Di Lella, A.G., Kwok, S.C.M., Ledley, F.D., Marvit, J. & Woo, S.L.C. (1986): Molecular structure and polymorphic map of the human phenylalanine hydroxylase gene. *Biochemistry* **25**, 743–749.

Di Lella, A.G., Marvit, J., Brayton, K. & Woo, S.L.C. (1987): An amino acid substitution involved in phenylketonuria is in tight linkage with DNA haplotype 2. *Nature* **327**, 333–338.

Eiken, H.G., Odland, E., Boman, H., Skjelkvale, L., Engebretsen, L.F. & Apold, J. (1991): Application of natural and amplification created restriction sites for the diagnosis of PKU mutations. *Nucl. Acids Res.* **19**, 1427–1430.

Eisensmith, R.C., Okano, I., Dasovich, M., Wang, T., Guttler, F., Lou, H., Guldberg, P., Lichter-Konecki, U., Konecki, D.S., Svensson, E., Hagenfeldt, L., Rey, F., Munnich, A., Lyonnet, S., Cockburn, F., Connor, J.M., Pembrey, M.E., Smith, I., Gitzelmann, R., Steinmann, B., Apold, J., Eiken, H.G., Giovannini, M., Riva, E., Longhi, R., Romano, C., Cerone, R., Naughten, E.R., Mullins, C., Cahalane, S., Ozalp, I., Fekete, G., Schuler, D., Berecsi, G.Y., Nasz, I., Brdicka, R., Kamaryt, J., Pijackova, A., Cabalska, B., Boszkowa, K., Schwartz, E., Kalinin, V.N., Jin, L., Chakraborty, R. & Woo, S.L.C. (1992): Multiple origins for phenylketonuria in Europe. *Am. J. Hum. Genet.* **51**, 1355–1365.

Goltsov, A.A., Eisensmith, R.C., Konecki, D.S., Lichter-Konecki, U. & Woo, S.L.C. (1992): Associations between mutations and a VNTR in the human phenylalanine hydroxylase gene. *Am. J. Hum. Genet.* **51**, 627–636.

Goltsov, A.A., Eisensmith, R.C., Naughton, E.R., Jin, L., Chakraborty, R. & Woo, S.L.C. (1993): A single polymorphic STR system in the human phenylalanine hydroxylase gene permits rapid prenatal diagnosis and carrier screening for phenylketonuria. *Hum. Mol. Genet.* **5**, 577–581.

Guldberg, P., Romano, V., Ceratto, N., Bosco, P., Ciuna, M., Indelicato, A., Mollica, F., Meli, C., Giovannini, M., Riva, E., Biasucci, G., Henriksen, K.F. & Guttler, F. (1993): Mutational spectrum of phenylalanine hydroxylase deficiency in Sicily: implications for diagnosis of hyperphenylalaninemia in Southern Europe. *Hum. Mol. Genet.* **2**, 1703–1707.

Güttler, F., Ledley, F.D., Lidski, A.S., DiLella, A.G., Sullivan, S.E. & Woo, S.L.C. (1987): Correlation between polymorphic DNA haplotypes at phenylalanine hydroxylase locus and clinical phenotypes of phenylketonuria. *J. Pediatr.* **110**, 68–71.

Güttler, F., Guldberg, P., & Henriksen, K.F., Mikkelsen, I., Olsen, B. & Lou, H. (1993a): Molecular basis for the phenotypical diversity of phenylketonuria and related hyperphenylalaninaemias. *J. Inherit. Metab. Dis.* **16**, 602–604.

Güttler, F., Guldberg, P., & Henriksen, K.F., Mikkelsen, I., Olsen, B., & Lou, H. (1993b): Mutation genotype of mentally retarded patients with phenylketonuria. *Dev. Brain Dysfunct.* **6**, 92–96.

Jennings, I.G., Kemp, B.E. & Cotton, R.G.H. (1991): Localisation of cofactor binding sites with monoclonal anti-idiotype antibodies: phenylalanine hydroxylase. *Proc. Natl. Acad. Sci. USA* **88**, 5734–5738.

Kleiman, S., Vanagaite, L., Bernstein, J., Schwartz, G., Brand, N., Elitzur, A., Woo, S.L.C. & Shiloh, Y. (1993): Phenylketonuria: variable phenotypic outcomes of the R261Q mutation and maternal PKU in the offspring of a healthy homozygote. *J. Med. Genet.* **30**, 284–288.

Konecki, D.S. & Lichter-Konecki, U. (1991): The phenylketonuria locus: current knowledge about alleles and mutation of the phenylalanine hydroxylase gene in various populations. *Hum. Genet.* **87**, 377–388.

Konecki, D.S., Schweitzer-Krantz, S., Byrd, D., Trefz, F.K. & Lichter-Konecki, U. (1993): Facilitation of hyperphenylalaninemia phenotype assessment by genotype analysis. *Pediatr. Res.* **152**, 1048–1049.

Kwok, S.C.M., Ledley, F.D., DiLella, A.G., Robson, K.J.H. & Woo, S.L.C. (1985): Nucleotide sequence of a full-length complementary DNA clone and amino acid sequence of human phenylalanine hydroxylase. *Biochemistry* **24**, 556–561.

Howells, D.W., Forrest, S.M., Dahl, H-H.M. & Cotton, R.G.H. (1990): Insertion of an extra codon for threonine is a cause of dihydropteridine reductase deficiency. *Am. J. Hum. Genet.* **47**, 279–285.

Marvit, J., DiLella, A.G., Brayton, K., Ledley, F.D., Robson, K.J.H. & Woo, S.L.C. (1987): GT to AT transition at a splice donor site causes skipping of the preceding exon in phenylketonuria. *Nucl. Acids Res.* **15**, 5613–5628.

Okano, Y., Eisensmith, R.C., Guttler, F., Lichter- Konecki, U., Konecki, D.S., Trefz, F.K., Dasovich, M., Wang, T., Henriksen, K., Lou, H. & Woo, S.L.C. (1991): Molecular basis of phenotypic heterogeneity in phenylketonuria. *N. Engl. J. Med.* **324**, 1232–1238.

Piazza, A., Cappello, N., Olivetti, E. & Rendine, S. (1988): A genetic history of Italy. *Ann. Hum. Genet.* **52**, 203–213.

Piazza, A. (1993): Who are the Europeans? *Science* **260**, 1767–1769.

Ramus, S.J., Forrest, S.M., Pitt, D.B., Saleeba, J.A. & Cotton, R.G.H. (1993): Comparison of genotype and intellectual phenotype in untreated PKU patients. *J. Med. Genet.* **30,** 401–405.

Rey, F., Abadie, V., Lyonnet, S., Berthelon, M., Caillaud, D., Melle, D., Labrune, P., Saudubray, J.M., Munnich, A., & Rey, J. (1992): Expression phénotypique de 12 mutations du gène de la phénylalanine hydroxylase. *Arch. Fr. Pediatr.* **49,** 705–710.

Saiki, R.K. (1987): Genetic analysis of enzymatically amplified B globin and HLA-DQ alpha genomic DNA with allele specific oligonucleotide probes. *Nature* **324,** 163–166.

Scriver, C.R. (1994): *PKU Mutation Analysis Consortium Database,* November.

Scriver, C.R., Kaufman, S. & Woo, S.L.C. (1989): The hyperphenylalaninemias. In: *The metabolic basis of inherited disease,* eds. C.R. Scriver, A.L. Beaudet, W.S. Sly, D. Valle. pp. 495–546. New York: McGraw Hill.

Schuster Gibbs, B. & Benkovic, S.J. (1991): Affinity labeling of the active site and the reactive sulfhydryl associated with activation of rat liver phenylalanine hydroxylase. *Biochemistry* **30,** 6795–6802.

Smooker, P.M., Howells, D.W. & Cotton, R.G.H. (1993): Identification and *in vitro* expression of mutations causing dihydropteridine reductase deficiency. *Biochemistry* **32,** 6443–6449.

Sullivan, S.E., Lidski, A.S., Brayton, K., DiLella, A.G., King, M., Connor, M. & Woo, S.L.C. (1985): Phenylalanine hydroxylase deletion mutant from a patient with classical PKU. *Am. J. Hum. Genet.* **37,** A177.

Svensson, E., von Dobeln, U., Eisensmith, R.C., Hagenfeldt, L. & Woo, S.L.C. (1993): Relation between genotype and phenotype in Swedish phenylketonuria and hyperphenylalaninemia patients. *Eur. J. Pediatr.* **152,** 132–139.

Togari, A., Ichinose, H., Matsumoto, S., Fujita, K. & Nagatsu, T. (1992): Multiple mRNA forms of human GTP cyclohydrolase I. *Biochem. Biophys. Res. Commun.* **187,** 359–365.

Thöny, B., Leimbacher, W., Burgisser, D. & Heizmann, C.W. (1992): Human 6-pyruvoyltetrahydropterin synthase: cDNA cloning and heterologous expression of the recombinant enzyme. *Biochem. Biophys. Res. Commun.* **189,** 1437–1443.

Chapter 7

Diagnosis of metabolic disorders with acute neonatal onset

Florence Poggi-Travert, Marco Spada, Thierry Billette de Villemeur, Philippe Hubert, Christiane Charpentier, Daniel Rabier, Pierre Kamoun and Jean-Marie Saudubray

Departments of Pediatrics and Biochemistry, Hôpital des Enfants-Malades, 149 rue de Sèvres, 75015 Paris, France

Summary

There are hitherto about 100 human diseases due to inborn errors of metabolism which can be revealed in the neonatal period or in very early infancy. These disorders have become a major cause of neonatal pathology, as the classical causes of neonatal distress have been markedly diminished by advances in obstetric, prenatal and perinatal management. Their incidence may well be underestimated as diagnostic errors are frequent. Many of them present early in the neonatal period, have a rapid fatal course and, as a whole, cannot be recognized by systematic screening tests which are too slow, too expensive and unreliable. This makes it an absolute necessity to teach primary care physicians a simple method of clinical screening before making decisions about sophisticated biochemical investigations.

As far as physiopathology is concerned, all metabolic disorders can be divided into three groups which can be helpful for diagnostic purposes: (1) diseases which disturb the synthesis or catabolism of complex molecules. All lysosomal disorders belong to this category. Only a few are clinically expressed in the neonatal period. By contrast, most of peroxisomal disorders clinically strike in the neonatal period. Another group of disorders is formed by mutations involving intracellular trafficking and processing of secretory proteins such as α-1-antitrypsin deficiency or the more recently described carbohydrate deficient glycoprotein syndrome. (2) Inborn errors of intermediary metabolism which lead to an acute or progressive endogenous intoxication secondary to an accumulation of toxic compounds proximal to the metabolic block. Amino-acidopathies, most of the organic acidurias, congenital urea cycle defects, and sugar intolerances belong to this group. (3) Inborn errors of intermediary metabolism in which the symptoms are at least partly due to deficiency in energy production or utilization processes. Congenital lactic acidaemias, fatty acid oxidation defects, and mitochondrial respiratory chain disorders belong to this group.

Since 1968, more than 300 newborns with inborn errors of intermediary metabolism, presenting with acute symptoms within the first month of life, have been evaluated by the metabolic and genetic service at Hôpital des Enfants-Malades, Paris. From this experience, a method of initial clinical evaluation and management has been developed. Acute neonatal forms of inherited errors of intermediary metabolism can be diagnosed or strongly suspected and assigned to one of five schematical bioclinical groups on the basis of the clinical history, physical examination, and readily available laboratory tests:

– Type I: neurological distress intoxication type with ketosis: maple syrup urine disease (MSUD).

– Type II: neurological distress intoxication type with ketoacidosis and hyperammonaemia: organic acidurias (MMA, PA, IVA) and long-chain fatty acid oxidation disorders (with cardiac symptoms).

– Type III: neurological deterioration energy deficiency type and hypotonia: congenital lactic acidosis (PC, PDH, respiratory chain deficiencies).

- Type IV: divided into three subtypes:
   (a) neurological distress intoxication type and seizures with hyperammonaemia and without ketoacidosis: urea cycle defects and fatty acid oxidation disorders (cardiac symptoms);
   (b) neurological deterioration, severe hypotonia, seizures without ketoacidosis or hyper-ammonaemia: non-ketotic hyperglycinaemia, peroxisomal disorders, sulphite oxidase deficiency and pyridoxino-dependent seizures;
   (c) storage disorders: GM1 gangliosidosis, sialidosis, galactosialidosis, Niemann–Pick type C.
- Type V: hepatomegaly with liver dysfunction divided into four subtypes:
   (a) hepatomegaly, hypoglycaemia and seizures: glycogenosis types I and III, gluconeogenesis defects and hyperinsulinism;
   (b) liver failure syndrome: fructosaemia, galactosaemia, tyrosinosis type I (after 3 weeks), neonatal haemochromatosis and respiratory chain disorders;
   (c) cholestatic jaundice and failure to thrive: α-1-antitrypsin deficiency, Byler's disease, inborn errors of bile acids, peroxisomal disorders and Niemann–Pick type C, and carbohydrate deficient glycoprotein syndrome (CDG);
   (d) hepatosplenomegaly with coarse facies: storage disorders.

One must emphasize frequent difficulties in investigating patients with life-threatening distress and multivisceral failure. At an advanced state, many non-specific symptoms that are secondary consequences can disturb the primary biological and clinical pattern.

There are hitherto over 300 human diseases which are due to inborn errors of metabolism and this number is constantly growing as new concepts and new techniques become available for identifying biochemical phenotypes. Among them, about 100 can appear in the neonatal period or very early in infancy. These disorders have become a major cause of neonatal pathology, as the classical causes of neonatal distress have been markedly diminished by advances in obstetric, prenatal and perinatal management. Their incidence may well be underestimated as diagnostic errors are frequent. Nevertheless, accurate diagnosis is essential in order to provide genetic counselling and prenatal diagnosis of subsequent pregnancies and especially because some of these conditions have an excellent response to therapy (Saudubray et al., 1984).

Inborn errors of metabolism are individually rare but collectively numerous. Many of them present early in the neonatal period, have a rapid fatal course and, as a whole, cannot be recognized through systematic screening tests which are too slow, too expensive and unreliable. This makes it an absolute necessity to teach primary care physicians a simple method of clinical screening before making decisions about sophisticated biochemical investigations. Clinical diagnosis of inborn errors of metabolism in the newborn infant may at times be difficult. This is at least partly due to four reasons:

(1) Many physicians think that since individual inborn errors are rare, they should be considered only after more common conditions like sepsis have been excluded;

(2) In view of the large number of inborn errors, it might appear that their diagnosis requires precise knowledge of a large number of biochemical pathways and their inter-relationships. As a matter of fact an adequate diagnostic approach can be based on the proper use of only a few tests;

(3) The neonate has an apparently limited repertoire of responses to severe overwhelming illness and the predominant clinical signs and symptoms are non-specific: poor feeding, lethargy, failure to thrive, etc. It is certain that many patients with such defects succumb in the newborn period without having received a specific diagnosis, death often having been attributed to sepsis or some other common causes;

(4) Classical autopsy findings in such cases are often non-specific and unrevealing. Infection is often suspected as the cause of the death, whereas sepsis is the common accompaniment of metabolic disorders.

Since 1968, more than 300 newborns with inborn errors of intermediary metabolism, presenting with acute symptoms within the first month of life, have been evaluated by the metabolic and genetic service at Hôpital des Enfants-Malades, Paris. From this experience, a method of initial clinical evaluation and management has been developed (Saudubray et al., 1989). Acute neonatal forms of inherited errors of intermediary metabolism can be diagnosed or strongly suspected and assigned to one of five schematical bioclinical groups on the basis of the clinical history, physical examination, and readily available laboratory tests. Prospectively, this method has proved to be a useful tool in the approach to ill newborns. Our data suggest that a clinically-oriented screening is more cost-efficient and more reasonable than a mass screening programme for rare inborn errors of metabolism.

General pathophysiological considerations

As far as physiopathology is concerned, all metabolic disorders can be divided into three groups which can be helpful for diagnostic purposes:

(1) diseases which disturb the synthesis or catabolism of complex molecules. In this first group of disorders, symptoms are permanent, progressive, independent of intercurrent events, and are not related to food intake.

All lysosomal disorders belong to this category in which deficiencies lead to the progressive accumulation of undigested substrates, usually complex polymers that cannot be hydrolysed normally. Only few lysosomal disorders are clinically expressed in neonatal period.

In peroxisomal biogenesis disorders, many anabolic functions are disturbed including plasmalogen (a major myelin constituent), cholesterol, bile acid biosynthesis and generalized peroxisomal beta-oxidation defects. These multiple and complex biochemical abnormalities result in a striking disorder of neuronal migration with malformations and severe neurological dysfunction. Most of peroxisomal disorders clinically strike in the neonatal period.

Another group of disorders is formed by mutations involving intracellular trafficking and processing of secretory proteins such as α-1-antitrypsin deficiency or the more recently described carbohydrate deficient glycoprotein syndrome (Jaeken et al., 1991). Such mutations are difficult to demonstrate because they do not manifest simply as enzyme deficiency states. Their diagnosis lies on the measurement of specific protein(s) in plasma, like α-1-antitrypsin, glycosylated transferrin, thyroid binding globulin, or total serum glycoproteins.

(2) Inborn errors of intermediary metabolism which lead to an acute or progressive endogenous intoxication secondary to an accumulation of toxic compounds proximal to the metabolic block. Symptoms are directly correlated to food intake and to nutritional state.

Amino-acidopathies (such as maple syrup urine disease or tyrosinaemia type I), most of the organic acidurias (methylmalonic, propionic, isovaleric, etc.), congenital urea cycle defects, and sugar intolerances (galactosaemia, fructosaemia) belong to this group. All the conditions in this group present clinical similarities including a symptom-free interval, clinical signs of 'intoxication' (such as vomiting, lethargy, coma, liver failure) and frequent humoral disturbances (acidosis, ketosis, hyperammonaemia, etc ...). The biological diagnosis is easy and mostly relies on plasma and urine amino acid or organic acid chromatography. Treatment of these disorders requires the removal of toxins (blood exchange transfusion or haemodialysis, peritoneal dialysis, special diets).

(3) Inborn errors of intermediary metabolism in which symptoms are at least partly due to the deficiency in energy production or utilization processes, ensuing distally from a defect in liver, myocardium, muscle, or brain.

Congenital lactic acidaemias (pyruvate carboxylase, pyruvate dehydrogenase deficiency), fatty acid oxidation defects, and mitochondrial respiratory chain disorders belong to this group. These diseases present an overlapping clinical spectrum which sometimes results also in part from the accumulation of toxic compounds in addition to the deficiency in energy production. Frequent symptoms common to this group include hypoglycaemia, hyperlactacidaemia, severe generalized hypotonia, myopathy, cardiomyopathy, failure to thrive, cardiac failure, circulatory collapse, sudden infant death syndrome, and malformations, the latter suggesting that the abnormal processes affected the foetal energetic pathways (Clayton & Thompson, 1988). The recent abundance of reports on inborn errors of respiratory chain which emphasize the amazing clinical diversity of these disorders illustrates the ubiquitous role of energetic processes at every age and in every organ (Munnich et al., 1992). Treatment of these disorders, if there is one, would need adequate energy replacement.

Identification of neonates 'at risk'

The clinical diagnosis can be schematized into three steps:

(1) Presenting signs: apparently non-specific symptoms

The neonate has a limited repertoire of responses to severe illness and at first glance presents unspecific symptoms such as respiratory disorders, hypotonia, poor sucking reflex, vomiting, diarrhoea, dehydration, lethargy, seizures, hepatic, cardiac or digestive injury ... all symptoms which could be easily attributed to infection or some other common cause. If they have occurred, the deaths of affected siblings may have been falsely attributed to sepsis, heart failure, or intraventricular haemorrhage, and it is important to review clinical records and autopsy reports critically when they are available.

(2) These apparently non-specific symptoms are actually included in a very evocative clinical context.

In the 'intoxication' type of metabolic distress, an extremely evocative clinical setting is the course of a full-term baby born after a normal pregnancy and delivery who, after an initial symptom-free period during which the baby is completely normal, deteriorates relentlessly for no apparent reason and does not respond to symptomatic therapy. The interval between birth and clinical symptoms may range from hours to weeks, depending on the nature of the metabolic block and the environment. In organic acidaemias and urea cycle defects, the duration of the interval is not necessarily correlated to the protein content of the feeding.

Investigations routinely performed in all sick neonates, including chest X-ray, CSF examination, bacteriological studies, and cerebral ultrasound yield normal results. This unexpected and 'mysterious' deterioration of a child after a normal initial period is the most important signal of the presence of an inherited disease of the 'intoxication type'. If present, careful re-evaluation of the child's condition is mandatory. Signs previously interpreted as non-specific manifestations of neonatal hypoxia, infection, or other common diagnoses take on new significance in this context.

In 'energy deficiencies' however, the clinical presentation is less evocative and displays variable severity. A careful reappraisal of the child is always warranted.

(3) Reappraisal of the child: clinical approach to inborn errors according to the main presenting sign.

Neurological deterioration

Indeed, many inborn errors of intermediary metabolism 'intoxication' type or 'energy deficiency' type are brought to a doctor's attention because of neurological deterioration. In the 'intoxication' type of metabolic distress, the initial symptom-free interval varies in duration between the conditions. Typically, the first reported sign is poor sucking and feeding, after which the child sinks into an unexplained coma despite supportive measures. At a more advanced state neurovegetative problems with respiratory disorders, hiccups, apnoeas, bradycardia, and hypothermia can appear. In the comatose state, many of these conditions have characteristic changes in muscle tone and involuntary movements. Generalized hypertonic episodes with opisthotonus are frequent, and boxing or pedalling movements as well as slow limb elevations, spontaneously or upon stimulation, are observed. Another neurological pattern suggesting metabolic disease is axial hypotonia and limb hypertonia with large amplitude tremors and myoclonic jerks which are often mistaken for convulsion.

In 'energy deficiencies', the clinical presentation is less evocative and displays a more variable severity. In many conditions, there is no free interval. The most frequent symptoms are a severe generalized hypotonia, hypertrophic cardiomyopathy, rapidly progressive neurological deterioration, possible dysmorphia, or malformations. In contrast to the 'intoxication' group, lethargy and coma are rarely inaugural signs. Hyperlactacidaemia with or without metabolic acidosis is a very frequent symptom.

Only few lysosomal disorders with 'storage' symptoms are expressed in the neonatal period. By contrast, most of peroxisomal disorders present immediately after birth with dysmorphia and severe neurological dysfunction.

Seizures

True convulsions occur late and inconsistently in inborn errors of intermediary metabolism with the exception of pyridoxine-dependent seizures (Bankier *et al.*, 1983) and some cases of non ketotic hyperglycinaemia, sulphite oxidase deficiency (Mises *et al.*, 1982; Wadman *et al.*, 1983), and peroxisomal disorders where they may be important inaugural elements in the clinical presentation. In contrast, newborns with MSUD, organic acidurias and urea cycle defects rarely experience seizures in the absence of pre-existing stupor or coma, or hypoglycaemia. The EEG often shows a periodic pattern in which bursts of intense activity alternate with nearly flat segments (Mises *et al.*, 1982).

Hypotonia

Hypotonia is a very common symptom in sick neonates. Whereas many non-metabolic inherited diseases can give rise to severe generalized neonatal hypotonia (mainly all severe fetal neuromuscular disorders), only a few inborn errors of metabolism present in neonates with isolated or predominant hypotonia. The most severe metabolic hypotonias are observed in hereditary hyperlactacidaemias, respiratory chain disorders, urea cycle defects, non-ketotic hyperglycinaemia (NKH), sulphite oxidase deficiency (SO) and peroxisomal disorders (PZO). In all these circumstances, the diagnosis is mostly based upon the association with the central hypotonia of lethargy, coma, seizures and neurological symptoms in NKH, SO, PZO, and of characteristic metabolic changes in congenital lactic acidosis and urea cycle disorders (hyperammonaemia). Severe forms of Pompe's disease (α-glucosidase deficiency) can mimic at first respiratory chain disorders when generalized hypotonia is associated to cardiomyopathy. Evocative cranio-facial dysmorphism is present only in typical Zellweger's syndrome but can be very moderate or even absent in variant forms of peroxisomal disorders. Lowe's syndrome should be systematically considered in boys who present with congenital cataracts, tubulopathy and minor facial dysmorphism.

'Hepatic' presentation

Four main clinical groups of hepatic symptoms can be identified:
(1) Hepatomegaly with hypoglycaemia and seizures suggest glycogenosis type I and III, and gluconeogenesis defects, or severe hyperinsulinism;
(2) Liver failure syndrome (jaundice, haemorrhagic syndrome, hepatocellular necrosis with elevated transaminases and hypoglycaemia with ascites and oedema) suggest fructosaemia, galactosaemia, tyrosinosis type I (after 3 weeks), neonatal haemochromatosis (Barnard & Manci, 1991) and respiratory chain disorders (Cormier *et al.*, 1991);

(3) Predominant cholestatic jaundice with failure to thrive is observed in α-1-antitrypsin deficiency, Byler's disease, inborn errors of bile acid metabolism (Clayton, 1991), peroxisomal disorders (Poll-Thé *et al.*, 1987), Niemann Pick–type C, and CDG syndrome (Jaeken *et al.*, 1991);

(4) Hepatosplenomegaly with coarse facies, multiplex dysostosis, cherry red spots, vacuolated lymphocytes and non-immune hydrops fetalis, suggest lysosomal disorders (GM1 gangliosidosis, Niemann–Pick types A and C, galactosialidosis, sialidosis type II, mucopolysaccharidosis type VII).

In our experience, hepatic presentations of inherited fatty acid oxidation disorders and urea cycle defects consist of acute steatosis or Reye's syndrome with normal bilirubin, only slightly prolonged prothrombin time and moderate elevation of transaminases rather than true liver failure with ascites and oedema (Saudubray *et al.*, 1992).

One must emphasize frequent difficulties in investigating patients with severe hepatic failure. At an advanced state, many unspecific symptoms that are secondary consequences of disturbances of liver intermediary metabolism can be present. Melituria (galactosuria, glycosuria, fructosuria), hyperammonaemia, hyperlactacidaemia, short-fast hypoglycaemia, hypertyrosinaemia (200 μmol/l), and hypermethioninaemia (sometimes higher than 500 μmol/l) are the signs mostly encountered in very advanced hepatocellular insufficiencies. Investigation of the parents can be very helpful for diagnosis of galactosaemias, mainly when the patient has been transfused.

'Cardiac' presentation

Sometimes metabolic distress can strike with predominant cardiac symptoms. Cardiac failure revealing or accompanying a cardiomyopathy (dilated hypertrophic) and most often associated with hypotonia, muscle weakness and failure to thrive suggest respiratory chain disorders, Pompe's disease, fatty acid oxidation disorders and phosphorylase β-kinase deficiency. Recent observations suggest that some respiratory chain disorders are tissue specific and are only expressed in myocardium as they are already found in phosphorylase-β-kinase deficiency (Servidei *et al.*, 1988). This highlights the importance of measuring respiratory chain enzymes activities directly on endomyocardium biopsy each time it is possible. The new multisystemic disorder carbohydrate-deficient glycoprotein syndrome can sometimes present in infancy with cardiac failure due to pericardial effusions and cardiac tamponade (Jaeken *et al.*, 1991). Among the hitherto known hereditary defects of fatty acid oxidation, seven can be revealed by cardiomyopathy and/or heart beat disorders (auriculo-ventricular block, bundle branch blocks, ventricular tachycardia) (Saudubray *et al.*, 1992). In general, severe forms of multiple acylCoA dehydrogenase (glutaric aciduria type II due to ETF or ETFDH deficiency) and long-chain fatty acid disorders involving CPT II, translocase, LCAD, LCHAD and trifunctional enzyme are severe, begin early in infancy or even in the neonatal period, and can be revealed by neonatal death, cardiac arrest or collapsus which can be easily misdiagnosed as toxic shock or idiopathic sudden infant death syndrome. The diagnostic work up of fatty acid oxidation lies in the urinary organic acid profile, plasma and urine carnitine, and acylcarnitine determination, loading tests, fasting tests, and whole fatty acid oxidation studies on fresh lymphocytes or intact fibroblasts.

Initial biological approach

Once clinical suspicion of an inborn metabolic error is aroused, general supportive measures and laboratory investigations must be undertaken immediately (Table 1). Abnormal urine odours can best be detected on a drying filter paper or by opening a container of urine which has been closed at room temperature for a few minutes. Although serum ketone bodies reach 0.5–1 mmol/l in early neonatal life, acetonuria is an important sign of a metabolic disease and is rarely, if ever, observed in a normal newborn. Its presence is always abnormal in neonates. The dinitrophenylhydrasine

(DNPH) test screens for the presence of alpha-keto acids such as seen in MSUD. The DNPH test can be considered significant only in the absence of glucosuria and acetonuria, which also react with DNPH. Hypocalcaemia and elevated or reduced blood glucose are frequently present in metabolic diseases. The physician should be wary of attributing marked neurological dysfunction merely to these findings.

Table 1. Initial investigations

	Basic investigations	Specific investigations
Urine	– Smell (special odour) – Look (special colour) – Acetone (Acetest, Ames) – Reducing substances (Clinitest, Ames) – Keto acids (DNPH) – pH (pHstix, Merck) – Sulfitest (Merck) – Brand reaction – Electrolytes (Na, K) – Uric acid (search for *hypo*uricuria)	– Urine collection: collect separately each fresh micturition and put it in the fridge – Freezing: Freeze at –20 °C samples collected before treatment and, afterwards, an aliquot of 24 h collection on treatment – Do not use them without having taken expert metabolic advice
Blood	– Blood cell count – Electrolytes (search for anion gap) – Glucose, calcium – Blood gases (pH, pCO$_2$, HCO$_3$, pO$_2$) – Uric acid (search for *hypo*uricaemia) – Prothrombin time – Transaminases (and other 'liver tests') – Ammonaemia – Lactic, pyruvic acids – 3OHbutyrate, acetoacetate – Free fatty acids	– Plasma heparinized 5 ml at –20° C – Blood on filter paper (as 'Guthrie' test) – Whole blood 10–15 ml collected on EDTA and frozen (for molecular biology studies)
Miscellaneous	– Lumbar puncture – Chest X-ray – Cardiac echography, ECG – Cerebral ultrasound, EEG	– Skin biopsy (fibroblast culture) – CSF 1 ml frozen – Post mortem: liver, muscle biopsies (macroscopic fragment frozen at –70° C) – Autopsy

The metabolic acidosis of organic acidurias is usually accompanied by an elevated anion gap. The urine pH should be below 5; otherwise, renal acidosis is a consideration. Ammonia and lactic acid should be determined systematically in newborns at risk. An elevated ammonia level in itself can induce respiratory alkalosis; hyperammonaemia with ketoacidosis suggests an underlying organic acidaemia. Elevated lactic acid levels in the absence of infection or tissue hypoxia are a significant finding. Moderate elevations (3-6 mmol/l) are often observed in organic acidaemias and in the hyperammonaemias; levels greater than 10 mmol/l are frequent in hypoxia. A normal serum pH does not exclude hyperlactacidaemia as a neutral pH is usually maintained until levels of 5 mmol/l are present. It is important to measure, as often as possible, lactate (L), pyruvate (P), 3-hydroxybutyrate (3OHB), and acetoacetate (AA) on a plasma sample immediately deproteinized at the bedside, in order to appreciate cytoplasmic and mitochondrial redox states through the measurement of L/P and 3OHB/AA ratios, respectively. Some organic acidurias induce granulocytopenia and thrombocytopenia, which may be mistaken for sepsis.

The storage of adequate amounts of plasma urine and CSF is an important element in diagnosis.

The utilization of these precious samples should be carefully planned after taking advice from specialists in inborn errors of metabolism. Although not available in most hospital laboratories, some sophisticated investigations (such as amino acid or organic acid chromatography) are available in many places. It is important to insist, however, that any reference laboratory used for this purpose should not only provide prompt test results and reference ranges, but also an interpretation of abnormal results (Burton, 1987).

If the child dies, adequate diagnosis is nonetheless important in order to make adequate genetic counselling possible. A postmortem protocol for the diagnosis of genetic disease has been proposed which includes the taking of urine and serum samples, fibroblasts culture (premortem if possible), and muscle and liver biopsies (three or more samples of 1 cm^3 of each, stored frozen on dry ice or in liquid nitrogen) (Kronick et al., 1983).

Once the above clinical and laboratory data have been assembled, specific therapeutic recommendations can be made. This process is completed within 2 or 4 h and often precludes long waiting periods for sophisticated diagnostic results. On the basis of this evaluation, most patients can be classified into five groups (Table 2) (Saudubray et al., 1989).

Clinical approach to aetiologies

According to the major clinical presentations (neurological deterioration of 'intoxication' type, neurological deterioration of 'energy deficiency' type, storage disorders, cardiac injury and liver dysfunction), and according to the proper use of the laboratory data described above, most patients can be assigned to one of five schematical syndromes (Table 2). In our experience, type I (MSUD), type II (organic acidurias), type IVa (urea cycle defects) and non-ketotic hyperglycinaemia (the most common disease in type IVb) encompass more than 65 per cent of the newborn infants with inborn errors of intermediary metabolism. The experienced clinician will, of course, have to carefully interpret the metabolic data, especially in relation to the time when they were collected and the treatments which were used. It is important to insist on the need to collect, at the same time, all the biological data listed in Table 1. Some very significant symptoms (such as metabolic acidosis, and especially ketosis) can be moderate and transient, largely depending on the symptomatic therapy. Conversely, at an advanced stage, many non-specific abnormalities (such as respiratory acidosis, severe hyperlactacidaemia, secondary hyperammonaemia) can disturb the primitive truth of the biological pattern. This is particularly true in disorders with a rapid fatal course, like urea cycle disorders in which the initial near constant presentation of hyperammonaemia with respiratory alkalosis and without ketosis shifts rapidly to a rather non-specific picture associating acidosis and hyperlactacidaemia (Saudubray et al., 1989).

Type I : Neurological distress of 'intoxication type' with ketosis

Type I is represented by MSUD. It is one of the commonest amino-acidopathies. After a symptom-free interval of 4 to 5 days, feeding difficulties develop and the child gradually becomes comatose with generalized hypertonic episodes, opisthotonus and boxing and pedalling movements. The diagnosis is confirmed by serum amino acid chromatography which displays an elevation of the branched-chain amino acids leucine (usually higher than 2 mmol/l), valine, isoleucine, and the presence of alloisoleucine.

Type II : Neurological distress of 'intoxication type' with ketoacidosis

Type II, neurological distress of 'intoxication type' with ketoacidosis and hyperammonaemia, encompasses many of the organic acidurias. Between the ages of 1 and 4 days, these children develop feeding difficulties and deteriorate into a coma over hours to days. They are acutely ill, dehydrated, acidotic with an increased anion gap and they are often hypothermic. Large amplitude tremors of limbs are the dominant abnormal movements. The urine in the acute phase is positive for ketones but this highly significant sign can be transient. Neutropenia and thrombocytopenia are

Table 2. Five neonatal types of inherited 'metabolic distress'

	Clinical type	Acidosis/ ketosis	Other signs	Diagnosis	Methods of investigation
I	Neuro distress 'intoxication' type Abnormal movements	Acidosis 0 DNPH +++ Acetest 0/±	NH3 N or ↑ ± Lactate N Glucose N	MSUD (special odour)	AAC (plasma, urine)
II	Neuro distress 'intoxication' type Dehydration	Acidosis ++ Acetest ++ DNPH 0/±	NH3 ↑+/++ Lactate N or ↑± Leucopaenia Thrombopaenia Glucose N or ↑	Organic acidurias (MMA, PA, IVA, MCD) Ketolytic defects	OAC (urine, plasma) Carnitine (plasma) Carnitine esters (urine, plasma)
	Neuro distress 'energy deficiency' Hepatic signs	Acidosis ++/+ Acetest 0 DNPH 0	NH3 ↑ Glucose N/↓	FAO and ketogenesis defects	Idem above Loading, fasting tests FAO studies (lymphocytes, fibroblasts)
III	Neuro distress 'energy deficiency' Polypnea	Acidosis +++/+ Acetest ++/+ Lactate +++/+	NH3 ↑/N Glucose N/↓	'Congenital lactic acidosis' (PC, PDH, Krebs cycle, MCD, respiratory chain)	L/P, 3OHB/AA ratios OAC (urine) Polarographic studies Enzyme assays (muscle, lymphocytes, fibroblasts)
IV					
(a)	Neuro distress 'intoxication' type Slight hepatocellular disturbances	Acidosis 0 (alcalosis) Acetest 0	NH3 ↑ ++ Lactate ↑ or N Glucose N	Urea cycle, triple H, FAO defects (GA II, CPT II, LCAD, LCHAD)	AAC (plasma, urine) Orotic acid (urine) Enzyme studies (liver, intestine)
(b)	Neuro distress Seizures Myoclonic jerks Severe hypotonia	Acidosis 0 Acetest 0	NH3 N Lactate N Glucose N	NKH SO ± XO Pyridoxino dependency Peroxisomal disorders	AAC (NKH, SO) VLCFA, phytanic acid in plasma (PZO)
(c)	Storage disorders Coarse facies HSM, Hydrops fetalis Cherry red spot	Acidosis 0 Acetest 0	Vacuolated lymphocytes Hepatic signs	GM1 gangliosidosis ISSD (Sialidosis Type II) MPS VII Galactosialidosis	Enzyme studies (lymphocytes, fibroblasts)
V					
(a)	Hepatomegaly Hypoglycaemia	Acidosis ++/+ Acetest +	Lactate ++/+ Glucose ↓ ++	Glycogenosis type I & III Fructose diphosphatase	Fasting, loading tests Loading studies (liver)
(b)	Liver failure Jaundice Ascitis	Acidosis +/0 Acetest +/0	Lactate ↑ ++/+ Glucose ↓ + or N	Fructosaemia; galactosaemia Tyrosinosis type I; neonatal haemochromatosis; Respiratory chain disorders	Enzyme studies Organic acids Enzyme studies
(c)	Cholestatic jaundice ± Failure to thrive ± Chronic diarrhoea Hepatomegaly	Acidosis 0 Ketosis 0		α-1-antitrypsin Inborn errors of bile acids metabolism Peroxisomal disorders; CDG	Protein electrophoresis OAC (plasma, urines) VLCFA, phytanic, pipecolic acid
(d)	HSM 'Storage' signs	Acidosis 0 Ketosis 0		Storage disorders	Oligosaccharides, MPS, SA, enzyme studies

N = normal; AAC = amino acid chromatography; FAO = fatty acid oxidation; HSM = hepatosplenomegaly; OAC = organic acids chromatography; MPS = mucopolysaccharides; SA = sialic acid; VLCFA = very long chain fatty acid. CDG = Carbohydrate deficiency glycoprotein syndrome. MSUD, MMA, PA, IVA, MCD, PC, PDH, L/P, 30HB/AA, CPT II, LCAD, LCHAD, NKH, SO-XO, GAII: see text for abbreviations.

also commonly observed and can contribute to the confusion with sepsis. Hyperammonaemia, sometimes as high as that observed in urea cycle defects, is a constant finding (Saudubray *et al.*, 1989). In some patients we have observed severe hyperglycaemia (greater than 15 mmol/l) with glycosuria before treatment with glucose.

In addition to methylmalonic, propionic and isovaleric acidurias, a large number of rare organic acidurias, presenting usually with neurological distress and metabolic acidosis, have been described in recent years as techniques for analysing organic acids have become more widely available and reliable (Saudubray *et al.*, 1989). Among them, glutaric aciduria type II or multiple acylCoA dehydrogenase deficiency (Goodman *et al.*, 1987) and hydroxymethylglutaryl-CoA lyase deficiency (Wysocki & Hahnel, 1986) have many similarities with methylmalonic, propionic and isovaleric acidurias except that ketosis is absent and hypoglycaemia is frequent. Very rare conditions in this group are succinylCoA transferase deficiency (Saudubray *et al.*, 1987), biotin-dependent multiple carboxylase defects due to holoenzyme synthetase deficiency (Burri *et al.*, 1981), short-chain fatty acylCoA dehydrogenase deficiency (Amendt *et al.*, 1987) and 3-methylglutaconicuria (Divry *et al.*, 1987) which all display ketoacidosis. Pyroglutamic aciduria is a rare condition which can start in the first days of life with a severe metabolic acidosis but without ketosis or abnormalities of blood glucose, lactate and ammonia.

The final diagnosis of all these organic acidurias is made by identifying specific abnormal metabolites by gas chromatography–mass spectrometry of blood and urine.

Type III : Lactic acidosis with neurological distress of 'energy deficiency' type

The clinical presentation of these children is very diverse. The main medical problem in group III patients is often the acidosis itself, which clinically may be surprisingly well tolerated and can at times be mild.

If a high lactic acid concentration is found, it is urgent to rule out readily treatable causes, especially hypoxia. Ketosis is present in most of the primary lactic acidaemias except pyruvate dehydrogenase deficiency. Ketosis is rarely if ever observed in lactic acidosis secondary to tissue hypoxia. Biotin-responsive multiple carboxylase deficiency may present as lactic acidosis and biotin therapy is indicated in all patients with lactic acidosis of unknown cause.

A definite diagnosis is often elusive and is attempted with specific enzyme assays and by considering metabolite levels, redox potential states and fluxes under fasting and fed conditions. The defects most frequently demonstrated are pyruvate carboxylase deficiency, pyruvate dehydrogenase deficiency, respiratory chain disorders (complex I and IV), and multiple carboxylase deficiency. Many cases remain unexplained.

Respiratory chain disorders are frequently observed in the neonatal period. Since the early descriptions (Van Biervliet *et al.*, 1977), a number of cases have been described (Di Mauro *et al.*, 1987). The most frequent symptoms are severe generalized hypotonia, dilated cardiomyopathy of hypokinetic type, rapid neurological deterioration, respiratory failure and severe lactic acidaemia. Some patients displayed facial dysmorphia and malformations, as have also been observed in infants with a deficiency of the pyruvate dehydrogenase complex (Clayton & Thompson, 1988; Aleck *et al.*, 1988).

Type IV

Type IVa: neurological distress of 'intoxication type' with hyperammonaemia and without ketoacidosis: urea cycle defects

Primary hyperammonaemias due to urea cycle defects have a variable symptom-free interval, sometimes only a matter of hours. A brief hypertonic period and hiccups may occur, after which a profound hypotonic coma rapidly develops and cardiocirculatory function may be compromised. The blood ammonia rises precipitously to levels of 400–2000 µmol/l or more. Respiratory alkalosis (pH 7.40) and moderate hyperlactacidaemia are frequently observed. An important diagnostic clue to separate urea cycle defects from organic acidurias with hyperammonaemia is the universal absence of ketonuria.

The two principal urea cycle disorders, which have non-diagnostic amino acid chromatograms are ornithine transcarbamylase deficiency (OTC) and carbamyl phosphate synthetase deficiency. The former is the only sex-linked congenital hyperammonaemia. Enzyme diagnosis by liver biopsy is the only definitive diagnostic technique. Citrullinaemia, arginosuccinic aciduria and argininaemia are diagnosed by amino acid chromatography which demonstrates the accumulation of citrulline, arginosuccinate and arginine respectively. In the 'triple H' syndrome, hyperammonaemia, hyperornithinaemia and homocitrullinaemia are present. An especially important diagnostic consideration is transient hyperammonaemia of the neonate.

Fatty acid oxidation disorders can also, though rarely, present in the neonatal period with hyperammonaemia and mimic urea cycle disorders (Demaugre et al., 1991; Pande et al., 1993).

Type IVb: neurological deterioration of 'energy deficiency' type without ketoacidosis and without hyperammonaemia

Non-ketotic hyperglycinaemia displays a very typical, although non-pathognomic, pattern. It is characterized by coma, hypotonia and myoclonic jerks appearing at birth or after a few hours in a child who did not experience perinatal hypoxia. A burst suppression EEG pattern (Mises et al., 1982) is always present. The diagnosis rests upon the demonstration of elevated serum glycine levels and especially an elevated CSF/serum glycine ratio.

The clinical spectrum of sulphite oxidase and combined sulphite and xanthine oxidase deficiencies includes hypotonia, seizures, myoclonic jerks, microcephaly and dysmorphic features. Lens dislocation may occasionally be noted as early as the first month of life. In combined sulphite and xanthine oxidase deficiencies due to an abnormal molybdenum cofactor, uric acid concentration is very low in plasma and urine. Sulphites are found in fresh urine at high concentrations (test with Sulfitest, Merck). Amino acid chromatography shows a specific profile with high sulphite concentrations in the form of sulphocysteine, whereas cystine concentration is close to zero (Wadman et al., 1983).

The common symptoms of peroxisomal disorders presenting in the neonatal period are an absence of a symptom-free interval, severe generalized hypotonia, early onset epileptic seizures and craniofacial dysmorphism (Poll-Thé et al., 1987). Some patients can display inaugural signs of hepatomegaly, jaundice, liver failure and failure to thrive without marked neurological dysfunction. Retinitis pigmentosa should be systematically searched for. Diagnosis requires special investigations including determination of very-long-chain fatty acid, plasmalogen, phytanic, bile acids and pipecolic acid in plasma, urine and fibroblasts. The most frequent conditions are Zellweger's syndrome and neonatal adrenoleucodystrophy. Many other rare variants have been recently described.

In most diseases of intermediary metabolism, convulsions are a late manifestation. However, they may be important elements in the clinical presentation of most patients with non-ketotic hyperglycinaemia, sulphite oxidase deficiency, and peroxisomal disorders described above.

Type IV c: storage disorders without metabolic disturbances

Only few lysosomal disorders are expressed clinically in the neonatal period. They can be associated with hydrops fetalis, neonatal ascites and oedema (GM1 gangliosidosis, Gaucher's disease, mucopolysaccharidosis type VII, sialidosis, galactosialidosis, sialuria, Niemann–Pick type C).

(5) Type V: Hepatomegaly and liver dysfunction

In this type, four main clinical groups of hepatic symptoms lead to the diagnosis of more than 20 inborn errors of metabolism already considered, under the heading 'Hepatic presentation' (p. 80).

Conclusion

Using our programmed approach of screening for inborn errors of intermediary metabolism, we have been able to diagnose about 300 affected neonates. The course of their diseases was so startling and they became ill so early in life that they were admitted to the local hospital and properly managed before any mass screening could be performed.

References

Aleck, K.A., Kaplan, A.M., Sherwood, W.G. & Robinson, B.H. (1988): *In utero* central nervous system damage in pyruvate dehydrogenase deficiency. *Arch. Neurol.* **45**, 987–989.

Amendt, B.A., Greene, C., Sweetman, L., Cloherty, J., Shih, V., Moon, A., Teel, L. & Rhead, W.J (1987): Short-chain acyl-CoA dehydrogenase deficiency. Clinical and biochemical studies in two patients. *J. Clin. Invest.* **79**, 1303–1309.

Bankier, A., Turner, M. & Hopkins, I.J (1983): Pyridoxine dependent seizures. A wider clinical spectrum. *Arch. Dis. Child.* **58**, 415–418.

Barnard, J.A. III & Manci, E. (1991): Idiopathic neonatal iron-storage disease. *Gastroenterology* **101**, 1420–1427.

Burri, B.J., Sweetman, L. & Nyhan, W.L. (1981): Mutant holocarboxylase synthetase: evidence for the enzyme defect in early biotin-responsive multiple carboxylase deficiency. *J. Clin. Invest.* **68**, 1491–1495.

Burton, B.K (1987): Inborn errors of metabolism: the clinical diagnosis in early infancy. *Pediatrics* **79**, 359–369.

Clayton, P.T. (1991): Inborn errors of bile acid metabolism. *J. Inherit. Metab. Dis.* **14**, 478–496.

Clayton, P.T. & Thompson, E. (1988): Dysmorphic syndromes with demonstrable biochemical abnormalities. *J. Med. Genet.* **25**, 463–472.

Cormier, V., Rustin, P., Bonnefont, J.P., Rambaud, C., Vassault, A., Rabier, D., Parvy, P., Couderc, S., Parrot-Roulaud, F., Carré, M., Risse, J.C., Cahuzac, C., Saudubray, J.M., Rötig, A., Hubert, P. & Munnich, A. (1991): Hepatic failure in disorders of oxidative phosphorylation with neonatal onset. *J. Pediatr.* **119**, 951–954.

Demaugre, F., Bonnefont, J.P., Colonna, M., Cepanec, C., Leroux, J.P. & Saudubray, J.M. (1991): Infantile form of carnitine palmitoyltransferase II deficiency with hepatomuscular symptoms and sudden death: physiopathological approach to carnitine palmitoyltransferase II deficiencies. *J. Clin. Invest.* **87**, 859–864.

Di Mauro, S., Bonilla, E., Zeviani, M., Servidei, S., De Vivo, D.C. & Schon, E.A. (1987): Mitochondrial myopathies. *J. Inherit. Metab. Dis.* **10 (Suppl 1)**, 113–128.

Divry, P., Vianey-Liaud, C., Mory, O. & Ravussin, S.S. (1987): A methylglutaconic aciduria familial neonatal form with fatal onset. *J. Inherit. Metab. Dis.* **10 (Suppl.)**, 286–289.

Goodman, S.I., Frerman, F.E. & Loehr, J.P. (1987): Recent progress in understanding glutaric acidemias. *Enzyme* **38**, 76–79.

Jaeken, J., Stibler, H. & Hagberg, B. (1991): The carbohydrate-deficient glycoprotein syndrome: a new inherited multisystemic disease with severe nervous system involvement. *Acta Paediatr. Scand.* **375 (Suppl)**, 5–71.

Kronick, J.B., Scriver, C.R., Goodyer, P.R. & Kaplan, P.B. (1983): A perimortem protocol for suspected genetic disease. *Pediatrics* **71**, 960–963.

Mises, J., Moussalli-Salefranque, F., Laroque, M.L., Ogier, H., Coudé, F.X., Charpentier, C. & Saudubray, J.M. (1982): EEG findings as an aid to the diagnosis of neonatal non ketotic hyperglycinemia. *J. Inherit. Metab. Dis.* **5 (Suppl.)**, 117–120.

Munnich, A., Rustin, P., Rötig, A., Chretien, D., Bonnefont, J.P., Nuttin, C., Cormier, V., Vassault, A., Parvy, P., Bardet, J., Charpentier, C., Rabier, D. & Saudubray, J.M. (1992): Clinical aspects of mitochondrial disorders. *J. Inherit. Metab. Dis.* **15**, 448–455.

Pande, S.V., Brivet, M., Slama, A., Demaugre, F., Aufrant, C. & Saudubray, J.M. (1993): Carnitine-acylcarnitine translocase deficiency with severe hypoglycemia and auriculo ventricular block. *J. Clin. Invest.* **91**, 1247–1252.

Poll-Thé, B.T., Saudubray, J.M., Ogier, H., Lombes, A., Munnich, A. & Frézal, J. (1987): Clinical approach to inherited peroxisomal disorders. In: *Human genetics*, eds. F. Vogel & K. Sperling, pp. 345–351. Berlin: Springer.

Saudubray, J.M., Ogier, H., Charpentier, C., Depondt, E., Coudé, F.X., Munnich, A., Mitchell, G., Rey, F., Rey, J. & Frézal, J. (1984): Neonatal management of organic acidurias. Clinical update. *J. Inherit. Metab. Dis.* **7**, 2–9.

Saudubray, J.M., Specola, N., Middleton, B., Lombes, A., Bonnefont, J.P., Jakobs, C., Vassault, A., Charpentier, C. & Day, R. (1987): Hyperketotic states due to inherited defects of ketolysis. *Enzyme* **38**, 80–90.

Saudubray, J.M., Ogier, H., Bonnefont, J.P., Munnich, A., Lombes, A., Hervé, F., Mitchell, G., Poll-The, B.T., Specola, N., Parvy, P., Bardet, J., Rabier, D., Coudé, M., Charpentier, C. & Frézal, J. (1989): Clinical approach to inherited metabolic diseases in the neonatal period: a 20-year survey. *J. Inherit. Metab. Dis.* **12 (Suppl.)**, 25–41.

Saudubray, J.M., Mitchell, G., Bonnefont, J.P., Schwartz, G., Nuttin, C., Munnich, A., Brivet, M., Vassault, A., Demaugre, F., Rabier, D. & Charpentier, C. (1992): Approach to the patient with a fatty acid oxidation disorder. In: *Proceedings of the fatty acid oxidation symposium of Philadelphia*, eds. P. Coates & K. Tanaka, pp. 271–288. New York: John Wiley–Alan R. Liss.

Servidei, S., Metlay, L.A., Chodosh, J. & Di Mauro, S. (1988): Fatal infantile cardiomyopathy caused by phosphorylase b kinase deficiency. *J. Pediatr.* **113,** 82–85.

Van Biervliet, J.P.G.M., Bruinvis, L., Ketting, D., De Bree, P.K., Van Der Heiden, C., Wadman, S.K., Willems, J.L., Brookelman, H., Van Haelst, U. & Monnens, L.A.H. (1977): Hereditary mitochondrial myopathy with lactic acidemia, a DeToni–Fanconi–Debré syndrome and a defective respiratory chain in voluntary muscle. *Pediatr. Res.* **1,** 1088–1093.

Wadman, S.K., Duran, M., Breemer, F.A., Cats, B.P., Johnson, J.L., Rajagopalan, K.V., Saudubray, J.M., Ogier, H., Charpentier, C., Berger, R., Smith, G.P.A., Wilson, J. & Krywawych, S. (1983): Absence of hepatic molybdenum cofactor: an inborn error of metabolism leading to a combined deficiency of sulphite oxidase and xanthine dehydrogenase. *J. Inherit. Metab. Dis.* **6,** 78–83.

Wysocki, S.J. & Hahnel, R. (1986): 3-Hydroxy-3-methylglutaryl-coenzyme A lyase deficiency. *J. Inherit. Metab. Dis.* **9,** 225–233.

Chapter 8

Multisystem involvement in lysinuric protein intolerance: a study on 20 Italian patients

Giancarlo Parenti[*], Barbara Incerti[*], Maria Rosaria Larocca[*], Carla Borrone[†], Maja Di Rocco[†], Rossella Parini[‡], Irma Dianzani[§], Alberto Ponzone[§], Pietro Strisciuglio[¶], Domenico Sperlì[¶], Carlo Dionisi Vici[**], Gianfranco Rizzoni[**] and Generoso Andria[*]

Departments of Pediatrics, [*]Federico II University, Naples, [†]Giannina Gaslini Institute, Genoa, [‡]University of Milan, [§]University of Turin, [¶]University of Reggio Calabria, Catanzaro, [**]Bambino Gesù Hospital, Rome, Italy

Summary

We report on 20 patients from 14 families, affected by lysinuric protein intolerance, observed in six Italian referral centres for the study of inborn errors of metabolism. All patients originated from Southern Italy. Some patients displayed unique clinical features, such as bone marrow abnormalities and pancreatitis. We also observed a frequent occurrence of severe complications, such as kidney and lung involvement, known to affect the clinical course and the outcome of the disease.

Introduction

Lysinuric protein intolerance (LPI) is an inborn error of metabolism due to defective transport of cationic amino acids at the basolateral membrane of enterocytes, renal tubular cells, hepatocytes and fibroblasts (Rajantie *et al.*, 1980; Smith *et al.*, 1987). The decreased intestinal absorption and the increased renal clearance cause a depletion of the plasmatic pools of these amino acids; this leads to an impaired functioning of urea cycle with consequent hyperammonaemic crises, mostly occurring after meals, an aversion to protein-rich food, protein malnutrition, visceromegaly and osteoporosis.

Approximately 80 patients affected by LPI have been so far reported in the literature; about half of them have been observed in Finland, where the frequency of the disease has been estimated as 1:60–80 000. In other populations the disease is much rarer and only sporadic cases have been reported (Simell, 1989). Italy, however, seems to have a relatively higher frequency of the disease: in a recent multicentre study we collected 17 Italian patients (Incerti *et al.*, 1993); three further patients have recently come to our attention.

Here we report on the clinical findings observed in the Italian patients. Some features observed among our patients appear unique and suggest a multisystem involvement in LPI.

Patients

Twenty patients from 14 families were observed in six referral centres for the study of inborn errors of metabolism over a period of 14 years. Seventeen of these patients have been reported previously (Quattrin, 1971; Andria et al., 1981, 1982; Di Rocco et al., 1984, 1993; Dianzani et al., 1986; Parenti et al., 1995; Parini et al., 1991.

Table 1 summarizes the patients' sex, age range at onset of symptoms, age range at diagnosis and the present age range. Sixteen patients are presently alive, four died at ages ranging from 18 months to 11 years.

Table 1. General clinical features and outcome of the Italian patients with lysinuric protein intolerance (LPI)

Sex (n)	17 males/3 females
Mean age at onset (range)	2+4/12 y (1m–4y)
Mean age at diagnosis (range)	7+1/12 y (1m–21y)
Dead (n) (age of death)	4 (18m, 6y, 10y, 11y)
Alive (n) (range of present age)	16 (4y–29y)

Geographic origin

All patients originated from the Southern part of Italy, most of them coming from Campania (eight cases), Calabria (six cases) and Puglia (three cases) (Fig. 1). In particular, a cluster of patients has been found in a small area around Naples, where we diagnosed seven cases from five families. Parental consanguineity is reported in six families.

Diagnosis

LPI diagnosis was based both on the clinical picture and on biochemical data. In all patients at least three of the following biochemical findings were observed: low plasma levels of cationic amino acids; increased orotic aciduria; hyperammonaemia and orotic aciduria after protein loading tests, both prevented by oral administration of citrulline; reduced intestinal absorption of cationic amino acids after oral loading tests. Routine biochemical tests were in all cases consistent with those observed in LPI, including elevated blood LDH, ferritin and T_4.

Clinical presentations

Table 2 summarizes the presenting clinical features in our patients. Most of them presented with typical signs of LPI such as visceromegaly, failure to thrive and an aversion to protein-rich food. In some cases neurological crises, probably due to metabolic decompensation, were misdiagnosed as seizures.

Table 2. Presenting clinical features in the Italian patients with LPI

	n
Visceromegaly	18/20
Protein aversion	13/20
Failure to thrive	14/20
Hyperammonaemia	6/20

Atypical features

A variety of other signs have occasionally been observed in association with the classical picture of the disease (Table 3). Particularly, bone marrow abnormalities, featuring erythroblastophagocytosis, were detected in eight patients. Bone marrow abnormalities seem to be typical of the Italian patients; they have never been observed among the Finnish patients and, to our knowledge, they have been found only in one other case, of Turkish origin (Behbehani et al., 1983).

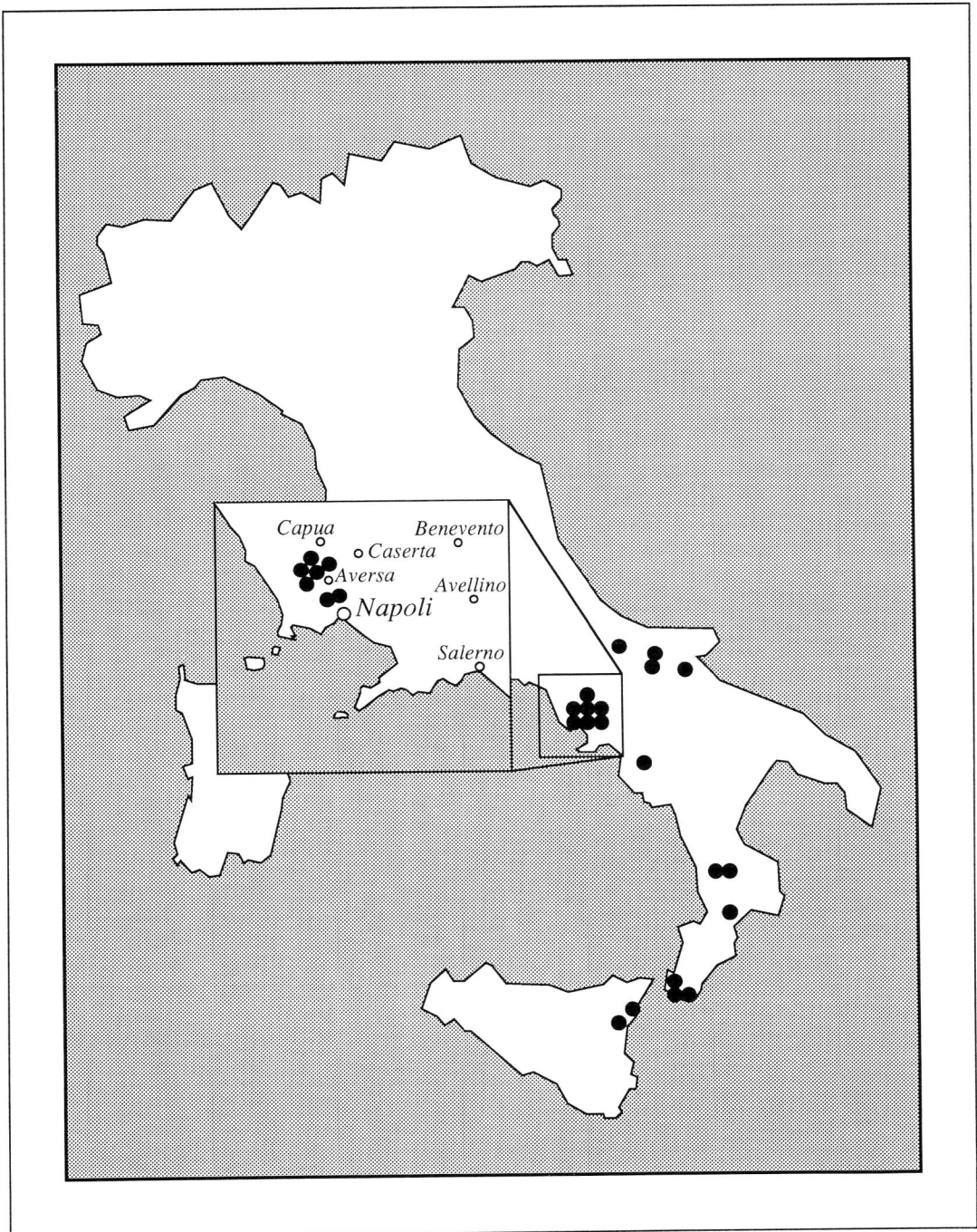

Fig. 1. Geographic origin of the Italian patients with LPI. Solid circles indicate the geographic origin of each patient. All patients originated from Southern Italy. A cluster of patients has been observed in a small area close to Naples (insert).

Table 3. Atypical signs in the Italian patients with LPI

	n
Bone marrow abnormalities	8/20
Kidney involvement	9/20
Lung involvement	11/20
Pancreatitis	2/20

Neuromuscular involvement was found in two patients. In one a diagnosis of myopathy was initially suspected, based on the presence of muscular hypotonia, elevated blood LDH and CK, and non-specific histological abnormalities. In the same patient seizures and mild mental retardation (IQ 61) were also observed. In the other patient mild mental retardation was present.

Initial misdiagnoses

In patients with atypical presentations a different diagnosis was initially suspected (Table 4). In most cases the presence of signs like visceromegaly, bone marrow abnormalities and reticulonodular lung opacities initially suggested a lysosomal storage disorder, such as Gaucher's disease, Niemann–Pick disease type B or mucopolysaccharidosis.

Table 4. Initial misdiagnoses in the Italian patients with LPI

	n
Gaucher disease	3
Niemann–Pick disease type B	1
Atypical mucopolysaccharidosis	2
Undefined lysosomal storage disease	1
Glycogen storage disease	1
Mitochondrial myopathy	1
Undefined haematological disease	1

Complications

An unusual feature of the Italian LPI patients is the occurrence of pancreatitis. Two of our patients experienced this complication. In one, surgical treatment was required and laparatomy showed both pancreatic fibrosis, suggesting chronic involvement, and liponecrosis, pointing to acute damage. In the other, pancreatitis recurred twice. The possible occurrence of pancreatitis has not been emphasized in previous reports and, to our knowledge, there is only a single autoptic observation of pancreatic involvement characterized by intraductal accumulation of PAS-positive material (Parto et al., 1994).

Kidney involvement has been observed in nine patients and ranged from mild proteinuria to chronic renal failure with both glomerular and tubular damage (Table 5). Generalized amino aciduria, detected in patients with tubular involvement, was particularly misleading in the initial diagnostic work-up, overshadowing cationic amino aciduria. Renal damage may dramatically affect the quality of life and the final outcome of patients with LPI: its presence, therefore, should be carefully evaluated.

Table 5. Kidney involvement in the Italian patients with LPI

	n
Proteinuria	5/9
Tubular dysfunction	4/9
Glomerular dysfunction	4/9
Microhaematuria	1/9

Lung involvement is a potentially life-threatening complication of LPI. During the past few years clinical reports have appeared (Di Rocco et al., 1993; Kerem et al., 1993; Parto et al., 1993; Parenti et al., 1995), pointing to its occurrence. The degree of lung disease is variable and ranges from subclinical involvement to interstitial pneumonia and fatal alveolar proteinosis (Table 6). Four of our patients presented with clinically overt lung involvement. In two of them respiratory disease was fatal. When investigated in nine asymptomatic patients by high resolution lung CT scan or radionuclide imaging evidence of subclinical lung involvement was found in six.

Table 6. Lung involvement in the Italian patients with LPI

	n
Symptomatic respiratory disease	4/11
Abnormal standard X-ray	9/11
Abnormal CT scan	6/11
Abnormal histology	1/11
Alveolar proteinosis	2/11

Therapy

All patients who are currently alive are treated with a low-protein diet and citrulline. Four patients were initially treated with arginine, later replaced by citrulline. In one case, who died at the age of 6y 6m, no treatment was started, since the diagnosis was retrospective.

Conclusions

LPI seems to have a relatively high frequency in Southern Italy. A cluster of seven patients, from five families, has been observed in a small area around Naples.

The paternal ancestors of an American patient also originated from the same area (Carpenter et al., 1985). In the ancestries of these patients common surnames recur, thus suggesting that a founder effect might be responsible for the higher incidence of the disease near Naples.

LPI's clinical picture has been delineated over the past few decades: most of the symptoms appear clearly related to the basic defect and the consequent metabolic derangement observed in the disease. However, recent clinical observations (Di Rocco et al., 1993; Parto et al., 1993; Parenti et al., 1995) have pointed to the occurrence of other manifestations, such as kidney and lung involvement, in patients with LPI. The present study suggests that these manifestations are frequent among the Italian patients. Moreover, our patients display unique features which have never been reported in subjects of different ethnic origin. Thanks to these observations, it has become clear that LPI is a multisystem disease.

The prognosis of the disease is strongly influenced by the possible occurrence of severe complications, such as alveolar proteinosis, chronic renal failure or pancreatitis. The occurrence of these complications is not apparently related to a good compliance to a low-protein diet and citrulline supplementation.

Acknowledgements

The financial support of Telethon, Italy (grant No E.09) is gratefully acknowledged.

References

Andria, G., Sebastio, G., Strisciuglio, P. & Del Giudice, E. (1981): Lysinuric protein intolerance: possible genetic heterogeneity? *J. Inherit. Metab. Dis.* **4**, 151–152.

Andria, G., Sebastio, G., Sartorio, R., Parenti, G., De Rosa, L., Strisciuglio, P. & Poggi, V. (1982): Un caso di intolleranza alle proteine con lisinuria con presentazione e anomalie ematologiche atipiche. *Ital. J. Pediatr.* **8**, 634A.

Behbehani, A.W., Gahr, M. & Schroter, W. (1983): Lysinuric protein intolerance. *Monatsschr. Kinderheilkd.* **131**, 784.

Carpenter, T.O., Levy, H.L., Holtrop, M.E., Shih, V.E. & Anast, C.S. (1985): Lysinuric protein intolerance presenting as childhood osteoporosis. *N. Engl. J. Med.* **31**, 290–294.

Dianzani, I., Bonetti, G., Cerutti, F., Guidoni, C., Marengo, M. & Bracco, G. (1986): Intolleranza alle proteine con lisinuria (LPI): presentazione di due casi. Congresso Straordinario Società Italiana di Pediatria, Sorrento 28–31 Oct.

Di Rocco, M., Cerone, R. & Caruso, U. (1984): Intolleranza alle proteine con lisinuria: un caso di difficile inquadramento diagnostico. *Ital. J. Pediatr.* **10**, 95–97.

Di Rocco, M., Garibotto, G., Rossi, G.A., Caruso, U., Taccone, A., Picco, P. & Borrone, C. (1993): Role of haematological, pulmonary and renal complications in the long-term prognosis of patients with lysinuric protein intolerance. *Eur. J. Pediatr.* **152**, 437–440.

Incerti, B., Andria, G., Parenti, G., Sebastio, G., Ghezzi, M., Strisciuglio, P., Sperli, D., Di Rocco, M., Borrone, C., Parini, R., Dianzani, I. & Ponzone, A. (1993): Lysinuric protein intolerance: studies on 17 Italian patients. *Am. J. Hum. Genet.* **53 (Suppl)**, 908A.

Kerem, E., Elpeg, O.N., Shalev, R.S., Rosenman, E., Bar Ziv, Y. & Branski, D. (1993): Lysinuric protein intolerance with chronic interstitial lung disease and pulmonary cholesterol granulomas at onset. *J. Pediatr.* **123**, 275–278.

Parenti, G., Sebastio, G., Strisciuglio P., Incerti, B., Pecoraro C., Terracciano L., Andria, G. (1995): LPI characterized by bone marrow abnormalities and severe clinical course. *J. Pediat.* **126**, 246–251.

Parini, R., Vegni, M., Pontiggia, M., Melotti, D., Corbetta, C., Rossi, A. & Piceni Sereni, L. (1991): A difficult diagnosis of lysinuric protein intolerance: association with glucose-6-phosphate dehydrogenase deficiency. *J. Inherit. Metab. Dis.* **14**, 833–834.

Parto, K., Svedstrom, E., Majurin, M.L., Harkonen, R. & Simell, O. (1993): Pulmonary manifestations in lysinuric protein intolerance. *Chest* **104**, 1176–1182.

Parto, K., Kallajoki, M., Aho, H. & Simell, O. (1994): Pulmonary alveolar proteinosis and glomerulonephritis in lysinuric protein intolerance: case reports and autopsy finding of four pediatric patients. *Human Pathol.*, **25**, 400–407.

Quattrin, N. (1971): Una nuova malattia tesaurismosica: mucopolisaccaridosi genotipica disemopoietica. *Min. Pediatr.* **23**, 672–686.

Rajantie, J., Simell, O. & Perheentupa, J. (1980): Basolateral membrane transport defect for lysine in lysinuric protein intolerance. *Lancet* **i**, 1219–1221.

Simmell, O. (1989): Lysinuric protein intolerance and other cationic amino acidurias. In: *The metabolic basis of inherited disease*, eds. C.R. Scriver, A.L. Beaudet, W.S. Sly & D. Valle, pp. 2497–2513. New York: McGraw-Hill.

Smith, D.W., Scriver, C.R., Tenenhouse, H.S. & Simell, O. (1987): Lysinuric protein intolerance mutation is expressed in the plasma membrane of cultured skin fibroblasts. *Proc. Natl. Acad. Sci. USA* **84**, 7711–7715.

Chapter 9

Variable clinical presentation is a characteristic feature of late-onset hyperammonaemias

Rossella Parini[*], Carlo Corbetta[†], Antonio Bastone[‡] and Mario Salmona[‡]

[*]Second Department of Pediatrics of the University of Milan, via della Commenda 9, 20122 Milan,; [†]Clinical Research Laboratory, Istituti Clinici di Perfezionamento, Milan; [‡]Istituto di Ricerche Farmacologiche Mario Negri, Milano, Italy

Summary

Late-onset hyperammonaemias are characterized by highly variable clinical symptoms and severity of disease, which may make the diagnosis very difficult. In this chapter we will deal with the clinical signs and symptoms seen in these patients and with problems of clinical and biochemical diagnosis. The rational bases for the chronic treatment are also given.

Introduction

The expression 'late-onset hyperammonaemias' is commonly used to indicate those patients who are affected by late-onset defects of the urea cycle. Lysinuric protein intolerance and hyperornithinaemia-hyperammonaemia-homocitrullinuria (HHH) syndrome often have a clinical picture that mimicks urea cycle defects and may be included in this group. The common sign, which is often the hallmark of these diseases, is hyperammonaemia.

Table 1 lists these disorders, their underlying defects, inheritance and the main biochemical findings. Altogether, their frequency as a group is 1:30,000 (Beaudet et al., 1989). It becomes higher among inbred populations and particular groups of patients such as psychiatric and mentally retarded patients.

The whole group is constituted by inherited diseases, which often have an acute onset in the neonatal age or in the first few months of life, but may also have a later, more insidious onset in infancy, adolescence or adulthood.

While in newborns physicians are always faced with a severely affected neonate with ever worsening neurological distress, the clinical picture in subsequent ages is greatly variable in severity, and only one, or very few, signs and symptoms of the disease may reveal themselves when the patient comes to the medical attention. These may also appear intermittently, between periods completely free of symptoms which may last a few days, months or years. Between the attacks, the diagnostic biochemical tests may be completely normal (Saudubray & Ogier, 1990).

Table 1. List of diseases treated in this chapter, with indication of enzyme defect (when known), inheritance and main biochemical findings

Disease/enzyme deficit	Inheritance	Main biochemical findings	
		Blood	Urine
Urea cycle defects			
Carbamylphosphate synthetase (CPS) deficiency	AR	↑ ammonia	
Ornithine transcarbamylase (OTC) deficiency	X-linked	↑ ammonia	↑ orotic acid
Argininosuccinate synthetase (ASS) deficiency – Citrullinaemia	AR	↑ ammonia, ↑ citrulline	
Argininosuccinate lyase (ASL) deficiency – Argininosuccinic aciduria	AR	↑ ammonia, ↑ citrulline	↑ argininosuccinic aciduria
Arginase (AS) deficiency – Argininaemia	AR	↑ arginine	
Lysinuric protein intolerance (LPI)	AR	↑ ferritin, ↑ LDH, ↑ ammonia, ↓ arginine, ↓ ornithine, ↓ lysine	↑ orotic acid, ↑ lysine, ↑ arginine, ↑ ornithine
Hyperornithinaemia-hyperammonaemia-homocitrullinuria (HHH) syndrome	AR	↑ ammonia, ↑ ornithine	↑ ornithine

It appears clear why many patients go unrecognized for years, and others die without a diagnosis. A high index of suspicion is needed, in some cases, to reach the diagnosis, mainly when biochemical data are normal, and stress or loading tests are necessary to reveal pathological findings.

It has to be underlined that older patients, once recognized, usually have an easier treatment and a better prognosis than the patients in the neonatal group. In fact, some late-onset patients have residual enzymatic activity. So, we could say that these are both the less treated (because unrecognized) and *the more treatable* patients.

The urea cycle

Nitrogen, which is derived from protein metabolism, cannot be stored in the organism. In mammals, it has two possible destinations: being retained for net biosynthetic purposes or being incorporated into urea, through the urea cycle, which is the waste nitrogen product. The urea cycle also allows *de novo* synthesis of arginine. A defect in ureagenesis then leads to two main consequences: the patient develops hyperammonaemia, because ammonia is not detoxified into urea, and arginine (except in arginase deficiency) becomes an essential amino acid. A schematic representation of the urea cycle is shown in Fig. 1. The process starts with the formation of carbamylphosphate from ammonia, bicarbonate and phosphate, through the activity of the enzyme carbamylphosphate synthetase (CPS). The carbamylphosphate enters the cycle and reacts with ornithine giving citrulline (enzyme, ornithine transcarbamylase (OTC)) which, in its turn, reacts with aspartic acid to form argininosuccinate (enzyme, argininosuccinate synthetase (ASS)). Argininosuccinic acid is then metabolized to arginine by the enzyme argininosuccinate lyase (ASL); in the subsequent step (enzyme, arginase (AS)) arginine gives rise to urea, which is eliminated, and to ornithine, which enters the cycle again (Brusilow & Horwitch, 1989).

Lysinuric protein intolerance (LPI) and hyperornithinaemia-hyperammonaemia-homocitrullinuria (HHH) syndrome are two distinct autosomal recessive disorders with clinical symptoms resembling those of the urea cycle defects. The pathophysiology involves defective transport of amino acids participating in the urea cycle (Simell, 1989; Valle & Simell, 1989). In LPI, a defect in the transport of cationic amino acids is found. It is probably expressed in many tissues, but the main features of the disease depend on its expression in kidney tubules and intestine, where the efflux of lysine, arginine and ornithine through the basolateral (antiluminal) membrane of the epithelial cells is impaired. As a consequence, these amino acids accumulate in the cells and escape through the luminal membrane into urine, thus depleting the plasma amino acid pool. A deficiency of arginine is the main cause of postprandial hyperammonaemia and orotic aciduria found in this disorder (Simell, 1989).

In HHH syndrome the transport of ornithine into mitochondria is diminished, with ornithine accu-

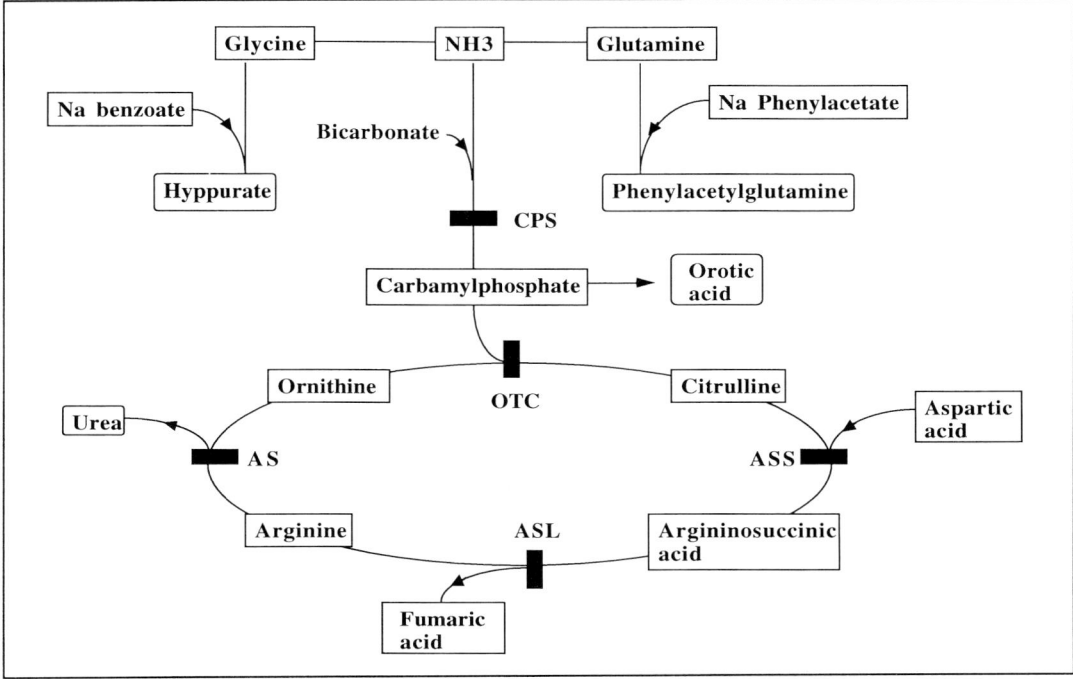

Fig. 1. Schematic representation of urea cycle. NH_3 = ammonia; CPS = carbamylphosphate synthetase; OTC = ornithine transcarbamylase; ASS = argininosuccinate synthetase; ASL = argininosuccinate lyase; AS = arginase (from Brusilow, 1986, modified).

mulating in the cytoplasm and reduced in the mitochondria, causing impaired ureagenesis, hyperammonaemia and orotic aciduria (Valle & Simell, 1989).

History and clinical patterns

The most common late presentations of these diseases are listed in Table 2. OTC deficiency and argininosuccinic aciduria are, by far, the most frequently encountered. The patient's history may reveal consanguineous parents or undiagnosed similar diseases in other members of the family. X-

Table 2. Most common clinical picture of late-onset hyperammonaemias

Anorexia, recurrent vomiting
Headache, ataxia, aggressive or apathetic behaviour, confusional state
Hemiplegia, hemiparesis
Stroke
Coma
Acute or chronic liver disease
Delayed growth
Delayed puberty
Mental retardation
Psychiatric symptoms
Hepatosplenomegaly (LPI)
Osteoporosis (LPI)

linked transmission of a lethal disease in male neonates and variable degrees of severity of the disease in females suggests OTC deficiency. Different degrees of protein intolerance in females depend on the X-inactivation pattern of the liver cells that happens by chance (Beaudet *et al.*, 1989).

The neonatal presentation of urea cycle defects is quite stereotyped, since it is dominated by the consequence of severe hyperammonaemia which leads to cerebral oedema (Brusilow & Horwitch, 1989): a few hours after birth the newborn starts showing progressive neurological distress, and falls into a severe coma within 24–48 h. Death is the natural consequence within few days, unless treatment is started.

Conversely, the late-onset forms may have many different clinical presentations with a wide spectrum of severity. The clinical picture may be dominated by recurrent crises with no or very few symptoms between the attacks, or by chronic symptoms only, ranging from mild to very severe (Brusilow & Horwitch, 1989; Bachmann, 1990; Saudubray & Ogier, 1990).

The intermittent form may range in severity from periodic migraine or cyclic vomiting, to severe recurrent episodes of stupor and coma, sometimes associated to hemiparesis or acute stroke (Kendall *et al.*, 1983; Parini *et al.*, 1987; de Grauw *et al.*, 1990; Mamourian & DuPlessis, 1991; Christodoulou *et al.*, 1993). The milder attacks may have a spontaneous resolution with self-selection of low-protein food, but the more severe episodes worsen progressively if treatment is not undertaken (Batshaw *et al.*, 1986; Coskun *et al.*, 1987; Stockler *et al.*, 1987; Brusilow & Horwitch, 1989; Finkelstein *et al.*, 1990).

The chronic form may vary from mild to severe chronic hepatitis, and from mild growth retardation and borderline mental development to very severe mental retardation and psychiatric symptoms (Krieger *et al.*, 1979; Brusilow & Horwitch, 1989; Lagas & Ruokonen, 1991). Quite frequently, patients who for years had only chronic symptoms may have an acute crisis, provoked by physical stress (sport, menstruation, puerperium), fasting, intercurrent diseases, new dietary habits (introduction of more proteins) or new treatments (e.g. valproate) (Batshaw *et al.*, 1986; Morgan *et al.*, 1987; Bachmann, 1990; Hawks Arn *et al.*, 1990; Honeycutt *et al.*, 1992). Conversely, patients who seem to have only acute attacks, are often not completely free of symptoms in between: they may have a mild mental retardation, mild gastrointestinal signs, anorexia, reduced height and weight gain, delayed pubertal development, hepatomegaly, and splenomegaly in LPI.

Laboratory features

The biochemical tests necessary for the diagnosis are listed in Table 3.

The plasma acid–base status and urinary organic acids have to be tested to exclude the diagnosis of organic acidaemia. Methylmalonic and propionic acidaemia and other rarer organic acidurias may seldom have a late onset with hyperammonaemia, but other findings are metabolic acidosis, ketosis, and a particular urine organic acid pattern. By contrast, in urea cycle disorders, metabolic acidosis and ketosis are rare and the urine organic acid pattern is aspecific.

Ferritin and LDH are typically elevated in lysinuric protein intolerance and may help in the first diagnostic evaluation.

Plasma ammonia may chronically be slightly/moderately elevated or may be increased during postprandial time only (2–4 h after the meals).

Plasma amino acid analysis may show too low or too high concentrations of citrulline, ornithine and arginine (see Fig. 1 and Table 1). Citrulline concentrations are usually elevated in ASS deficiency and may be high in ASL deficiency; in this last case the diagnosis is confirmed by the finding of high concentrations of argininosuccinic acid in plasma and urine. CPS and OTC are the two enzymes which contribute to citrulline formation: when these are defective, the citrulline concentration is usually low. Ornithine is high in plasma in HHH syndrome and low in LPI. Arginine levels may be low in CPS, OTC, ASS and ASL deficiency and high in AS deficiency.

Table 3. Tests necessary for diagnosis of late-onset hyperammonaemias

First step	
Blood	Urine
Ammonia	Amino acids
Acid–base status	Argininosuccinic acid
Glucose	Orotic acid
Transaminases	Organic acids
Urea	
Amino acids	
Ferritin	
LDH	

Second step
Allopurinol challenge test
Acute protein-loading test
24 h protein-loading test

When decompensation is developing slowly, glutamine plasma concentrations may be increased when those of ammonia are still normal: as demonstrated by Maestri et al. (1992), glutamine may in fact represent a storage site for nitrogen accumulation. In some cases, however, both plasma ammonia and amino acids may also be completely normal.

Urinary orotic acid levels are usually elevated in OTC deficiency, LPI, HHH syndrome, and may also be increased in citrullinaemia and argininaemia (Bachmann & Colombo, 1980). Orotic acid is an intermediate metabolite of pyrimidine synthesis and is synthesized from carbamylphosphate; its synthesis is stimulated by an increased concentration of carbamylphosphate in the cytosol. Orotic-aciduria then indicates a block after the CPS step (Fig. 1). Many OTC deficient females may have normal blood ammonia and amino acids, but increased excretion of orotic acid (Hokanson et al., 1978).

There are a number of OTC-deficient females who also have normal values of urinary orotic acid in basal conditions (Hokanson et al., 1978). The protein-loading test is the classic test used to reveal latent hyperammonaemia. It is usually performed with 1–2 g/kg/meal depending on the age and weight of the subject. Basal and 1, 2, 4 and 6 hour blood samples are taken to measure plasma ammonia and amino acids. Urine is collected 24 h before the test and in four separate 6 h urine collections after the meal for the orotic acid assay. This test has mainly been used in the last 20 years to detect asymptomatic OTC-deficient females for genetic counselling and antenatal diagnostic purposes (Hokanson et al., 1978). While only a small proportion of asymptomatic obligate carrier females have hyperammonaemia after a high-protein meal, about 90 per cent of them may be identified by increased excretion of orotic acid, suggesting that this test has only a 10 per cent false-negative rate (Brusilow & Horwitch, 1989). However, the test bears the risk of developing iatrogenic hyperammonaemia and has to be performed in specialized departments by physicians who are expert in the field. It has recently been partially replaced by a challenge test with allopurinol which allows the detection of a pathological excretion of orotic acid and orotidine without provoking hyperammonaemia (Hauser et al., 1990; Burlina et al., 1992). It is based on two observations: (1) OTC-deficient patients have an increased pyrimidine biosynthesis, (2) oxipurinol ribonucleotide, the in vivo reaction product of allopurinol, has an inhibitory effect on orotidine monophosphate decarboxylase (Fig. 2). As a consequence, after a single dose of allopurinol, subjects with OTC deficiency excrete large amounts of orotidine in the urine. This test has approximately the same false-negative rate as the single-meal protein-loading test, but is safer and more convenient.

In extreme situations, a 24 h protein-loading test may be necessary (Spada et al., 1994) to reach a diagnosis in patients with intermittent clinical and biochemical abnormalities suggesting urea cycle disorder.

Clinical case reports

The following case reports are a series of observations made in our department in the last 12 years, each illustrating the different clinical pictures presented in Table 2.

1. MP was the second daughter of healthy non-consanguineous parents. The first daughter died at the age of 2 years with a presumptive diagnosis of encephalitis. M. was healthy until the age of 2y 10m when she started having bimonthly episodes of refusal of food, persistent vomiting, obnubilation and hypersomnia with spontaneous resolution. The recognition of chronically elevated transaminases (2–10-fold of the normal values) with no signs of infection led to the diagnosis of non-A, non-B chronic hepatitis.

At 7 years, a metabolic investigation led to the finding of increased excretion of orotic acid in the urine and a diagnosis of OTC deficiency was made. Treatment with arginine first and citrulline later was started, associated with a hypoproteic diet. Afterwards the patient never presented episodes of vomiting and hypersomnia, her transaminases normalized in 2 months and her growth velocity had a remarkable increase in the 2 following years: at diagnosis (7 years) she weighed 19 kg (–2 SD) and was 113 cm (–2 SD) high; at 9 years, her weight was 26 kg (–0.36 SD) and her height was 130 cm (0 SD). Now, at 16 years, she has normal physical (height 170 cm = +2 SD; weight 52 kg= –1 SD) and mental development (WISC-R IQ 130) and is attending the high school; liver function tests are normal.

2. MV: The family history of this young woman showed two brothers who died in the first week of life, one sister who died at 7 years of age due to an unexplained coma, after repeated episodes of recurrent vomiting and ketosis, and two apparently healthy sisters and one healthy brother. Her first child, a boy, died with severe hyperammonaemia at 4 days of age. She came to our department at the age of 27, for genetic counselling in view of future possible pregnancies. Her personal history revealed that she did not like meat and had occasional episodes of headache and refusal of food. The dietary enquiry revealed that anyway she ate about 50 g of protein/day, which represents a normoproteic diet. Levels of ammonia and amino acids in plasma and of orotic acid excretion were normal. A protein-loading test (1 g/kg) was then performed, which yielded hyperammonaemia (maximum 173 μmol/l at the 6th h) and abnormal orotic acid excretion (maximum 13 μmol/mmol creatinine between the 4th and the 8th h).

Although well informed about her heterozygous OTC deficiency, she refused our suggestion to start citrulline treatment and to follow a moderately hypoproteic diet. An explanatory letter was given to her and her husband. Two months later she was admitted, obnubilated and hemiparetic, to a neurological department near Milan and was not able to explain her genetic condition nor to show our letter. When at last the situation was understood, it was too late for her, as she had died in irreversible coma.

3. CD: This case has already been partially reported (Parini et al., 1987). He was the second son of healthy non-consanguineous parents. The first child was healthy. From 8 months of age, he had episodes of refusal of food, vomiting and hypersomnia lasting 2–3 days and spontaneously abating, with an approximately monthly frequency. At 2 years he was admitted to our hospital with right-sided hemiparesis following 2 days of his usual periodic illness. Liver function tests were normal. Orotic acid was elevated in the urine (1000 μmol/24 h) and the diagnosis of late-onset OTC deficiency in a male was made. The CT scan revealed only a mild brain atrophy. Hemiparesis receded after 2 days of treatment which consisted of arginine supplementation, later substituted with citrulline and a mildly hypoproteic diet (1 g/kg protein/day). No further crises were observed in

subsequent years. The patient is now 12 years old and has a normal physical (weight 32 kg: −1 SD; height 149 cm: +1 SD) and mental development (IQ 120 WISC-R).

4. VD is the first son of healthy non-consanguineous parents. In the neonatal period hypotonia and hypokinesis were observed, which receded in a few days. The EEG was aspecific. The baby was discharged at 15 days of age without a clear diagnosis.

At 3 years he was admitted to our hospital with repeated seizures during a febrile illness. In spite of anticonvulsant therapy with phenobarbital, he had five episodes in the first day and two in the second day and was obnubilated in between. In the fourth day, when he seemed to recover, psychomotor retardation and intermittent ataxia were noted and a metabolic evaluation was undertaken. It showed argininosuccinic aciduria (12.07 g/20 h) and hypercitrullinaemia (196 µmol/l). The diagnosis of argininosuccinic aciduria was made and confirmed with the direct measurement of enzyme activity in the red cells (0.086 nmol/h/mg Hb–control 16.18). The parents and the brother had values consistent with a heterozygous condition (father 6.95, mother 4.83, brother 5.23). He was then treated with arginine and a moderately hypoproteic diet. He never had further episodes of ataxia or obnubilation. He is now 14 years old with normal physical development and mild mental retardation (IQ 73 WISC-R).

5. NF is the first daughter of healthy non-consanguineous parents. Her history showed normal psychomotor development until 2 years of age when, during an infectious illness, she had repeated seizures. From then on, she developed a mild psychomotor retardation and psychiatric symptoms. At 34 years of age during a gynaecological examination which necessitated fasting for anaesthesia, she fell down in a coma from which she recovered a few days later after intensive care. In that period a metabolic disease was suspected and the diagnosis was made of argininosuccinic aciduria on the basis of abnormal excretion of argininosuccinic acid (4g/24 h) and elevated plasma citrulline levels (127 µmol/l). Arginine treatment was started. Afterwards she never had any more episodes of coma although no other amelioration was seen in her clinical state.

6. FM: This boy is the second child of healthy non-consanguineous parents. The first child, a daughter, is healthy. The maternal uncle had died at 15 years of age with a diagnosis of encephalitis. The patient was healthy until 3 years of age when he developed anorexia, recurrent vomiting and lethargy followed by repeated seizures and coma. He was hospitalized in a paediatric department in Milan where a diagnosis of encephalitis was made. Between 3 and 7 years of age he had five other analogous episodes but a clear diagnosis was not reached although at each episode he was hospitalized in paediatric or neuropaediatric departments. At the age of 7 years, while he was in Japan with his family, he developed another episode and was hospitalized in the paediatric department of the Kobe Kaisei Hospital in Japan. There, an increase of plasma ammonia was demonstrated after a protein-loading test. OTC activity, measured in a biopsy sample of the liver was 0.27 µmol/mg of protein. A moderately hypoproteic diet was prescribed and the child did not have any other crises in subsequent years.

At 23 years of age he came to our department asking if there were other possible treatments for his disease. His physical and mental development were completely normal. He plays many sports and is attending the second year of the Faculty of Law at the University of Milan. We simply gave him a low-dose citrulline treatment and suggested a yearly check of biochemical tests.

7. GL was the third daughter of healthy non-consanguineous parents. A brother died in neonatal age. A sister died at the age of 18 after the seventh episode of confusion, obnubilation, lethargy and coma (Perini et al., 1993). The diagnosis of OTC deficiency was made post-mortem (1.04 µmol/h per mg of protein; control 13.4; CPS 2.1; control 2.99). Two other sisters are healthy. G. was normal until puberty but a self-selected low-protein diet was reported in the history. After puberty she developed periodic aggressive and restless behaviour, and mild mental retardation was recognized. Twice she was hospitalized with a mild coma. She was referred to our observation after the second coma by the neurologist who raised the suspicion of OTC deficiency, on the basis of her sister's

history – she had died some time before. On arrival the patient looked healthy and all the first-step tests were normal (plasma ammonia, plasma arginine and citrulline, and urinary orotic acid) except for plasma glutamine which was elevated (1570 µmol/l). An allopurinol challenge test was performed and a significant increase of orotic acid was found in her urine (maximum value 86 µmol/mmol creatinine in the 6–12 h period). The mother also had abnormal results, while the two sisters, 24 and 10 years old, were normal. She was taught to continue her self-selected low-protein diet, completely avoiding protein-rich food (meat, fish, eggs, cheese) and to start treatment with citrulline and sodium benzoate. The dietary inquiry showed that her spontaneous protein intake per day was 20–25 g. In the following 3 years she never had other acute decompensations.

8. FS is the second child of healthy unrelated parents coming from the same village near Salerno (South Italy). The three other children of the couple are healthy. F. had suboptimal gain of height and weight since his first year of age and was frequently hospitalized from 3 years on, for hepatosplenomegaly of unknown origin. He came to our department at the age of 10. Self-selection of low-protein food was reported. His height was 117 cm (–5 SD) and his weight was 22 kg (–3 SD). His psychomotor development was normal. The clinical examination showed moderate hepatosplenomegaly. Abnormal values of LDH (2697 U/l, n.v. 230–460) and ferritin (1536 mg/dl, n.v. 8–300) were found. Plasma ammonia was normal. As this clinical and biochemical pattern is typical of LPI, the specific biochemical tests were done (plasma and urine amino acids and urinary orotic acid) which showed low plasma concentrations and increased urinary excretion of dibasic amino acids (ornithine, lysine, arginine) together with an increased excretion of orotic acid. Treatment with citrulline was started. One month later liver and spleen sizes were within normal limits. Now, at 14 years old, his height is 148 cm (–2 SD) and weight is 36 kg (–2 SD).

Treatment

Treatment of these patients is based on three main principles (Brusilow & Horwitch, 1989; Bachmann, 1990):

(1) reducing nitrogen intake. This is achieved with a low protein diet; in some cases natural proteins are partially substituted by artificial formulas of essential amino acids with the aim of giving enough for growth-essential amino acids and less nitrogen. This allows us to limit nitrogen catabolism through the urea cycle. Protein restriction is not the rule in LPI. Besides, endogenous protein catabolism has also to be minimized, avoiding prolonged fasting and insufficient caloric intake.

(2) supplying the deficient intermediates of urea synthesis: arginine, which is also an essential amino acid for these patients, or citrulline, which could substitute for arginine in CPS and OTC deficiency, HHH syndrome and LPI.

(3) treating with substances (sodium benzoate and sodium phenylacetate) which allow nitrogen elimination through alternative pathways (Fig. 1).

Outside the acute decompensation periods, the more common risk in these patients is to restrict the protein intake excessively. Because of this, in patients with a chronic pattern, we usually start with a protein intake close to the previous spontaneous one, which is assessed by the dietitian in an interview with the patient or his relatives. After evaluation of the metabolic balance reached with the administration of arginine or citrulline, we decide if the protein intake really has to be reduced.

Arginine and citrulline dosages (200–700 mg/kg/day) have to be individualized on the basis of the defect, age and weight of the patient, protein intake, levels of plasma ammonia and amino acids. The risk of excessive treatment has also to be considered. A general indication is that treatment should be adapted so that the preprandial arginine concentration lies between 100 and 150 µmol/l and the ammonia level is normal (Bachmann, 1990).

Sodium benzoate forms hippurate by binding with glycine (Fig. 1); hippurate is formed in the liver

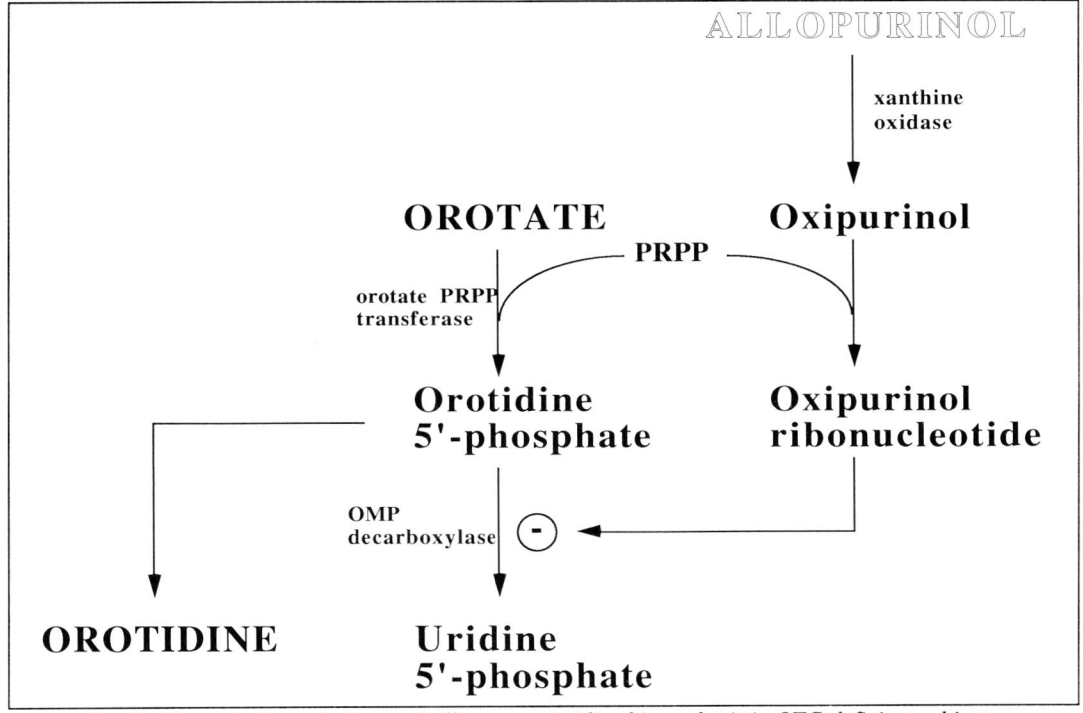

Fig. 2. *Allopurinol metabolism and effect on pyrimidine biosynthesis in OTC-deficient subjects.*

and excreted at a high clearance rate: one mole of hippurate binds one mole of nitrogen. Sodium phenylacetate and phenylbutyrate form phenylacetylglutamine in the kidney with binding of two moles of nitrogen (Fig. 1).

Other treatments are:

– enzyme supplementation by bimonthly erythrocyte transfusion in argininaemia (with the risk of immunological sensitization and infections!);

– liver transplantation: it has been performed in some OTC-deficient females who could not reach a satisfactory metabolic compensation and in CPS deficiency and citrullinaemia (Tuchman, 1989; Todo *et al.*, 1992).

Experimental studies are in progress on gene therapy (Grompe *et al.*, 1992; Demarquoy, 1993) which is probably a promising perspective for the future.

Discussion and conclusions

In conclusion, the extreme variability of symptoms and their severity is a characteristic of late-onset hyperammonaemic disorders. The consequence is that diagnostic delays and errors are common, with a median delay of diagnosis of 16 months (Brusilow & Horwitch, 1989). It is well exemplified by the series of clinical cases presented here. In our group of patients the time between first symptoms and diagnosis ranged between 13 months and 30 years.

In the all cases, a detailed analysis of the history revealed signs or symptoms which were not explained by the first diagnostic hypothesis. Furthermore, it was never supported by laboratory tests. It is in cases like these, when the diagnosis is not clear, that we have to make an effort to search for other hypotheses and test them. The history of the patient has to be reviewed critically with the aim of explaining the whole cluster of symptoms and signs. In most patients the specific biochemical tests give abnormal results and allow the diagnosis to be reached; in a few cases only, is a stress or loading test needed.

In the *patient's history* data that should elicit suspicion are: high-protein food avoidance, crises precipitated by abundant meals, recently started treatment with valproate, and, in women, recently completed puberty, menstruation (hormonal factors favouring tissue catabolism or increased need for energy), puerperium.

In the *clinical evaluation*, besides the well-known symptoms of hyperammonaemia, stroke-like episodes and hemiparesis have to be underlined. They are more and more frequently reported not only in urea cycle defects but also in other metabolic disorders (Vallée et al., 1994) and seem to be mostly attributable to localized ischaemia in brain tissue.

Diagnosis is more difficult if the patient is an adult because it is a common opinion that these genetic diseases have an earlier onset in life. If this patient also has normal standard biochemical tests, it is usually the rule for the physician to accept the normal results and try to explain symptoms in another way. At this point, a firm suspicion may be maintained only on the basis of knowledge and experience in this special field, and its exclusion rests on the performance of complicated, time-consuming, sometimes risky, tests. However, if the whole clinical and biochemical pattern is not fully explained, a further clinical study of the patient with the aid of specialists in the field is strongly indicated. It will probably enable the correct diagnosis in most of these patients affected by 'orphan' diseases. This is really worthwhile, because recognition of the disease is often the only means of guaranteeing a normal future life for the patient, by a few simple dietary measures and precautions. Furthermore, the correct diagnosis in one patient carries other additional advantages: the whole family may be studied and other patients recognized who are asymptomatic, and all the members of the family may receive adequate genetic counselling.

Acknowledgements

We thank Dr Gabriella Nebbia and Professor Vittorio Carnelli, Clinica Pediatrica I, Istituti Clinici di Perfezionamento, Milan and Dr Maria Gianelli, Clinica Neurologica, Novara, for having referred patients 1, 8 and 7 respectively. We also acknowledge the generous support of the Fondazione Pierfranco e Luisa Mariani, Milan (with a grant for promoting the prevention of mental retardation in metabolic diseases).

References

Bachmann, C. & Colombo, J.P. (1980): Diagnostic value of orotic acid excretion in heritable disorders of the urea cycle and in hyperammonemia due to organic acidurias. *Eur. J. Pediatr.* **134,** 109–113.

Bachmann, C. (1990): Urea cycle disorders. In: *Inborn metabolic diseases*, eds. J. Fernandes, J.-M. Saudubray & K. Tada, pp. 212–228. Berlin, Heidelberg: Springer.

Batshaw, M.L., Msall, M., Beaudet, A.L. & Trojak, J. (1986): Risk of serious illness in heterozygotes for ornithine transcarbamylase deficiency. *J. Pediatr.* **108,** 236–241.

Beaudet, A.L., Scriver, C.R., Sly, W.S., Valle, D., Cooper, D.N., McKusick, V.A. & Schmidke, J. (1989): Genetics and biochemistry of variant human phenotypes. In: *The metabolic basis of inherited disease*, eds. C.R. Scriver, A.L. Beaudet, W.S. Sly & D. Valle, pp. 3–163. New York: McGraw-Hill.

Brusilow S.W. (1986): Alterazioni del ciclo dell'urea. *Minuti Menarini*, 19–26 March.

Brusilow, S.W. & Horwich, A.L. (1989): Urea cycle enzymes. In: *The metabolic basis of inherited disease*, eds. C.R. Scriver, A.L. Beaudet, W.S. Sly, & D. Valle, pp. 629–663. New York: McGraw-Hill.

Burlina, A.B., Ferrari, V., Dionisi-Vici, C., Bordugo, A., Zacchello, F. & Tuchman, M. (1992): Allopurinol challenge test in children. *J. Inherit. Metab. Dis.* **15,** 707–712.

Christodoulou, J., Qureshi, I.A., McInnes, R.R. & Clarke, J.T.R. (1993): Ornithine transcarbamylase deficiency presenting with strokelike episodes. *J. Pediatr.* **122,** 423–425.

Coskun, T., Ozalp, I., Monch, S. & Kneer, J. (1987): Lethal hyperammonaemic coma due to ornithine transcarbamylase deficiency presenting as brain encephalitis in a previously asymptomatic ten-year-old boy. *J. Inherit. Metab. Dis.* **10**, 271.

de Grauw, T.J., Smith, L.M.E., Brockstedt, M., Meijer, Y., van der Kleivan Moorsel, J. & Jakobs, C. (1990): Acute hemiparesis as the presenting sign in a heterozygote for ornithine transcabamylase deficiency. *Neuropediatrics* **21**, 133–135.

Demarquoy, J. (1993): Retroviral-mediated gene therapy for the treatment of citrullinemia. Transfer and expression of argininosuccinate synthetase in human hematopoietic cells. *Experientia* **49**, 345–348.

Finkelstein, J.E., Hauser, E.R., Leonard, C.O. & Brusilow, S.W. (1990): Late-onset ornithine transcarbamylase deficiency in male patients. *J. Pediatr.* **117**, 897–902.

Grompe, M., Jones, S.N., Loulseged, H. & Caskey, C.T. (1992): Retroviral-mediated gene transfer of human ornithine transcarbamylase into primary hepatocytes of *spf* and *spf-ash* mice. *Hum. Gene Ther.* **3**, 35–44.

Hauser, E.R., Finkelstein, J.E., Valle, D. & Brusilow, S.W. (1990): Allopurinol-induced orotidinuria. A test for mutations at the ornithine carbamoyltransferase locus in women. *N. Engl. J. Med.* **322**, 1641–1645.

Hawks Arn, P., Hauser, E.R., Thomas, G.H., Herman, G., Hess, D. & Brusilow, S. (1990): Hyperammonemia in women with a mutation at the ornithine carbamoyltransferase locus. A cause of postpartum coma. *N. Engl. J. Med.* **322**, 1652–1655.

Hokanson, J.T., O'Brien, W.E., Idemoto, J. & Schafer, I.A. (1978): Carrier detection in ornithine transcarbamylase deficiency. *J. Pediatr.* **93**, 75–78.

Honeycutt, D., Callahan, K., Rutledge, L. & Evans, B. (1992): Heterozygote ornithine transcarbamylase deficiency presenting as symptomatic hyperammonemia during initiation of valproate therapy. *Neurology* **42**, 666–668.

Kendall, B.E., Kingsley, D.P.E., Leonard, J.V., Lingam, S. & Oberholzer, V.G. (1983): Neurological features and computed tomography of the brain in children with ornithine carbamoyl transferase deficiency. *J. Neurol. Neurosurg. Psychiatry* **46**, 28–34.

Krieger I., Snodgrass, P.J. & Roskamp, J. (1979): Atypical clinical course of ornithine transcarbamylase deficiency due to a new mutant (comparison with Reye disease). *J. Clin. Endocrinol. Metab.* **48**, 388–392.

Lagas, P.A. & Ruokonen A. (1991): Late onset argininosuccinic aciduria in a paranoid retardate. *Biol. Psychiatry* **30**, 1229–1232.

Maestri, N.E., McGowan, K.D. & Brusilow, S.W. (1992): Plasma glutamine concentration: a guide in the management of urea cycle disorders. *J. Pediatr.* **121**, 259–261.

Mamourian, A.C. & DuPlessis, A. (1991): Urea cycle defect: a case with MR and CT findings resembling infarct. *Pediatr. Radiol.* **21**, 594–595.

Morgan, H.B., Swaiman, K.F. & Johnson B.D. (1987): Diagnosis of argininosuccinic aciduria after valproic acid-induced hyperammonemia. *Neurology* **37**, 886–887.

Parini, R., Corbetta, C., Bardelli, P., Careddu, P., Cathelineau, L., Delcò, A., Ronchi, M.T. & Piceni Sereni, L. (1987): Partial OTC deficiency in a male. Follow-up and family study. *Perspect. Inherit. Metabol. Dis.* **7**, 13–18.

Perini, M., Zarcone, D. & Corbetta, C. (1993): Hyperammonemic coma in an adolescent girl: an unusual case of ornithine transcarbamylase deficiency. *Ital. J. Neurol. Sci.* **14**, 461–464.

Saudubray, J.-M. & Ogier, H. (1990): Clinical approach to inherited metabolic disorders. In: *Inborn metabolic diseases*, eds. J. Fernandes, J.-M. Saudubray & K. Tada, pp. 3–25. Berlin, Heidelberg: Springer.

Simell, O. (1989): Lysinuric protein intolerance and other cationic amino acidurias. In: *The metabolic basis of inherited disease*, eds. C.R. Scriver, A.L. Beaudet, W.S. Sly & D. Valle, pp. 2497–2513. New York: McGraw-Hill.

Spada, M., Guardamagna, O., Rabier, D., van der Meer, S.B., Parvy, P., Bardet, J., Ponzone, A. & Saudubray, J.M. (1994): Recurrent episodes of bizarre behavior in a boy with ornithine transcarbamylase deficiency: diagnostic failure of protein loading and allopurinol challenge tests. *J. Pediatr.* **125**, 249–251.

Stockler, S., Grossschadl, F., Bachmann, C. & Roscher, A. (1987): Ornithine transcarbamylase variant in a male patient. *J. Inherit. Metab. Dis.* **10**, 272.

Todo, S., Starzl, T.E., Tzakis, A., Benkov, K.J., Kalousek, F., Saheki, T., Tanikawa, K. & Fenton, W.A. (1992): Orthotopic liver transplantation for urea cycle enzyme deficiency. *Hepatology* **15**, 419–22.

Tuchman, M. (1989): Persistent acitrullinemia after liver transplantation for carbamylphosphate synthetase deficiency (letter). *N. Engl. J. Med.* **320**, 1498–1499.

Valle, D. & Simell, O. (1989): The hyperornithinemias. In: *The metabolic basis of inherited disease*, eds. C.R. Scriver, A.L. Beaudet, W.S. Sly, D. & Valle, pp. 599–627. New York: McGraw-Hill.

Vallée, L., Fontaine, M., Nuyts, J.-P., Ricart, G., Krivosic, I., Divry, P., Vianey-Saban, C., Lhermitte, M. & Vamecq, J. (1994): Stroke, hemiparesis, and deficient mitochondrial beta-oxidation. *Eur. J. Pediatr.* **153,** 598–603.

Chapter 10

Treatment of organic acidurias

Alberto B. Burlina

Department of Pediatrics, University of Padua, Via Giustiniani 3, 35128 Padua, Italy

Summary

The major recent advances in disorders of amino acids and organic acids have been in their management. Treatment regimens for many disorders have been improved and standardized. Treatment options commonly used in organic aciduria include: (a) substitution, elimination or restriction of a substrate(s) (dietary treatment); (b) cofactor replacement; (c) enhancing alternative pathways or increasing excretion of toxic metabolites; (d) gene therapy (organ transplant). It is important to realize that real efforts do have to be made not only initially at diagnosis but also in long-term management, to reach the goal of preventing mental and physical handicap.

Introduction

Organic acidurias are inherited disorders of the catabolism of amino acids, carbohydrates and fatty acid oxidation characterized by the accumulation and excretion of non-amino organic acids in the urine. Disorders of fatty acid β-oxidation are dealt with in the chapter by Uziel (Ch. 2) while defects in the metabolism of carbohydrates are covered by De Vivo's (Ch. 4).

Organic acidurias have the reputation of being associated with the urinary excretion of huge amounts of metabolites; for example, in propionic acidaemia, patients typically excrete large amounts of 3-hydroxypropionic acid and methylcitric acid; those with isovaleric acidaemia excrete large amounts of 3-hydroxyisovaleric acid and isovalerylglycine.

Many of the organic acids that accumulate in this type of disorder are relatively strong and will accordingly give rise to changes in the acid–base status of the blood plasma. The extent of the acid–base changes is highly dependent on the concentration of their organic acids, but on the other hand, it cannot be overlooked that some organic acidurias are characterized by moderate (or even low) excretions of abnormal organic acids (i.e. 4-hydroxybutyric aciduria, tyrosinaemia type I, and 3 methylglutaconic aciduria type II) and for this reason many patients with organic acidaemia do not have a metabolic acidosis. For all these reasons, the diagnosis is still difficult (Duran et al., 1991). Moreover, specific reagents for the detection of organic acids do not exist and diagnosis in infants and children is performed by demonstrating specific abnormal organic acids in urine, usually by combined gas chromatography-mass spectrometry (GC-MS) (Burlina, 1986).

The most frequent organic acidurias susceptible to treatment are reported in Table 1. Some of these disorders have more than one cause. For example, multiple carboxylase deficiency may be due to defects of biotinidase or holocarboxylase synthetase; methylmalonic acidaemia may be due to defects of methylmalony-CoA mutase or of any of several enzymes involved in the synthesis of the mutase coenzyme, such as adenosyl-B_{12}.

Table 1. Organic acidurias capable of treatment

MSUD
Propionic aciduria
 Methylmalonic aciduria
 Glutaric aciduria type I
 3-Methylglutaconyl-CoA lyase
 Tyrosinaemia type I
 Isovaleric acidaemia
 β-ketothiolase deficiency
 Multiple carboxylase deficiency

Therapeutic protocols are therefore influenced by the pathophysiology and disease mechanism and good therapy has to be the result of a true symbiosis between the fields of human biochemical genetics and nutrition.

Therapeutic strategies for organic acidurias

The management of infants with organic acidurias is demanding (Nyhan, 1991). Treatment options commonly used include:

- substitution, elemination or restriction of a substrate(s) (dietary treatment);
- cofactor replacement;
- enhancing alternative pathway or increasing excretion of toxic metabolites;
- gene therapy (organ transplant).

Dietary treatment

The mainstay of treatment for most organic acidurias is dietary restriction of amino acid(s) that are not metabolized properly. The substrate must be provided, however, in adequate amounts to promote normal growth while avoiding excesses that are toxic (Ogier et al., 1990).

In many organic acidurias we are confronted with the problem that products of the catabolism of essential amino acids are highly toxic. Their accumulation leads to serious clinical illness and death. It has seemed intuitively reasonable to approach this problem with the rigid restriction of the intake of protein in all organic acidurias, except for maple syrup urine disease (MSUD) in which the natural protein is partially replaced with a synthetic amino acid mixture.

Often the best that can be done is to reduce the total protein intake to the minimum needed to maintain satisfactory growth whilst maintaining normal energy intake. Essential amino acids and other nutrients have to be maintained at the optimum level at which the offending amino acid or acids can be provided that will meet the anabolic needs for growth while keeping the accumulation of toxic intermediates at minimal levels. It requires careful monitoring of the levels of the accumulating amino acid or organic acid, rates of growth in weight, height and head circumference, and nitrogen balance.

In normal conditions it is expected that if the precursors are not provided in excess of requirements, the toxic metabolite will not accumulate. However, it is not as simple as this because during anabolism in the presence of minimal quantities of amino acids, even at quantities below requirements, these substrates are available to catabolic enzymes and therefore there is always a certain level of accumulation. This certainly is the case in disorders of propionate metabolism: in fact below a certain amino acid intake we would expect the catabolism of tissue proteins and an increased of accumulation of metabolites (Nyhan *et al.*, 1991). Similarly an appropriate intake of vitamins and minerals must be maintained.

During illness and fasting various metabolic adaptations occur and the diet may need to be altered. Metabolic stress precipitated by minor infections or surgery may lead to serious biochemical derangement (the rate of protein breakdown exceeds that of synthesis with a net production of amino acids and an increase in their irreversible catabolism) and to prevent such serious complications the diet is changed to an 'emergency regimen' (Dixon & Leonard, 1992). This consists of a high carbohydrate intake (a solution of glucose polymer), sometimes with the addition of a fat emulsion, to reduce endogenous protein metabolism and hence the accumulation of toxic intermediates.

The use of special metabolic formulas is still controversial. Those formulas which are free of the precursor amino acids are important factors in the treatment of these disorders because they provide a buffer of nitrogen, which is beneficial in the promotion of visceral and somatic protein synthesis. A low-protein diet that supplies only whole protein sources may not have sufficient nitrogen for synthesis. In addition, the use of special metabolic formulas allows the flexibility to decrease toxic amino acids, if clinically indicated, while supplying enough amino acids to promote growth and present catabolism (Queen *et al.*, 1981). Anyway, it is important to point out that the use of metabolic formulas is not accepted worldwide (Poggi *et al.*, 1993).

At the meeting of European Metabolic Group in Lausanne, 1992 (Milupa Scientific Information, 1994) a workshop was held in order to establish proposals for the follow up of patients with metabolic disorders. Biochemical indicators of overtreatment and insufficient treatment in organic acidurias are summarized in Table 2.

Table 2. Biochemical indicators of overtreatment and insufficient treatment in propionic and methylmalonic acidurias

Overtreatment	Insufficient treatment
Plasma protein ↓	Ketoacidosis (Acetest +)
Albumin ↓	Anaemia/thrombopenia
Prealbumin ↓	Lactate ↑
Trace elements ↓	Ammonia ↑
Essential amino acids ↓	OLCFA ↑
Transaminases ↑	Urinary metabolites ↑
Urinary metabolites ↑	Free carnitine ↓
	Acyl/free carnitine ↑

Clinically it is difficult to differentiate signs of overtreatment from insufficient treatment. Failure to thrive, oedemas, loss of appetite, vomiting, cardiomyopathy (Massaud & Leonard, 1993), pancreatitis (Burlina *et al.*, 1993) and in particular skin and hair abnormalities (De Raeve *et al.*, 1994) are common in both situations.

The frequency at which the treatment should be controlled will depend on the severity of the enzyme defect; it further depends on the compliance and on the extent of understanding of the disease shown by the parents, and the experience of the paediatricians with management of the specific disorder (Poggi *et al.*, 1993).

Cofactor replacement

In some organic acidurias there is altered binding of a vitamin cofactor to the mutant apoenzyme and it is often possible to provide a large excess of the cofactor and overcome this altered binding affinity.

The cofactor-responsive organic aciduria can be classified according to the mechanism by which the holoenzyme activity is increased. The mechanisms include defective processing of a vitamin or cofactor (cobalamin for methylmalonic aciduria, biotin for multiple carboxylase deficiency), defective binding of a cofactor (thiamine for MSUD), and undetermined mechanisms (riboflavine for β-oxidation defects) (Sweetman, 1991).

An example of defective processing of a vitamin-related organic aciduria is represented by biotinidase deficiency. The treatment of biotinidase deficiency is essentially the administration of pharmacological doses of biotin. The customary dose is 10 mg of biotin/day given orally, but doses as high as 30–60 mg/day have been given either orally or intravenously. The optimum amount has not yet been established. For most patients the response is immediate and dramatic, with correction of biochemical markers (lactic acidosis) and clinical signs (skin rash, alopecia, neurological symptoms), and development becomes normal. Some patients have developed nerve deafness and optic atrophy while being treated with biotin. These problems have not occurred in any patients with holocarboxylase synthetase deficiency (the other defect in which biotin can be used) while being treated with biotin, and may be due to the toxicity of biocytin in the patients with biotinidase deficiency (Wolf & Heard, 1990).

Several important points must be emphasized in vitamin-responsive organic acidurias (Leonard & Daish, 1985).

(a) The requirement of pharmacological doses of the cofactor to produce a therapeutic response is very high (1000 μg/day) compared with the recommended daily allowance (25 μg/day);

(b) it is desirable to demonstrate a reproducible improvement in specifically aberrant clinical chemical values whether or not the precise defect in the reaction mechanism is known, so as to identify candidates for such therapeutic approaches;

(c) The ultimate designation of 'responsiveness' must be derived from observations of the clinical efficacy of therapy rather than from measurements of reaction precursors or products.

Increasing excretion of toxic metabolites or enhancing alternative pathways

Carnitine

Treatment of organic acidurias by means of conjugation of potentially hazardous substances are nowadays frequently used. Originally it was thought that only glycine conjugates were formed (i.e. isovalerylglycine in isovaleric acidaemia) but now other conjugating substrates such as carnitine and glucuronic acid are well recognized.

A secondary deficiency of carnitine occurs widely in patients with organic acidaemias. These include propionic acidaemia, methylmalonic acidaemia, isovaleric acidaemia, glutaric acidaemia type I, 3-hydroxy-3-methyl-glutaryl CoAHMG-CoA lyase deficiency and the fatty acyl-CoA dehydrogenase deficiencies (Roe et al., 1991). In these patients, acyl coenzyme A compounds accumulate in the mitochondria and cause inhibition of many of the respiratory enzymes. They are removed by forming an acyl–carnitine complex that is excreted in the urine. The use of carnitine for 'buffering' acyl coenzyme A compounds leads to loss of tissue carnitine and the development of a secondary carnitine deficiency. The clinical complications can be prevented by carnitine supplementation (Winter et al., 1992), treating patients with these disorders are persuaded that this is a real advance in management, above all when the patients are in catabolic state or are faced with intercurrent infections or surgery. Anyway, it is still difficult to document the physiological effects of treatment because therapy in these patients is not only by administering carnitine. Theoretically, the maximum benefit should accrue not simply when the free carnitine level in the blood is normal, but when urinary esters are maximal; however, it is difficult to achieve this status despite progressive increases in carnitine dosage.

The customary dose is 100 mg/kg/b.w. by mouth but doses as high as 400 mg/kg/b.w. have been suggested. This compound is virtually non-toxic, but the amount that can be tolerated is limited by the production of diarrhoea at higher doses. The effectiveness of replenishing deficient stores can be readily assessed by measuring the concentration of acyl and free carnitine in the blood and urine.

Metronidazole

Different antibiotics have a markedly greater effect on fecal propionate concentrations but they also have a high incidence of side-effects. Metronidazole has recently been chosen because there is a low risk of complications and because the antibacterial mechanism of action is specific for anaerobes, the bacterial subgroup to which propionate production capacity is most closely linked (Brain et al., 1988).

Studies by Walter et al. (1988) and Thompson et al. (1990) have shown that a dose of metronidazole varying from 10 to 20 mg/kg resulted in a fall in the excretion of all metabolites in methylmalonic (MMA) and propionic (PA) patients, and in clinical improvement (increased alertness, increased activity and improved appetite).

The optimal method of administering metronidazole in MMA and PA has not yet been determined. At the moment such therapy should be approached with some caution and with careful monitoring for side-effects (including gastrointestinal disturbances, leucopoenia and peripheral neuropathy) until safety has been reached in these disorders. It is possible that continuing metronidazole treatment at a dose of 10 mg/kg per day may lead to the appearance of resistant strains of anaerobic bacteria, which are the major bacterial source of propionate. Alternatively, the use of metronidazole intermittently, or by rotation with other antibiotics, may decrease the likelihood of developing resistant strains . Our preliminary results (unpublished observations) in five patients with MMA have shown that the breath hydrogen test remains negative after 6 months' treatment with metronidazole and clinically an apparent improvement in appetite was present. This effect may be attributable to lowering of the plasma propionate concentration, particularly in the portal vein. In sheep, infusion of propionate into the portal vein markedly inhibits feeding, an effect apparently mediated through hepatic receptors (Amil & Forbers, 1980), and it would implicate increased propionate concentrations as a cause of poor appetite in disorders of propionate metabolism.

While current studies underline the importance of bacterial propionate production in the gut in disorders of propionate metabolism, the optimal long-term therapeutic approach remains to be determined. A large study aimed at better delineation of the best approach to therapy with metronidazole in PA and MMA patients has recently been done and will be soon published (Thompson, in press).

NTBC

Treatment with a diet restricted in phenylalanine and tyrosine may prevent or alleviate the kidney damage, but does not prevent a fatal outcome in patients affected with tyrosinaemia type I. At present, liver transplantation is the only effective therapy but one of the major problems of follow-up studies of tyrosinaemia is predicting the moment at which hepatocellular carcinoma will develop and the time of the liver transplantation (Kvittingen, 1991). Today there are no reliable biochemical parameters able to predict the correct time. Recently Lindstedt et al. (1992) reported treating one acute and four subacute-chronic cases with 2-(2-nitro-4-trifluoro-methylbenzoyl)-1,3-cyclohexanedione (NTBC), a potent inhibitor of 4-hydroxylphenylpyruvate dioxygenase, to prevent the formation of maleylacetoacetate and fumarylacetoacetate and their saturated derivatives. The oral daily dose was 0.1–0.6 mg/kg and the biochemical data showed decreased excretion of succynilacetoacetate succynilactone and α-fetoprotein. Improved liver function was reflected by normal concentrations of prothrombin complex and in decreased activities of alkaline phosphatase and γ-glutamintransferase in serum. Computed tomography revealed regression of hepatic abnormalities in three patients. No side-effects were encountered.

A large trial, including more than 10 centres, is currently in progress to confirm if this type of treatment may thus offer an alternative to liver transplantation in hereditary tryosinaemia type I.

Gene therapy (organ transplant)

The ultimate goal of treatment of organic aciduria, as of many genetic diseases, is repair of the genetic defect, i.e. gene therapy. Recent advances in the technology of gene transfer, and in particular the use of modified viruses to carry genetic material, have turned what was previously a distant prospect into an immediate reality. There are currently more than 40 approved human gene therapy protocols, including for organic acidurias, with more being approved constantly (Levine & Friedman, 1993).

Liver transplantation has become a realistic alternative for the treatment of some organic acidurias such as tyrosinaemia type I. The question is whether we have to restrict this type of therapy to organic acidurias that are mainly or completely confined to the liver or whether we can extend it to those affecting not only the liver but other tissues as well. For example in propionic aciduria and methylmalonic aciduria the enzyme is ubiquitous, but the main site of production of the toxic compound is muscles while for the catabolism it is the liver. For this reason, patients who present with propionic or methylmalonic acidurias that are difficult to control with conventional therapy could benefit because a transplanted liver may well be able to clear all toxic metabolites.

At the moment little information is available (J.-M. Saudubray, personal observations) but this problem will be one of the main topics for the next future on treatment of organic acidurias.

References

Amil, M.M. & Forbers, J.M. (1980): Feeding in sheep during intraportal infusions of short-chain fatty acids and the effect of liver denervation. *J. Physiol.* **298,** 407–414.

Brain, M.D., Jones, M. & Borrielo, S.P. (1988): Contribution of gut bacterial metabolism to human metabolic disease. *Lancet* **i,** 1078–1079.

Burlina, A.B. (1986): The role of urinary organic acid analysis in the detection and management of inherited metabolic diseases. *Riv. Ital. Ped. (IJP)* **12,** 541–551.

Burlina, A.B., Bordugo, A., Da Dalt, L., Zacchello, F., Shenwood, G. & Bennett, M. (1993): Pancreatitis in propionic acidemia. *Ped. Res.* **33,** 190A.

De Raeve, L., De Meirler, L., Ranet, J., Vandenplas, Y. & Gerlo, E. (1994): Acreodermatitis enteropathic-like cutaneous lesions in organic aciduria. *J. Pediatr.* **124,** 416–420.

Dixon, M.A. & Leonard, J.V. (1992): Intercurrent illness in inborn errors of intermediary metabolism. *Arch. Dis. Child.* **67,** 1387–1391.

Duran, M., Dorland, L., Bruineis, L., Ketting, D. & Von Spong, F.J. (1991): Organic aciduria. In: *Inborn errors of metabolism*, eds. J. Schaub, F. Von Hoof & M. Vis, pp. 93–108, Nestlé Nutrition. New York: Raven Press.

European Metabolic Group (1994): *Monitoring of treatment of inborn errors of metabolism*, meeting, Lausanne, 1992. Milupa Scientific AG, Friedrichsdorf.

Kvittingen, E.A. (1991): Tyrosinemia type I – an update: *J. Inherit. Metab. Dis.* **14,** 554–562.

Leonard, J.V. & Daish, P. (1985): Evaluation of cofactor responsiveness. *J. Inherit. Metab. Dis.* **8,** (Suppl.), 17–19.

Levine, F. & Friedmann, T. (1993): Gene therapy. *Am. J. Dis. Child.* **147,** 1167–1171.

Lindstedt, S., Holme, E., Lock, E., Hjalmarson, O. & Strandvi, K. (1992): Treatment of hereditary tyrosinaemia type I by inhibition of 4-hydroxyphenylpyruvate dioxygenase. *Lancet* **310,** 813–815.

Massaud, A.F. & Leonard, J.V. (1993): Cardiomyopathy in propionic acidemia. *Eur. J. Pediatr.* **152,** 441–445.

Nyhan, W.L. (1991): Classic approaches to the treatment of inherited metabolic disease. In: *Therapy for genetic disease*, ed. T. Friedmann, pp. 2–33. New York: Oxford University Press.

Nyhan, W.L., Riu-Asaro, M. & Acosta, P. (1991): Advances in treatment of amino acid and organic acid disorders. In: *Treatment of genetic diseases*, ed. R.J. Desnick, pp. 30–43. New York: Churchill Livingstone.

Ogier, H., Charpantier, C. & Saudubray, J.M. (1990): Organic acidemias. In: *Inborn metabolic diseases*, eds. J. Fernandes, J.M. Saudubray & K. Tada, pp. 271–299. Berlin: Springer.

Poggi, F., Depondt, E. & Saudubray, J.M. (1993): Nutrition et maladies héréditaires. In: *Traité de nutrition pédiatrique*, eds. C. Ricour, J. Ghisolfi, G. Putet & O. Goulet, pp. 779–828. Paris: Maloine.

Queen, P.M., Fernhoff, P.M. & Acosta, P.B. (1981): Protein and essential amino acid requirements in a child with propionic acidemia. *J. Am. Diet. Assoc.* **79,** 562–565.

Roe, C., Millington, D., Kahler Kodo, N. & Norwood, J. (1991): Carnitine and organic acidurias. In: *Inborn errors of metabolism*, eds. J. Schaub, F. Van Hoof & H. Vis, pp. 57–70. Nestlé Nutrition, New York: Raven Press.

Sweetman, L. (1991): Cofactor replacement. In: *Therapy for genetic disease*, ed. T. Friedmann, pp. 34–61. New York: Oxford University Press.

Thompson, G.N., Choluvers, R.A., Walter, J.M., Bresson, J.L., Lyonnet, S.L., Reld, P.J., Saudubray, J.M., Leonard, J.V. & Hallidat, D. (1990): The use of metronidazole in management of methylmalonic and propionic acidemias. *Eur. J. Pediatr.* **149,** 792–796.

Walter, J.M., Leonard, J.V., Thompson, G.N., Holliday, D. & Barlet, T. (1988): Propionate production from the gut in propionic acidemia. *Lancet* **ii,** 226.

Winter, S.C., Hugh Vance, W., Zorn, M.E. & Vance, C.K. (1992): Carnitine deficiency in paediatrics: experience at Vally Children's Hospital. In: *L-Carnitine*, eds R. Ferrari, S. Di Mauro & G. Sherwood, pp. 209–222. London: Academic Press.

Wolf, B. & Heard, G.S. (1990): Biotinidase deficiency. *Adv. Hum. Genet.* **18,** 1–21.

Chapter 11

Lysosomal storage diseases

Rosanna Gatti

Third Paediatric Division, Istituto Giannina Gaslini, Largo G. Gaslini 5, 16147 Genova, Italy

Summary

The classic definition of lysosomal storage disease – the abnormal deposit of substrate within vacuoles related to lysosomes resulting from the deficiency of a specific lysosomal enzyme – can be modified to include a deficiency of proteins necessary for lysosomal function, such as protective and activator proteins. Lysosomal diseases without lysosomal enzyme deficiency also result from genetic disorders of lysosomal transport. Cystinosis, sialic acid storage disease, Niemann–Pick disease type C and cobalamin F mutation are currently classified as lysosomal membrane transport defects. The lysosomal storage diseases are probably far commoner than we realize and an overall incidence of not less than 1:5000 newborns is reported.

Because of an extensive heterogeneity, the enzymatic diagnosis must be associated with the evidence of lysosomal, storage. On the other hand, significant evidence of lysosomal storage but none of enzyme deficiency needs chemical analysis of biological fluids and/or biopsy tissue. A comprehensive approach is useful because it helps one to remember the range of diagnostic possibilities and it will aid in identifying specific diseases.

The relationship between genotypes and phenotypes provided by molecular analyses is of major clinical and therapeutic importance as exemplified by Gaucher's disease and metachromatic leucodystrophy.

Treatment of lysosomal storage diseases with bone marrow transplantation (BMT) is cautious and data prospective study will provide more specific recommendations for the future. Successful BMT results appear to be essential for somatic gene therapy by autologous engineered haematopoietic stem cells infusion.

Introduction

In the past, lysosomal storage diseases were considered only as rare and academic diseases. Increasing clinical awareness and improved diagnostic techniques have led to an ever-increasing number of patients diagnosed with them. With the exception of some ethnic groups, no reliable data are available concerning the incidence of each of the inherited lysosomal diseases, but overall incidence is probably not less than 1:5000 newborns.

The increasing interest shown in these disorders by basic and clinical scientists results from their contribution to the knowledge of lysosomal biology and the strong feeling that treatment is now part of the clinical scene.

Definition and classification

The demonstration of lysosomal accumulation of glycogen as the result of α-glucosidase deficiency and data from other disorders led Hers (1963) to define an inborn lysosomal disease as one in which a single lysosomal enzyme is deficient and abnormal deposits of the natural substrate for that enzyme are present within vacuoles related to lysosomes. The original concept of single lysosomal enzyme deficiency–lysosomal substrate storage has been modified owing to progress in the knowledge of the biology of lysosomes.

The lysosomal enzymes are glycoproteins which are synthesized in ribosomes bound to the endoplasmic reticulum. The initial product of protein synthesis undergoes extensive modifications including the acquisition of oligosaccharide chains and the introduction in some of these of mannose-6-phosphate (Man-6-P), the marker for the lysosomal destination. Within the lysosomes newly synthesized acid hydrolases undergo a maturational process that involves one or more proteolytic cleavage steps.

Recent studies have provided evidence that non-enzymic proteins with protective or activator functions are required for the activity of some lysosomal enzymes. A 32-kDa protective protein is necessary to protect β-galactosidase and neuraminidase against intralysosomal proteolytic degradation (D'Azzo et al., 1982). Sphingolipid activator proteins (SAP) or saposins are cofactors which cooperate in sphingolipid catabolism with sphingolipid-degrading hydrolases (Table 1).

Table 1. SAP (sphingolipid activator proteins) or saposins

Nomenclature	Prevalent enzyme/substrate specificities
SAP A	
SAP B (SAP-1)	Sulphatide
SAP C (SAP-2)	β-Glucosidase and glucosylceramide
SAP D (SAP-3, SAP hex)	GM_2 ganglioside and β-hexosaminidase A

Furst & Sandhoff (1992) and Kishimoto et al. (1992) have demonstrated that the four saposins derive from a single precursor protein (prosaposin) which is processed to four peptides. The specificities of the SAP types are quite different; the GM_2 ganglioside activator (SAP-3) is highly specific for this ganglioside and β-hexosaminidase A, whereas the others have broader enzyme/substrate specificities.

An inborn lysosomal disease can result not only from mutations within the gene encoding specific acid hydrolases but also from mutations affecting the genes that code other proteins necessary for lysosomal function.

In mucolipidosis II and III, the primary defect of the phosphotransferase that equips the acid hydrolases with mannose-6-P markers for their delivery to lysosomes results in deficiency in many acid hydrolases.

Mutations outside the structural genes for the enzyme resulting in multiple lysosomal deficiency were demonstrated in galactosialidosis and suggested in multiple sulphatase deficiency. The patients with galactosialidosis have a severe deficiency of the 32-kDa protein that gives rise to a secondary deficiency of β-galactosidase and neuraminidase (Shimmoto et al., 1990).

A deficiency of SAPs has been identified in patients with GM_2 gangliosidosis (Conzelman & Sandhoff, 1987), metachromatic leucodystrophy (MLD)(Schlote et al., 1991), Gaucher's disease (Schnabel et al., 1991) and combined sphingolipidosis which could not be accounted for by a loss of enzyme activity (Harzer et al., 1989).

The other group of lysosomal storage diseases without lysosomal enzyme deficiency is that of inborn errors of lysosomal membrane transport. Four inherited diseases are currently classified as lysosomal membrane transport defects: cystinosis, sialic acid storage disease (SASD), Niemann–Pick disease type C and cobalamin F mutation. Among these only cystinosis and SASD have been directly demonstrated to be monogenic disorders caused by a primary defect of a lysosomal carrier (Gahl et al., 1989; Mancini et al., 1991).

The evidence that Niemann–Pick disease type C represents a lysosomal transport defect is still indirect. Several lines of evidence indicate that cholesterol derived from lysosomal degradation of low-density lipoproteins is not available for esterification in the endoplasmic reticulum. Therefore the metabolic defect could reside in a blockage of transport of cholesterol from the lysosome to the endoplasmic reticulum/Golgi apparatus (Vanier et al., 1991; Roff et al., 1991).

The cobalamin F mutation is one of the complementation group found in genetic defects of Vitamin B_{12} metabolism. The intralysosomal accumulation of cyanocobalamin in cultured fibroblasts of patients suggests the absence of a putative cobalamin membrane transporter to transfer cobalamin from the lysosomes to the cytosol (Vassiliadis et al., 1991). This leads to cellular deficiency of the active coenzymes methylcobalamin and adenocobalamin. There are two other congenital disorders, a subtype of glycogenosis type II (Ullrich et al., 1989) and lipofuscinosis (Hall et al., 1991) which are lysosomal disorders with a possible involvement of membrane component.

Currently lysosomal storage diseases are classified according to the prevalently accumulated substrate into three broad groups: the sphingolipidoses, the mucopolysaccaridoses and the glycoproteinoses. The disorders of glycoprotein degradation resulting in the accumulation and urinary excretion of oligosaccharides and glycopeptides are more usually called oligosaccharidoses (Cantz & Ullrich-Bott, 1990). During the past few years two new genetic defects in the enzymes cleaving the oligosaccharide chain of glycoproteins have been described: β-mannosidase (Dorland et al., 1988) and α-N-acetylgalactosaminidase (Schindler et al., 1989). Mucolipidosis is a term restricted to mucolipidosis II, III and IV that present clinical and/or biochemical features of mucopolysaccharidoses and sphingolipidoses. Glycogenosis II and acid lipase deficiency are separate lysosomal storage diseases because of the different nature of the accumulated substrate.

Diagnosis

A lysosomal storage disease is normally suspected on the basis of progressive neurological dysfunction, visceromegaly, skeletal dysostosis or other more specific findings such as coarse facies, pulmonary infiltrates, angiokeratoma etc. Any approach to diagnosis relies to some degree on experience and intuition. Some patients can be diagnosed with reasonable accuracy on the basis of history and physical examination alone. In adults the diagnosis of lysosomal storage disease is difficult, in the face of insidious, slowly progressive neurological and psychiatric symptoms.

Preliminary diagnostic studies in patients potentially affected by lysosomal storage disease should include examination of a peripheral blood smear for vacuolated or granulated leucocytes, urinary screening for mucopolysaccharidoses and oligosaccharidoses, a radiological bone survey and neurophysiological studies. On the grounds of the above information it is possible to select specific enzyme assays in serum, leucocytes or cultured fibroblasts. The widespread use of synthetic substrates for measuring lysosomal enzyme activities has facilitated but also somehow complicated the diagnosis of lysosomal diseases. These substrates can measure enzyme-related activities toward different substrates. But then, β-galactosidase activity with an artificial substrate may represent the sum of different β-galactosidases encoded by different structural genes and having different substrate specificities. Moreover the mutant enzyme can hydrolyze the artificial substrate and not the natural substrate, as exemplified by the GM_2 gangliosidosis B_1 variant (Suzuki & Vanier, 1991), or vice versa. The condition of normal individuals found to have lysosomal enzyme deficiency using artificial substrates is named 'pseudodeficiency', and is known for β-hexosaminidase (Navon et al., 1973), α-galactosidase A (Bach et al., 1982), α-glucosidase (Nishimoto et al., 1988), arylsulphatase A and galactocerebrosidase (Wenger & Louie, 1991). These phenomena have considerable significance for the diagnosis of affected patients, heterozygote screening and prenatal diagnosis. They indicate the need to associate artificial-substrate enzyme assays with other chemical and/or morphological evidence of lysosomal storage or its absence.

Heterogeneity

There is considerable phenotypic and genotypic heterogeneity in lysosomal storage diseases. The variability in time course and in symptomatology is related to different allelic or non-allelic mutations in loci controlling the activity of acid hydrolases. Usually the phenotypes are classified as infantile, late infantile, juvenile and adult with reference to the course, and severe or mild and neuronopathic or non-neuronopathic with reference to the symptoms. There are nevertheless many patients who appear aberrant or intermediate compared with the classical phenotypes. On account of the recessive nature of most of the lysosomal diseases and of the possibility of different mutations, these patients are compound heterozygotes rather that true homozygotes in the strict sense. The combination of different alleles can explain the large variability in severity and in combinations of visceral, ocular, neurological and other manifestations.

Different primary defects at the DNA levels explain the observed phenotypic variability but they are not sufficient to understand which factors determine the course and the symptoms of the diseases. For GM_2 gangliosidosis and MLD, Conzelman & Sandhoff (1991) proposed a simple kinetic model to correlate onset, progression and severity with residual enzyme activity. A total lack of enzyme blocks the catabolism of the substrate which accumulates, giving rise to a rapidly progressive early-onset form. Some residual activity is sufficient to degrade most of the substrate, giving rise to slower accumulation which is responsible for less severe forms with late onset and slow evolution.

Different gene defects can underlie a homogeneous clinical entity as is shown by MPS III A, B, C and D which are very similar disorders caused by different enzyme deficiencies involved in heparan sulphate degradation.

Molecular analysis

Many of the lysosomal genes have been cloned. Molecular diagnosis is likely to correlate the phenotype with specific homozygous or compound heterozygous genotypes and to supplement enzymatic diagnosis in some circumstances such as prenatal diagnosis, heterozygous detection and pseudodeficiency.

Genotype–phenotype correlations have relevant implications for prognosis and treatment as exemplified by Gaucher's disease and MLD.

Gaucher's disease has been traditionally divided into three clinical forms: type 1, non-neuronopathic, the most common form with a high prevalence in Ashkenazi Jews; types 2 and 3, neuronopathic, without ethnic prevalence and distinguished by differing life expectancies, longer in type 3. Most Gaucher patients suffer from mutations within the glucocerebrosidase gene while only a few have saposin-C deficiency. To date 36 different acid-β-glucosidase disease mutations have been identified (Horowitz & Zimran, 1994). Four mutations (N370S, 84GG, IVS2(1+), L444P or NciI) account for 94–97 per cent of the disease mutations in Ashkenazi Jews. In the non-Jewish population, N370S and NciI mutations account for 65–75 per cent of the mutations, the 84GG mutation was not found and rarer mutations appear. A review of molecular diagnostic informations reveals a clear relationship between genotypes and phenotypes. Type 1 patients had at least one allele carrying the N370S mutation. Most patients homozygous for this mutation were mildly affected. Patients with the genotype N370S/NciI, N370S/recNciI developed moderate to severe type 1 disease and patients with the genotype N370S/? had a disease whose severity depended on the nature of the unknown allele.

NciI homozygosity was found only in neuronopathic types 2 and 3. In the more severely affected patients, classified as type 2, the allele carrying the NciI mutation was frequently associated with an allele carrying rare or unknown mutations.

The distribution of genotypes among the different phenotypes of 42 Gaucher patients that we examined is illustrated in Table 2.

Table 2. Prevalence of genotypes according to clinical types among 42 Gaucher patients

Clinical type	Genotype									Total
	370/?	370/370	370/NciI	370/IVS10⁻¹GA	NciI/?	NciI/IVS10⁻¹GA	NciI/NciI	370/recNciI	?/?	
I	10	2	8	1	1			3	1	26
II					4	1			2	7
III							8		1	9
Total	10	2	8	1	5	1	8	3	4	42
%	23.8	4.76	19.04	2.38	11.90	2.38	19.04	7.14	9.52	100.0

A heterozygosity of a novel splicing abnormality only reported previously in a Japanese patient (Ohshima et al., 1993) was demonstrated in two of our patients. The patient with the genotype N370S/IVS10⁻¹GA had a moderate type 1 disease while the patient with the genotype NciI/IVS10⁻¹GA had a severe lethal type 2 variant.

Based on genotypic analyses, persons with Gaucher's disease and parents at risk for this disease can then be informed about appropriate therapy and reproductive decisions.

A clear correlation was demonstrated between the arylsulphatase A (ARSA) genotype and the clinical phenotype. Allelic mutations at the ARSA locus cause deficiencies of this lysosomal enzyme whose clinical outcome is different forms of MLD or, more frequently, the so-called 'pseudodeficiency' (PD) which has no apparent clinical consequence.

Polten et al. (1991) have identified two alleles termed allele I and A that account for about half of all ARSA alleles in patients with MLD. The heterozygosity of allele I is associated with no residual ARSA activity and predisposes for the severe late infantile form. Allele A encodes for an unstable but active ARSA. One copy of allele A produces the juvenile form and two copies allow the mildest adult type of MLD. Patients with juvenile and adult forms should be better candidates for bone marrow transplantation than those with the late infantile form because they have a residual ARSA activity.

ARSA pseudodeficiency is caused by homozygosity for the PD allele that encodes for a reduced and structurally altered ARSA activity but sufficient for normal sulphatide catabolism *in vivo* (Gieselman et al., 1989). The frequency of the PD gene is about 7–15 per cent in the general population predicting that 0.5–2 per cent will have low ARSA activity. Also compound heterozygotes for MLD and PD have low ARSA activity. Because PD is so frequent and because enzymatic analysis cannot distinguish between MLD and PD it is not unusual that patients who are PD homozygotes and MLD/PD compound heterozygotes with neurological symptoms of unknown origin are misdiagnosed as suffering from MLD (Penzien et al., 1993). Genotype molecular analysis is obligatory for reliability of the diagnosis and genetic counselling (Li et al., 1992). The existence of mutations in the PD allele causing MLD (Gieselman et al., 1991) and of PD allele variants (Shen et al., 1993) gives rise to complex genotypes that need critical evaluation of the molecular techniques used. Sequence analysis of the ARSA gene in a PD heterozygote individual shows the normal allele and the PD allele with the A1620G transition (Fig. 1).

After the diagnosis

Once the diagnosis of lysosomal storage disease has been confirmed, what can be done? Counselling is undertaken to assist the parents in planning for the child and in future family planning. The

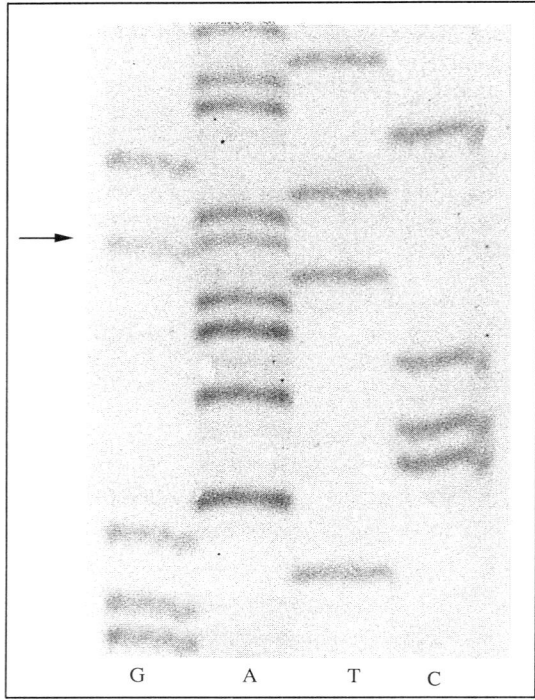

Fig. 1. Sequencing gel of the ARSA cDNA showing the normal allele and the pseudodeficiency (pd) with the A1620G transition.

most common questions, i.e. what is the course of the disease? how is the disease treatable? do not have a simple answer. The considerable heterogeneity of any of the lysosomal storage diseases is an obstacle to correctly informating the parents on these points. It is to be hoped that prognostic DNA testing, as is now being done for Gaucher's disease and MLD, will be available within a very short time for the other diseases. Nevertheless it is imperative that parents be told the probable course of the disease, the present status of therapeutic approaches and prevention through carrier screening and prenatal diagnosis.

Those physicians who have great experience in lysosomal diseases are the most qualified to use their knowledge for counselling parents. Pilot parent groups or simply other parents with children with similar disorders are often far more supportive.

Most of the lysosomal disorders are autosomal recessive. The frequency of the carrier state for these diseases in the general population is very low; however, relatives of an affected child are possible carriers and if there is a reliable test to detect them, they should be tested. In most instances the test's benefits are more psychological than effective in terms of disease prevention, but in families with a high degree of intermarriage and in families who have lived many generations in small villages, carrier detection in the extended family may indeed uncover other carrier couples. Detecting carriers should be not confined to families of affected children only in those diseases, such as Tay–Sachs disease and Gaucher's disease, with a high prevalence in ethnic groups.

Detecting carriers of Fabry's disease and Hunter's disease transmitted as X-linked or resulting from new mutations is difficult. For this reason all mothers and possible carrier females in the family are considered at risk for all pregnancies.

All lysosomal storage diseases can be diagnosed in the first or second trimester of fetal life by measuring enzymic activity on intact chorionic villi or cultured amniotic fluid cells, respectively. These techniques are highly reliable when done in a competent manner and no family with one affected child should be in fear of having another (Besley, 1992).

Owing to the advances in micromanipulation techniques and in DNA analysis of single cells, the preimplantation genetic diagnosis (PGD) will in the future be a reliable option for those couples who cannot accept prenatal diagnosis and the subsequent elective abortion of the affected fetus. The possibility of PGD for Tay–Sachs disease has been demonstrated by Verlinsky & Kuliev (1993).

The therapeutic approach to lysosomal diseases involves direct administration of the appropriate enzyme, transplantation of allografts capable of producing the normal gene product and gene replacement therapy. The limitations as well as the encouraging successes of these strategies have been the subject of recent reviews (Desnick, 1991; Hobbs & Riches, 1992).

The successes of β-glucosidase replacement in the non-neuronopathic type I Gaucher's disease have renewed the interest in this therapeutic strategy. The prerequisites for clinical application of enzyme supplementation may be summarized as follows: availability of adequate amounts of stable, sterile, human enzyme; absence of immunological complications; delivery of the enzyme to the major tissue and subcellular sites of pathology; appropriate serial biochemical and clinical methods to evaluate the efficacy of the treatment. The availability of an animal model of the lysosomal diseases could significantly contribute to perfecting enzyme therapy. Problems and actual experience with enzyme replacement therapy in Gaucher's disease are discussed in Chapter 12 of this volume.

The rationale for the use of bone marrow transplantation to treat lysosomal storage diseases is directly derived from the *in vitro* experiment of the clearing of abnormal lysosomes, when fibroblasts from a lysosomal disease are grown with normal fibroblasts (Neufeld & Cantz, 1971).

The bone marrow haematopoietic stem cell proliferation provides a normal donor set of macrophages, lymphocytes and monocytes that spreads into the reticuloendothelial system of the recipient. Macrophages from the donor's bone marrow invade the patient's brain parenchyma by diapedesis through the capillaries and become microglial cells. The cross-correction observed *in vitro* was confirmed *in vivo* by a decreased substrate concentration as measured biochemically and morphologically (Shull *et al.*, 1987; Hoogebrugge *et al.*, 1988).

Experimental data and clinical observations demonstrate that the clearance of accumulated substrate in the central nervous system is late, suggesting that the penetration of circulating monocytes in the central nervous system is slow.

There are contrasting opinions on the efficacy of bone marrow transplantation in lysosomal storage diseases. This dichotomy originates from the absence of homogeneous criteria of indication, limitations and long-term evaluation. On the one hand, bone marrow transplantation is considered with skepticism because of the considerable risk and high cost and there are expectations of enzyme replacement therapy. On the other, bone marrow transplantation has support from those who note that it is and will be the only readily available method of treatment for the next years. A consortium of 20 centres at which these transplantations have been done in the United States and Canada began a strict comparison of transplant and non-transplant patients whose results will indicate the most appropriate recommendations for the future care of these patients (Desnick, 1991).

At this moment it appears justified to limit bone marrow transplantation to asymptomatic patients or to subjects with mild neurological symptoms in the presence of histocompatible matches. The concept that enzyme replacement in the brain requires several months after full engraftment, contraindicates bone marrow transplantation in infantile neurological diseases. By contrast, juvenile and adult forms should be considered for bone marrow transplantation because the slow rate of disease progression offers a sufficient time for haematopoietic cells to enter the central nervous system and prevent or arrest the deterioration (Desnick, 1991).

Lysosomal storage diseases for which bone marrow transplantation has proved therapeutic are potential candidates for gene therapy. The introduction of a wild-type form of the specific enzyme gene into autologus haematopoietic stem cells and the infusion of these engineered cells into patients is an attractive prospect for treatment. Moullier *et al.* (1993) have demonstrated correction of mucopolysaccharide storage in the viscera of mice with deficiency of β-glucuronidase by implantation of genetically modified autologous fibroblasts. The correction of lysosomal enzyme deficiencies by retroviral-gene transfer has so far been reported for β-glucocerebrosidase deficiency (Ohashi *et al.*, 1992; Correl *et al.*, 1992), arylsulphatase B deficiency (Peters *et al.*, 1991) and arylsulphatase A deficiency (Rommerskirch *et al.*, 1991). If these studies prove safe and effective, the next step will be the transplantation of the patient's genetically modified bone marrow stem cells.

Conclusions

Our knowledge of lysosomal storage diseases has progressed from the diagnosis of single lysosomal enzyme deficiency to lysosomal diseases in absence of a lysosomal enzyme deficiency. Now we know of protective and activator proteins, multiple lysosomal enzyme deficiency and lysosomal transport disorders. In the last decade a large number of transporters has been characterized in the lysosomal membrane for the transport of amino acids, sugars, nucleosides, inorganic ions, vitamins and other miscellaneous compounds. Congenital defective transports for cystine, sialic acid and vitamin B_{12} have been detected. The clinical pictures of these transports disorders are quite polymorphic. Histological evidence of lysosomal storage is lacking cobalamin F mutation and typical features of most lysosomal storage diseases, such as visceromegaly or skeletal dysostosis, are absent in cystinosis and cobalamin F mutation. It seems, in general, that detectable lysosomal storage can be expected when the metabolite is produced in the lysosome at a relatively high rate and/or it represents a structural component rather than trace components like a vitamin or a hormone.

The emerging group of inborn errors of lysosomal transport has contributed to the understanding of how the lysosomes actively participate in complex subcellular mechanisms. Their role is not restricted to the catabolism of a wide variety of macromolecules but is essential for the fate of the products of catabolism. According to this extensive definition of lysosomal function, new lysosomal transport defects are predictable in hitherto unexplained genetic disorders, with or without evidence of lysosomal storage. The therapeutic role of thiols in cystinosis opens more hopeful therapeutical possibilities for lysosomal transport defects than for lysosomal disease caused by enzyme deficiencies.

Acknowledgements

The author thanks Miss Stefania Cabras for secretarial assistance. Molecular analyses in patients with Gaucher's disease and metachromatic leucodystrophy were supported by Telethon Grants A.25 and C.02 /1993.

References

Bach, G., Rosenmann, E., Karnic, A. & Cohen, T. (1982): Pseudodeficiency of alpha-galactosidase A. *Clin. Genet.* **221**, 59–64.

Besley, G.T.N. (1992): Enzyme analysis. In: *Prenatal diagnosis and screening*, eds. D.J.H. Brock, C.H. Rodeck & M.A. Ferguson-Smith, pp 127–145. Edinburgh: Churchill Livingstone.

Cantz, M. & Ullrich-Bott, B. (1990): Disorders of glycoprotein degradation. *J. Inherit. Metab. Dis.* **13**, 523–537.

Conzelmann, E. & Sandhoff, K. (1978): AB variant of infantile GM2 gangliosidosis: deficiency of a factor necessary for stimulation of hexosaminadase A-catalyzed degradation of ganglioside GM2 and glycolipid GA2. *Proc. Natl. Acad. Sci. USA* **75**, 3979–3983.

Conzelmann, E. & Sandhoff, K. (1991): Biochemical basis of late onset neurolipidoses. *Dev. Neurosci.* **132**, 197–204.

Correll, P.H., Colilla, S., Dave, M.P.G. & Karlsson, S. (1992): High levels of human alpha-glucocerebrosidase activity in macrophages of long-term reconstituted mice after retroviral infection of hematopoietic stem cells. *Blood* **80**, 331–336.

D'Azzo, A., Hoogeveen, A.T., Reuser, A.J.J., Robinson, D. & Galjaard, H. (1982): Molecular defect in combined β-galactosidase and neuraminidase deficiency in man. *Proc. Natl. Acad. Sci. USA* **79**, 4535–4539.

Desnick, R.J. (1991): *Treatment of genetic diseases*. New York: Churchill Livingstone.

Dorland, L., Duran, M., Hoefnagels, F.E.T., Breg, J.N., Fabery de Jonge, H., Cransberg, K., van Sprang, F.J. & van Diggelen, O.P. (1988): β-Mannosidase in two brothers with hearing loss. *J. Inherit. Metab. Dis.* **11**(Suppl. 2), 255–258.

Furst, W. & Sandhoff, K. (1992): Activator proteins and topology of lysosomal sphingolipid catabolism. *Biochem. Biophys. Acta* **1126**, 1–16.

Gahl, W.A., Renlund, M. & Thoene, J.G. (1989): Lysosomal transport disorders: cystinosis and sialic acid storage disorders. In: *The metabolic basis of inherited disease*, eds. C.R. Scriver, A.L. Beaudet, W.S. Sly & D. Valle, pp. 2619–2680. New York: McGraw-Hill.

Gieselman, V., Polten, A., Kreysing, J. & von Figura, K. (1989): Arylsulphatase A pseudodeficiency: loss of polyadenylation signal and a *N*-glycosylation site. *Proc. Natl. Acad. Sci. USA* **86**, 9436–9440.

Gieselman, V., Fluharty, A.L., Tønnesen, T. & von Figura, K. (1991): Mutations in the arylsulphatase A pseudodeficiency allele causing metachromatic leucodystrophy. *Am. J. Hum. Genet.* **49,** 407–413.

Hall, N.A., Lake, B.D., Dewji, N.N. & Patrick, A.D. (1991): Lysosomal storage of subunit c of mitochondrial ATP synthase in Batten's disease (ceroidolipofuscinosis). *Biochem. J.* **275,** 269–272.

Harzer, K., Paton, B.C., Poulos, A., Kustermann-Kuhn, B., Roggendorf, W., Grisar, T. & Popp, M. (1989): Sphingolipid activator protein deficiency in a 16-week-old atypical Gaucher disease patient and his fetal sibling: biochemical signs of combined sphingolipidoses. *Eur. J. Pediatr.* **149,** 31–39.

Hers, H.G. (1963): Alpha-glucosidase deficiency in generalized glycogen storage disease (Pompe's disease). *Biochem. J.* **86,** 11–16.

Hobbs, J.R. & Riches, P.S. (1992): *Correction of certain genetic diseases by transplantation.* Cogent II. London: Westminster Medical School.

Hoogebrugge, P.M., Poorthius, B.J.H.M., Romme, Ad.E., van de Kamp, J.J.P., Waggemaker, G. & van Bekkum, D.W. (1988): Effect of bone marrow transplantation on enzyme levels and clinical course in the neurologically affected witcher mouse. *J. Clin. Invest.* **81,** 1790–1794.

Horowitz, M. & Zimran, A. (1994): Mutations causing Gaucher disease. *Hum. Mut.* **3,** 1–11.

Kishimoto, Y., Hiraiwa, M. & O'Brien, J.S. (1992): Saposins: structure, function, distribution and molecular genetics. *J. Lipid Res.* **33,** 1255–1267.

Li, Z.G., Waye, J.S., Chang, P.L. et al. (1992): Diagnosis of arylsulphatase A deficiency. *Am. J. Med. Genet.* **43,** 976–982.

Mancini, G.N.S, Beerens, C.E.M.T., Aula, P.T. & Verheijen, F.W. (1991): A sialic acid storage diseases; multiple lysosomal transport defect for acidic monosaccharides. *J. Clin. Invest.* **87,** 1329–1335.

Moullier, P., Bohl, P., Heard, J.H. & Danos, O. (1993): Correction of lysosomal storage in liver and spleen of MPS VII mice by implantations of genetically modified fibroblasts. *Nature Genet.* **4,** 154–159.

Navon, R., Padch, B. & Adam, A. (1973): Apparent deficiency of hexosaminidase A in healthy members of a family with Tay–Sachs disease. *Am. J. Hum. Genet.* **25,** 287–293.

Neufeld, E.F. & Canzt, M.J. (1971): Connective factors for inborn errors of mucopolysaccharide metabolism. *Ann. NY Acad. Sci.* **179,** 580–587.

Nishimoto, J., Inui, K., Okada, S., Ishigami, W., Mirota S., Yamano, T. & Yabuuchi, H. (1988): A family with pseudodeficiency of acid alpha-glucosidase. *Clin. Genet.* **33,** 254–261.

Ohashi, T., Boggs, S., Robbins, P., Bahnson, A., Patrene, K., Wei, F.S., Wei, J.F., Li, J., Lucht, L., Fei, Y., Clark, S., Kimk, M., He, H., Mowery-Rushton, P. & Barranger, J.A. (1992): Efficient transfer and sustained high expression of the human glucocerebrosidase gene in mice and their functional macrophages following transplantation of bone marrow transduced by a retroviral vector. *Proc. Natl. Acad. Sci. USA* **89,** 11302–11336.

Ohshima, T., Sasaki, M., Matsuzaka, T. & Sakuragawa, N. (1993): A novel splicing abnormality in a Japanese patient with Gaucher's disease. *Hum. Mol. Genet.* **2,** 1497–1498.

Penzien, J.M., Kappler, J., Herschkowitz, N., Schuknecht, B., Leinekugel, P., Propping, P., Tønnesen, T., Lou, H., Moser, H., Zierz, S., Conzelmann, E. & Gieselmann, V. (1993): Compound heterozygosity for metachromatic leucodystrophy and arylsulfatase A pseudodeficiency alleles is not associated with progressive neurological disease. *Am. J. Hum. Genet.* **52,** 557–564.

Peters, C., Rommerskirch, W., Madoressi, S. & von Figura, K. (1991): Restoration of arylsulphatase B activity in human mucopolysaccharidosis-type-VI fibroblasts by retroviral-vector-mediated gene transfer. *Biochem. J.* **276,** 499–504.

Polten, A., Fluarthy, A.L., Fluarthy, C.B., Kappler, J, von Figura, K. & Gieselmann, V. (1991): Molecular basis of different forms of metachromatic leucodystrophy. *N. Engl. J. Med.* **324,** 18–22.

Roff, C.F., Goldin, E., Comly, M.E., Cooney, A., Brown, A., Vanier, M.T., Miller, S.P.F., Brady, R.S. & Pentchev, P.G. (1991): Type C Niemann–Pick disease: use of hydrophobic amines to study defective cholesterol transport. *Dev. Neurosci.* **13,** 315–319.

Rommerskirch, W., Fluarthy, A.L., Peters, C., von Figura, K. & Gieselman, V. (1991): Restoration of arylsulphatase A activity in human-metachromatic-leucodystrophy fibroblasts via retroviral-vector-mediated gene transfer. *Biochem. J.* **280,** 459–461.

Schindler, D., Bishop, D.F., Wolfe, D.E., Wang, A.M., Egge, H., Lemieux, R.U. & Desnick, R.J. (1989): Neuroaxonal dystrophy due to lysosomal α-N-acetylgalactosaminidase deficiency. *N. Engl. J. Med.* **320,** 1735–1740.

Schlote, W., Harzer, K., Christomanou, H., Paton, B.C., Kustermann-Kuhn, B., Schmid, B., Seeger, K., Beudt, U., Schuster, I. & Langenbeck, U. (1991): Sphingolipid activator protein 1 deficiency in metachromatic leucodystrophy with normal arylsulphatase A activity. A clinical, morphological, biochemical and immunologic storage. *Eur. J. Ped.* **150,** 584–591.

Schnabel, D., Schroder, M. & Sandhoff, K. (1991): Mutation in the sphingolipid activator protein 2 in a patient with a variant of Gaucher disease. *FEBS Lett.* **284,** 57–59.

Shen, N., Li, Z.G., Waye, J.S., Francis, G. & Chang, P.L. (1993): Complications in the genotypic molecular diagnosis of pseudo arylsulphatase A deficiency. *Am. J. Med. Genet.* **45,** 631–637.

Shimmoto, M., Takano, T., Fukuhara, Y., Oshima, A., Sakuraba, H. & Suzuki, Y. (1990): Japanese-type adult galactosialidosis: a unique and common splice junction mutations causing exon skipping in the protective protein/carboxypeptidase gene. *Proc. Jpn. Acad.* **668,** 217–222.

Shull, R.M., Hastings, N.E., Selcer, R.R., Jones, J.B., Smith, J.R., Cullen, W.C. & Costantopoulos, G. (1987): Bone marrow transplantation in canine mucopolysaccharidosis I: effects within the central nervous system. *J. Clin. Invest.* **79,** 435–443.

Suzuki, K. & Vanier, M.T. (1991): Biochemical and molecular aspects of late onset GM_2-gangliosidosis: B_1 variant as prototype. *Dev. Neurosci.* **13,** 288–294.

Ullrich, K., von Bassewitz, D., Shin, J., Korithenberg, R., Sewell, S. & von Figura, K. (1989): Lysosomal glycogen storage disease without deficiency of acid alpha-glucosidase. *Prog. Clin. Biol. Res.* **306,** 143–148.

Vanier, M.T., Pentchev, P., Rodriguez-Lafrasse, C. & Rousson, R. (1991): Niemann–Pick disease type C: an update. *J. Inherit. Metab. Dis.* **14,** 580–595.

Vassiliadis, A., Rosenblatt, D.S., Cooper, B.A. & Bergeron, J.J.M. (1991): Lysosomal cobalamin accumulation in fibroblasts from a patient with an inborn error of cobalamin metabolism (cbl F complementation group): visualization by electron microscopic radioautography. *Exp. Cell Res.* **195,** 295–302.

Verlinsky, Y. & Kuliev, A.M. (1993): Approaches to preimplantation genetic diagnosis. In: *Preimplantation diagnosis of genetic diseases*, eds. Y. Verlinsky & A.M. Kuliev, pp. 19–25. New York: Wiley–Liss.

Wenger, D.A. & Louie, E. (1991): Pseudodeficiencies of arylsulphatase A and galactocerebrosidase activities. *Dev. Neurosci.* **13,** 216–221.

Chapter 12

Enzyme replacement therapy for Gaucher's disease types 1, 2 and 3

Mario Carrozzi, Manuela Zanatta, Aldo Scabar and Bruno Bembi

Istituto per l'Infanzia IRCCS 'Burlo Garofolo', via dell'Istria 65/1, 34100 Trieste, Italy

Summary

Our experience in the treatment of Gaucher's disease with macrophage-targeted glucocerebrosidase is described. The analysis of the clinical data shows that the treatment is effective especially for non-neurological symptoms in Gaucher's disease types 1, 2 and 3.

Introduction

Gaucher's disease (GD) is the most frequent form of sphingolipidosis (Norman, 1970; Desnick, 1982; Barranger & Ginnis, 1989). This autosomic recessive disease may be due to:
- the absence of a lysosomal hydrolase (β-glucosidase);
- the absence of the enzyme's activator (Schnabel *et al.*, 1982);
- inefficient functioning of the enzyme.

Together these conditions result in an excessive intracellular storage of glycolipid glucocerebroside.

This heaped-up substance, resulting from the turnover of circulating erythrocytes and leucocytes, accumulates in the cells of the endothelial reticular system (ERS) or within the central nervous system (CNS) as in neurological forms. The incidence of the non-neurological form within populations of Caucasian origin is 1:50 000 newborns while the incidence in Ashkenazi Jews is 1:500–2000 newborns.

Three phenotypical forms of Gaucher disease are described:
- type 1: without neurological involvement;
- type 2: neurologically acute;
- type 3: neurologically subacute.

Clinical

Type 1

Gaucher's disease of the first type includes more than 80 per cent of the cases reported. Clinical symptomatology is characterized by splenomegaly (which generally precedes hepatomegaly), frequent haemorrhages, involvement of the bone structure with pain and typical deformity (Erlenmeyer flask-like deformity) and slowed growth. Laboratory examinations reveal pancytopenia, and involvement of the haemopoietic bone marrow; accumulation within the lung interstices, the lymphatic system and the kidney tissue is present (Barranger & Ginnis, 1989).

Type 2

Gaucher's disease of the second type was first described by Oberling and Woringer in 1927. It presents a rather stereotyped clinical picture, characterized by early and progressive neurological deterioration which leads to death within the first two years of life (Barranger & Ginnis, 1989). Its major clinical features are briefly summarized in Table 1.

Table 1. Gaucher's disease type 2: clinical features

	Gaucher's disease Type II
Age of onset	6–12 months
Neurological signs	Bulbar palsy with – head and neck hyperextension – dysphagia – trismus – strabismus – increased muscle tone – brisk stretch reflexes – positive Babinsky signs Epilepsy
Non-neurological signs	Splenomegaly Hypersplenism Hepatomegaly
Evolution	Death: – 90% in the first year – 10% in the second year

Type 3

The first description of type 3 Gaucher's disease was described by Hillborg in 1959. It affected a Swedish child from a small community in a town near the Arctic Circle. The clinical evolution is typically characterized by early onset in childhood with splenomegaly and later involvement of the central nervous system. This form is also known as the juvenile or subacute neuropathic form (Conradi *et al.*, 1984, 1991; Erikson, 1986).

Gaucher's disease type 3 has recently been divided in two subtypes: 3a and 3b (Brady *et al.*, 1993). The clinical findings in 3a patients include: myoclonic and generalized tonic–clonic seizures, horizontal supranuclear gaze palsy, spasticity, ataxia and dementia. The age of onset is during adolescence or childhood, and systemic involvement is not particulary severe. Progressive neurological deterioration leads to death after a variable length of time. The only neurological sign in patients with Gaucher's disease 3b is horizontal supranuclear gaze palsy, while systemic involvement is severe: important hepatomegaly, oesophageal varices and severe skeletal involvement. Death occurs from to hepatic or pulmonary complications.

A few considerations on neuropathology

The Gaucher cell is the marker of this disease even in the central nervous system (Norman, 1970; Barranger *et al.*, 1989). This cell derives from the histiocytes–monocytes, it is full of lipids and in the central nervous system it is typically organized in small clusters localized within the periadventitial spaces, within the Virchow–Robin spaces, or less frequently, as in the case of type 2 disease, it is found free within the ganglial and pyramidal layers of the cortex.

From a neuropathological viewpoint, the alterations characterized by loss of neurons and secondary gliosis may be: diffuse and non-selective or localized within the dentato-cerebellar, bulbar (as in the Type 2 of Gaucher's disease) and thalamo-cortical areas (Winkelmann *et al.*, 1983; Conradi *et al.*, 1984; Barranger *et al.*, 1989).

Regarding the mechanism which leads to neuron damage, intracellular accumulation has been shown in type 2 Gaucher's disease but data is not as convincing for type 3, where neuron damage mediated by a vascular insufficiency has been hypothesized (Brady *et al.*, 1993).

The ultimate cause, however, is still unknown. One hypothesis is a toxic effect of the lysophospholipids (in particular of the glucosylsphingosin) which may inhibit C protein kinase activity and disrupt cellular metabolism, as neuron lesions occur near G-cell clusters. Another hypothesis is that histiocytes may be unable to detoxify the surrounding microenvironment (Winkelmann *et al.*, 1983; Conradi *et al.*, 1984; Barranger *et al.*, 1989).

The glucocerebrosidase gene

Molecular biology studies have localized the gene on chromosome 1 (at band q 21), and have described the sequence of the structural gene and of the pseudogene (Levy *et al.*, 1991). The latter is situated 16 kDa from the structural gene. The mutations are generally point form, but insertions, deletions and recombinations between gene and pseudogene have also been found (Beutler, 1992).

The mutations found in Caucasians are different from those found in Ashkenazi Jews where four mutations account for 96 per cent of the mutated alleles. Table 2 compares the most prevalent types of mutation (with regard to the nucleotide positions in cellular cDNA) and their frequency in the two populations.

Table 2. Genetic mutations in Ashkenazi Jews and Caucasians

	Mutation	Frequency
Ashkenazi Jews	1226	75 %
	84GG	13 %
	1448	5 %
	ISV2+	3 %
Caucasians	1226	35 %
	1448	35 %
	Other mutations	25 %

Relation between genotype and clinical expression

Despite the difficulties presented by the number of mutations (about 30), Zimran *et al.* (1989) observed that:

— homozygosis 1448 is correlated with the most severe clinical form (types 2 and 3)

— heterozygosis 1226/1448 or 1226/other mutation is correlated with a clinical form of intermediate severity.

— homozygosis 1226/1226 is correlated with a mild Type 1 form.

Other combinations are correlated with rather severe clinical forms of the disease.

The study of the genome is of fundamental importance in the clinical definition of the disease. In one of our patients, the diagnosis of type 1 Gaucher's disease (without proven neurological symptomatology) had to be redefined as type 2 after the discovery of a 1448/1448 homozygosity. The EEG performed after this examination proved to be altered.

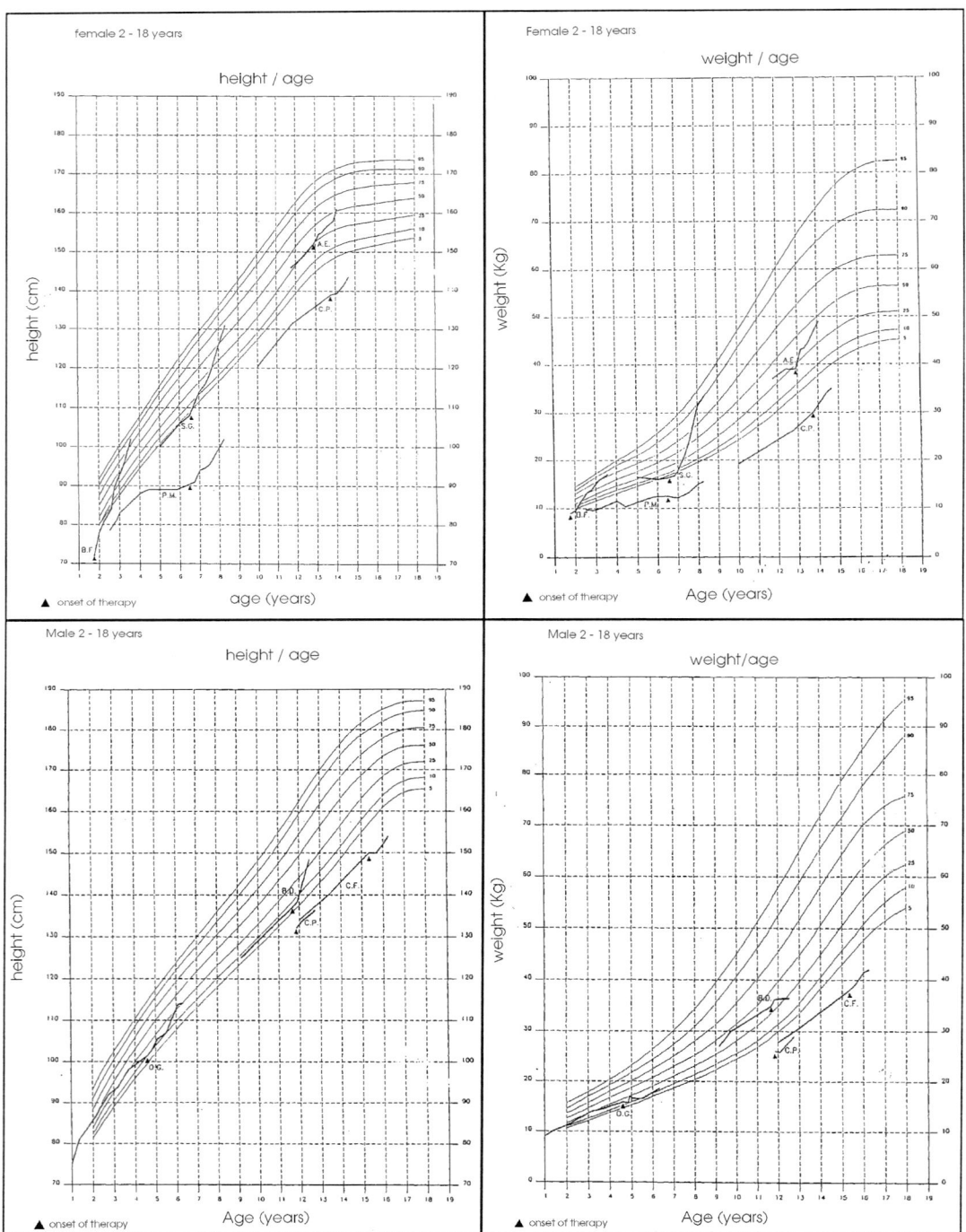

Fig. 1a–d. Growth and weight increase in male and female, before and after the onset (head of arrow) of substitutive therapy with macrophage-target glucocerebrosidase.

Substitutive enzymatic therapy

The enzyme is obtained from human placenta and can be separated by its hydrophobicity. In the 1980s the enzyme was purified but was of little effect, until it was realized that its functioning depends on the presence of a mannose residue (Brady & Barton, 1991). The modification is carried out when the residues preceding mannose are decomposed by three enzymes (deglycosylation). The enzyme thus modified (deglycosylate) enters the RES cells where it can function (Brady & Barton, 1991). As yet there is no evidence that the enzyme is able to bypass the blood–brain barrier (Brady et al., 1993).

Case studies

Table 3 shows patients who underwent substitution therapy. Hindered growth rate and hepatosplenomegaly were found in all the children; six patients were splenectomized and five showed involvement of the bone structure.

Table 3. Patients undergoing substitution therapy

	Children			Adults		
	Male	Female	Total	Male	Female	Total
Type 1	5	3	8	9	2	11
Type 2	2	–	2	–	–	–
Type 3	1	3	4	1	–	1

Therapeutic plan

High doses (70–120 U/kg/month) of enzyme infusion are given to paediatric patients with neurological involvement every week, while patients with type 1 Gaucher's disease receive 30–60 U/kg/month, every two weeks. Adult patients receive 30/U/kg/month without distinction to the type.

Results

Evolution of non-neurological symptoms

Clinical aspects

– increased growth (height and weight) (Figs. 1a–d);
– remarkable reduction of organomegaly especially of spleen (the reduction was less remarkable for liver) (Figs. 2 and 3);
– reduction of bone-structure symptomatology (disappearance of bone pains).

Laboratory examination

– normalization of haemoglobin level;
– increase of blood platelets;
– reduction of acid phosphatase and transaminase;
– proper bone reparation.

Evolution of neurological symptoms

Results for type 3 Gaucher's disease are shown in Table 4. The neurological signs, if present, modified only slightly. EEG findings were actually worse (Patient P.M. and B.F.); when faced with

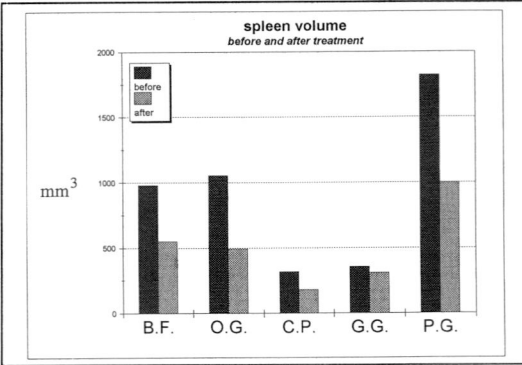

Fig. 2. Evolution of spleen volume before and after the onset of substitutive therapy with macrophage-target glucocerebrosidase.

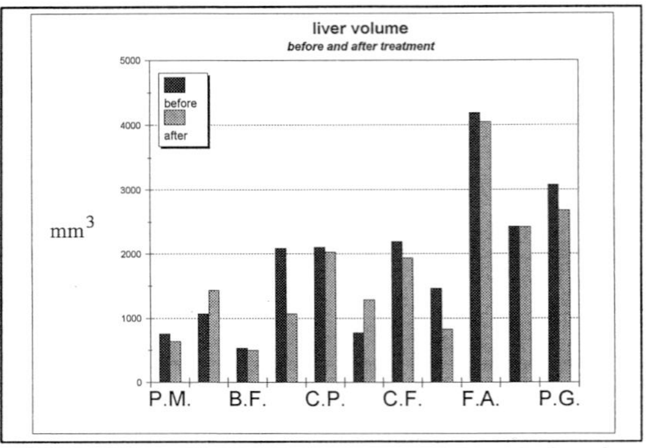

Fig. 3. Evolution of liver volume before and after the onset of substitutive therapy with macrophage-target glucocerebrosidase.

the necessity for pharmacological treatment (patient P.M.), the epilepsy responded to valproate. The major improvements were in behaviour: the patients became more sociable and active in their interactions, probably due to their better general health. Variations in the developmental quotients (IQ) probably reflect this aspect rather than an increase in cognitive abilities.

Table 4. Results and evolution in type 3 Gaucher's disease (all patients had genotype 1448/1448)

Patient	Sex	Age (years)	Onset of therapy (age)	Psychometric evaluations Terman-Merril Scale/WISC-R		Electroencephalographic findings
				Before	After	
P.M.	F	8	6+6/12	IQ = 30 IQ = 50	Slightly better (IQ = 40) IQ = 60	– Slowing of background activity – Right centrotemporal spikes – Generalized discharges of spikes and waves
S.G.	F	8+5/12	6+7/12	IQ = 79	NV	– Slowing of background activity – Left temporocentral spikes
B.F.	F	4	16m	IQ = 114	NV	– Bilateral asynchronous rolandic spikes

Patient	Sex	Age (years)	Onset of therapy (age)	Splenectomy	Neurological status	
					Before	After
P.M.	F	8	6+6/12	+	Spastic tetraparesis No autonomous walking Left 6th cranial nerve palsy Brisk stretch reflexes Poor social interaction	Reduction of hypertonus Began to walk NV NV Better social interaction
S.G.	F	8+5/12	6+7/12	+	Poor social interaction Slight dysmetria	Better social interaction NV
B.F.	F	4	16m	–	–	–

NV = no variation

Table 5. Results and evolution in type 2 Gaucher's disease

			Patient: A.V., 8 months					
Time	Substitutive therapy	Hb (g%)	M. tone	Lar. spasm	Trismus	Myoclonus	Seizure	EEG
0	100/2 days IV	10.4	Hypo++	±	No	±	No	Right posterior spikes in sleep
2	200/2 days IV	9.9	Hypo++	No	No	+	No	– Bilateral posterior spikes in wakefulness and sleep – No myoclonic epilepsy
4	400/4 days IV	10.5	Hypo+++	No	No	+++	Yes	– Slowing of background activity – Myoclonic epilepsy
6	Stop IV	8.4	Hypo+++	+	No	+++	Yes	– Slowing of background activity – Myoclonic epilepsy
			Patient: D.M., 7 months					
Time	Substitutive therapy	Hb (g%)	M. tone	Lar. spasm	Trismus	Myoclonus	Seizure	EEG
0	100/2 days IV	9.1	Hyper+++	+++	+++	No	No	– Slowing of background activity – Sporadic posterior sharp waves
2	200/2 days IV	11.1	Hyper+++	+++	+++	±	No	– Slowing of background activity – Generalized discharges of atypical sharp waves
4	600 weekly 40 IR	10.3	Hyper+++	+	+	±	Yes	– Slowing of background activity – Myoclonic epilepsy
6	600 weekly 10 IR	12.7	Hyper++	No	±	+	Yes	– Slowing of background activity – Myoclonic epilepsy

The results and evolution for type 2 disease are shown in Table 5. In patient D.M., drugs were given both systemically and intrarachidially. In January 1994, an intraventricular catheter was inserted and connected to a subcutaneous reservoir.

Conclusions

Treatment with deglycosylate enzyme has proved to be effective in Gaucher's disease types 1 and 3 especially for non-neurological symptoms. With respect to the neurologic symptoms, results are less comforting: their clinical progression may be slowed or arrested, but electrophysiological findings (EEG) suggest that despite treatment, the disease continues in its evolution.

Something else may be said about Type 2 disease which is invariably quickly fatal despite classic treatment, as in A.V.'s case.

The fact that D.M.'s symptoms were slowed, presumably by enzyme infusion into the cephalo-rachidian fluid, raises a few questions:

(a) does the enzyme pass the blood–brain barrier at all, or with difficulty?

(b) has this approach been effective in the treatment of Type 2 Gaucher's patients if begun before the appearance of neurologic symptoms?

(c) while new cures (for example genetic treatment) are awaited, may this type of enzyme treatment be considered a valid alternative?

(d) does the distress suffered by the patients and their families and the high cost justify the use of such an invasive treatment?

References

Barranger, J.A. & Ginnis, E.I. (1989): Glucosylceramide lipidoses: Gaucher disease. In: *The metabolic bases of inherited disease*, 6th edn, eds. C.R. Scriver, A.L. Beaudet, W.S. Sly & D. Valle, pp. 1677–1698. New York: McGraw-Hill.

Beutler, E. (1992): Gaucher disease: new molecular approaches to diagnosis and treatment. *Science* **256**, 794–799.

Brady, R.O. & Barton, N.W. (1991): Enzyme replacement therapy for type I Gaucher disease. In: *Treatment of genetic disease*, ed. R.J. Desnick, pp. 153–168. Edinburgh: Churchill Livingstone.

Brady, R.O., Barton, N.W. & Grabowsky, A. (1993): The role of neurogenetics in Gaucher disease. *Arch. Neurol.* **50**, 1212–1224.

Conradi, N.G., Sourander, P., Nilsson, O., Svennerholm, L. & Erikson, A. (1984): Neuropathology of the Norbottnian type of Gaucher's disease. *Acta Neuropathol.* **65**, 99–109.

Conradi, N., Kyllerman, M., Mansson, J.E., Percy, A.K. & Svennerholm, L. (1991): Late-infantile Gaucher disease in a child with myoclonus and bulbar signs: neuropathological and neurochemical findings. *Acta Neuropathol.* **82**, 152–157.

Erikson, A. (1986): Gaucher disease – Norbottnian type III – neuropediatric and neurobiological aspects of clinical patterns and treatment. *Acta Paediatr. Scand.* **326(Suppl.)**, 1–41.

Hillborg, P.O. (1959): Morbus Gaucher i Norbotten. *Nord Med.* **61**, 303.

Levy, H., Or, A., Eyal, N., Wilder, S., Widgerson, M., Kolodny, E.H., Zimran, A. & Horowitz, M. (1991): Molecular aspects of Gaucher disease. *Dev. Neurosci.* **13**, 352–362.

Norman, R.M. (1970): Gaucher's disease, In: *Handbook of clinical neurology*, Vol. 10, Ch. 21, eds. P.S. Winken & Bruyn, pp. 509–531. Amsterdam: North Holland Publishing.

Oberling, C. & Woringer, P. (1927): La maladie de Gaucher chez le nourisson. *Rev. Franc. de Pediat.* **3**, 475–532.

Resnick, R.J. (1982): Gaucher disease (1882–1982): centennial perspective on the most prevalent Jewish genetic disease. *Mt Sinai. J. Med.* **49,6**, 443–455.

Schnabel, D., Schröder, M. & Sandhoff, K. (1991): Mutation in the sphingolipid activator protein 2 in a patient with a variant of Gaucher disease. *Fed. Eur. Biochem. Soc.* **284**, 57–59.

Winkelmann, M.D., Banker, B.Q., Victor, M. & Moser, H.W. (1983): Non-infantile neuronopathic Gaucher's disease: a clinicopathologic study. *Neurology* **33**, 994–1008.

Zimran, A., Sorge, J., Gross, E., Kubitz, M., West, C. & Beutler, E. (1989): Prediction of severity of Gaucher's disease by identification of mutations at DNA level. *Lancet* **iv**, 349–352.

Chapter 13

Peroxisomal disorders: classification, diagnosis and treatment

Ruud B.H. Schutgens*, Peter G. Barth[†], Björn M. van Geel[†] and Ronald J.A. Wanders*

Divisions of Paediatric Clinical Biochemistry and [†]Neuropaediatrics, Department of Paediatrics, Emma Children's Hospital, Academic Medical Centre Amsterdam, Amsterdam, The Netherlands

Summary

At least 16 different genetic disorders resulting from a deficiency of one or more peroxisomal enzymes have been identified. Neurological involvement is found in 13. We describe the clinical and biochemical characteristics and present a tentative classification into three groups. In group I no functional peroxisomes, or only a limited number, are detectable in cells. This group is referred to as generalized peroxisome deficiency disorders. In group II peroxisomes are present in cells but the activities of multiple peroxisomal enzymes are deficient. In group III the biochemical defect is limited to a single enzyme defect. A remarkable phenotypic and genetic heterogeneity is found in most peroxisomal disorders. Recent developments in the clinical and biochemical diagnosis of peroxisomal disorders are presented and new options for therapy evaluated. We also discuss recent findings in molecular biological studies in different peroxisomal disorders.

Introduction

Peroxisomal disorders are genetic diseases resulting from a deficiency of one or more peroxisomal enzymes or from a defect at the level of one or more peroxisomal membrane proteins. In mammals, peroxisomes are organelles bounded by single membranes and containing catalase activity, a number of oxidase enzymes producing hydrogen peroxide and a variable set of about 40 other enzymes depending upon the species and the type of tissue. Peroxisomes do not contain DNA.

Peroxisomes are probably ubiquitous in animal cells, except mature erythrocytes. They are generally abundant in tissues active in lipid metabolism such as the liver, sebaceous glands and brown fat. In the nervous tissue of the rat they were found to be especially enriched in myelin-producing oligodendrocytes and most abundant in the oligodendrocyte processes adjacent to the growing myelin sheets (Holtzman, 1982; Adamo et al., 1986; Kamei et al., 1993).

Zellweger's (cerebro-hepato-renal) (ZS) syndrome is the prototype of the peroxisomal disorders. This multisystem disorder is characterized by embryofetopathy and regressive changes which continue into postnatal life.

At present we recognize at least 16 different peroxisomal disorders with neurological involvement in 13 (Table 1). A large genetic and phenotypic variability is found in most.

Table 1. Classification of peroxisomal disorders

Group I	Peroxisomes deficient, generalized loss of peroxisomal functions: – Cerebro-hepato-renal (Zellweger) syndrome; – Neonatal adrenoleucodystrophy (NALD); – Infantile Refsum disease; – Hyperpipecolic acidaemia.
Group II	Peroxisomes present, multiple loss of peroxisomal functions: – Rhizomelic chondrodysplasia punctata; – Zellweger-like syndrome.
Group III	Peroxisomes present, single loss of peroxisomal function: – X-linked adrenoleucodystrophy and variants; – Acyl-CoA oxidase deficiency (pseudo-NALD); – Bi(multi)-functional protein deficiency; – Peroxisomal thiolase deficiency (pseudo-Zellweger's syndrome); – Dihydroxyacetone phosphate acyltransferase deficiency; – Alkyl-dihydroxyacetone phosphate synthase deficiency; – Glutaryl-CoA oxidase deficiency; – Di- and trihydroxycholestanoic acidaemia; – Hyperoxaluria type I; – Mevalonate kinase deficiency.

The peroxisomal disorders identified so far are usually subdivided into three groups depending upon whether there is a generalized (group I), multiple (group II) or single loss (group III) of peroxisomal functions (Table 1).

In group I no functional peroxisomes, or only a limited number, are detectable in cells of the patients; in group II and III normal peroxisomes are present, at least in cultured skin fibroblasts of patients.

In this chapter we will summarize the essential clinical and biochemical findings in the more frequently encountered peroxisomal disorders. We will pay particular attention to the most recent developments in diagnosis and treatment and to the neurological and neuropathological characteristics of the different diseases. We refer to recent reviews for more detailed descriptions of specific aspects (Wanders *et al.*, 1989; van den Bosch *et al.*, 1992; Dimmick & Applegarth, 1993; Schutgens & Wanders, 1994; Lazarow & Moser, 1995).

Functions of peroxisomes in man

The major metabolic functions of peroxisomes which are of direct relevance to human diseases are summarized in Table 2.

Peroxisomal oxidation and respiration

Peroxisomes contain a simple respiratory pathway based upon the formation of hydrogen peroxide by a large collection of oxidases and the subsequent decomposition of this toxic compound by catalase (see van den Bosch *et al.*, 1992). Substrates for these oxidases vary from D- and L-amino acids, L-α-hydroxyacids, fatty acyl CoAs, glutaryl-CoA, oxalate, polyamines and pipecolic acid to intermediates in bile acid synthesis like di- and trihydroxycholestanoyl-CoA (DHCA-CoA and THCA-CoA) and pristanoyl-CoA.

Table 2. Major metabolic functions of peroxisomes in man

Catabolic functions
- Hydrogen peroxide-based cellular respiration
- β-oxidation of
  - *long-chain fatty acid (saturated/unsaturated)
  - *very long-chain (>C_{22}) fatty acid (saturated/unsaturated)
  - *Branched-chain fatty acids
  - *Prostaglandins
  - *Xenobiotics
- L-Pipecolic acid oxidation
- Ethanol oxidation
- Purine catabolism
- Polyamine catabolism

Anabolic functions
- Plasmalogen biosynthesis
- Cholesterol biosynthesis
- Bile acid biosynthesis
- Dolichol biosynthesis
- Glyoxylate transamination

Peroxisomal β-oxidation

One of the major functions of peroxisomes is the β-oxidative chain shortening of long-chain (C_{16}–C_{22}) and, very-long-chain (> C_{22}) saturated fatty acids, DHCA, THCA, branched chain fatty acid derivatives, prostaglandins (PG) like PG-F2, xenobiotics, long-chain dicarboxylic acids, certain mono- and polyunsaturated fatty acids, 12- and 15-hydroxyeicosatetraenoic acid and certain leucotrienes. Rather than being a functional duplicate of the mitochondrial β-oxidation system, peroxisomes are involved in the β-oxidation of a distinct set of substrates.

Activation of these compounds to CoA-derivatives precedes the actual β-oxidative chain shortening in the peroxisomes. A set of different synthases is active in these reactions.

Ether–phospholipid biosynthesis

A third major function of peroxisomes concerns their role in the biosynthesis of ether–phospholipids including the plasmalogens. The synthesis of these phospholipids involves a series of reactions both in the peroxisomes and in the endoplasmic reticulum. The two enzymes responsible for the introduction of the characteristic ether-linkage in these compounds i.e. dihydroxyacetone-phosphate acyltransferase (DHAP-AT) and alkyldihydroxyacetone phosphate synthase (alkyl-DHAP synthase) are localized in peroxisomes.

Ether-phospholipids are particularly abundant in membranes of electrically active tissues such as brain. Zoeller *et al.* (1988) reported that plasmalogens protect animal cell membranes against damage by reactive oxygen species such as singlet oxygen. Much still has to be learned about the functions of plasmalogens in membranes.

Other metabolic functions

In humans peroxisomes are essential in the detoxification of glyoxylate and in the metabolism of dolichols, polyamines and certain leucotrienes. Recently evidence was obtained for a role of peroxisomes in cholesterol synthesis. (see van den Bosch *et al.*, 1992).

From the information available on the enzyme content of peroxisomes it is clear that they have many more metabolic functions still to be unravelled.

Clinical characteristics of peroxisomal disorders with neurological involvement

Group I contains Zellweger's syndrome as the prototype, neonatal adrenoleucodystrophy (NALD) and the milder infantile type of Refsum's disease (IRD).

Newborn infants with 'classic Zellweger's syndrome' show both major and minor malformations (feto-embryopathy) such as a very large anterior fontanel, abnormal earlobes, hypoplastic supraorbital ridges, simian creases, cortical cysts in the kidneys, neuronal migration defects in the brain, as well as an active (ongoing) process in the brain (fat storage in astrocytes, dysmyelinogenesis), liver (fibrosis, cirrhosis) and retina (degeneration). The most threatening symptom at birth is severe hypotonia and paresis. These are the symptoms that usually prompt referral to neonatal intensive care units. Some of the symptoms are the direct result of these pareses: clubfeet, swallowing disorder and ventilatory insufficiency. External features in the newborn such as simian creases and the muscular hypotonia often suggest Down's syndrome as the highest ranking possibility. However, the severity of the muscular pareses should alert the attending (neuro)paediatrician to the possibility of Zellweger's syndrome. The accompanying cerebral malformations are probably in large part responsible for epileptic phenomena.

Radiological procedures may help the clinician to support a presumptive diagnosis of Zellweger's syndrome. A radiological survey of the skeleton may reveal periarticular calcifications.

Subsequently, psychomotor retardation, hearing deficits, hepatic cholestasis and fibrosis become evident. Both the visual evoked response and acoustic brainstem evoked response are severely disturbed. Characteristically, infants with classic Zellweger's syndrome rarely survive beyond the first few months of life. It has been shown that the defect of neuronal migration commences early in fetal development and can be identified in fetuses with the syndrome at 14 weeks gestation (Powers &Tummons, 1989).

Milder variants of classic Zellweger's syndrome have been described (Barth *et al.*, 1987). Patients exhibit some psychomotor development and survive beyond the first year of life.

In the syndrome, functional peroxisomes are strongly deficient in all cell types studied, including glial cells in the cerebral cortex and white matter (Kamei *et al.*, 1993).

A similar, but milder deficiency of peroxisomes is also found in the clinically milder disorders of group I which include NALD and especially IRD. Zellweger's syndrome, NALD and IRD share a combination of core symptoms: retinopathy, deafness, psychomotor retardation and liver disease. The finding of this rare combination should alert the paediatrician to the possibility of a peroxisomal disorder. It is important to mention that these core symptoms are also present in the peroxisomal β-oxidation defects belonging to group III. Kelley *et al.* (1988) have suggested criteria to discriminate between Zellweger's syndrome and NALD. Both are autosomal recessive disorders.

The clinical course of IRD is even milder than NALD, with no distinct abnormalities in the neonatal period, minor facial dysmorphism and often survival into the second decade of life (Poll-Thé *et al.*, 1987).

Hyperpipecolic acidaemia is a rare disorder resembling NALD clinically. It is doubtful whether this is a separate entity.

The severity of clinical abnormalities in group I disorders may reflect the extent of peroxisomal malfunction.

Group II comprises classic rhizomelic chondrodysplasia punctata (RCDP) and a rare disorder named Zellweger-like syndrome. RCDP is an autosomal recessive disorder and is clinically characterized by a disproportionately short stature due to symmetrical shortening of the proximal parts of the extremities, coronal clefting of the vertebrae and calcified stippling adjacent to ossified ischial and pubic bones. The calcifications decrease with age in affected children.

Typical craniofacial dysmorphism and sometimes cataracts are present. The hypotonic and hyporeflexic infants have seizures, severe growth retardation and severe psychomotor developmental failure. We diagnosed 49 RCDP patients including six fetuses by specific biochemical procedures. In our experience, most patients survive beyond their first year of life, sometimes even into their second decade.

In RCDP patients, peroxisomes are identifiable in cultured fibroblasts, but abnormally enlarged peroxisome structures are found in the liver (De Craemer et al., 1991; Hughes et al., 1992). In other types of chondrodysplasia punctata, like Conradi–Hünermann disease and X-linked dominant and X- linked recessive chondrodysplasia, no peroxisomal abnormalities have been found (Schutgens et al., 1988).

In the last two years we have identified several patients with all the clinical signs and symptoms of classic RCDP, but only a single deficiency of either DHAP-AT (Wanders et al., 1992; Barr et al., 1993; Caruso, 1993, Clayton et al., 1994) or alkyl-DHAP synthase (Wanders et al., 1994). These RCDP variants are listed in the group III disorders in Table 1 as only a single peroxisomal enzyme was found to be deficient.

Group III includes X-linked adrenoleucodystrophy (X-ALD) as the most frequent disorder. It has become clear that the clinical presentation of X-ALD is very diverse, ranging from the lethal childhood phenotype to one with adrenocortical insufficiency as the only manifestation (Table 3).

Table 3. Different phenotypes of X-linked adrenoleucodystrophy and their frequency in several countries

Phenotype	% of total		
	USA* (n = 1475)	France† (n = 185)	Netherlands (n = 78)
Childhood cerebral	48	⎫	29.5
Adolescent cerebral	5	⎬ 57	2.6
Adult cerebral	3	3	0.0
AMN	25	28	43.6
Addison only	10	8	20.5
Pre/Asymptomatic	8	4	3.8

*Phenotype distribution among male X-ALD patients in the Kennedy Krieger Institute, Baltimore, USA, as reported by Moser et al. (1994); † Phenotype distribution among French male X-ALD patients as reported by Aubourg & Chaussain (1990).

In childhood ALD, onset is before the age of 10 years after normal psychomotor development for several years. Deterioration usually starts with behavioural disturbances, and then affects vision, speech and gait. Often adrenocortical insufficiency, seizures and dementia develop. The cerebral demyelination results in a vegetative state or death in most cases within 3 years after onset. Next to the metachromatic leucodystrophies, X-ALD is probably the most common form of leucodystrophy.

Budka et al. (1976) were the first to recognize adult patients with myelopathy, peripheral neuropathy and adrenocortical insufficiency as suffering from another phenotype of this disorder known as adrenomyeloneuropathy (AMN). There are also reports of hypogonadism, sexual impotence, a tendency to fatigue, urinary bladder dysfunction and psychiatric symptoms in AMN (Assies et al., 1994).

Other phenotypes of X-ALD are listed in Table 3 together with their frequencies as found in studies in different countries. Different phenotypes may occur within the same pedigree.

In contrast to the findings reported by Moser et al. (1994) and Aubourg & Chaussain (1990), we found that in the Netherlands AMN is the most frequently encountered phenotype (about 44 per cent of total).

Heterozygous females of this X-linked inherited disorder may exhibit progressive spastic paraparesis and peripheral neuropathy with onset in the fourth or fifth decade and very rarely adrenal cortical insufficiency also (Moser et al., 1987).

Other disorders belonging to group III are acyl-CoA oxidase deficiency (pseudo-NALD), bi(multi)-functional protein deficiency and peroxisomal thiolase deficiency (pseudo-Zellweger's syndrome), all reported in a limited number of cases only. There is neurological involvement in these (rare) diseases.

Other disorders in this group are DHAP-AT deficiency (pseudo-RCDP) reported so far in five patients and the recently identified alkyl-DHAP synthase deficiency. The phenotype of both disorders is very much like classic RCDP.

Disorders in group III without neurological involvement include hyperoxaluria type I, and glutaric aciduria type III.

Finally, several patients have been recognized who are suspected to suffer from a peroxisomal disorder on clinical grounds, but with di- and trihydroxycholestanoic acidaemia as the only specific biochemical abnormality (Christensen et al., 1990; Przyrembel et al., 1990; Wanders et al., 1991).

Biochemical characteristics of peroxisomal disorders

In Group I disorders functional peroxisomes are absent or severely reduced in number in all cell-types studied. As a result, nearly all peroxisomal enzymes are deficient and metabolic functions in which peroxisomal enzymes play a role are impaired. These include the peroxisomal β-oxidation of saturated and unsaturated very-long-chain fatty acids like $C_{26:0}$ (cerotic acid) and $C_{24:6w3}$ (docosahexaenoic acid) fatty acid, DHCA and THCA, the metabolism of phytanic acid, pristanic acid, and pipecolic acid and the biosynthesis of etherphospholipids (Table 4). As a result several specific metabolites either accumulate in plasma, fibroblasts and in the chorionic villous cells of patients or are deficient, allowing the biochemical diagnosis of these disorders both prenatally and postnatally.

Table 4. Diagnostic parameters in peroxisomal disorders

Disorder	Zellweger NALD	RCDP	DHAP-AT deficiency	X-ALD/AMN
Plasma				
VLCFAs	↑↑	n	n	↑
Phytanic acid*	↑	↑↑	n	n
DHCA/THCA†	↑↑	n	n	n
DHA ($C_{22:6w3}$)	↓↓/↓	n	n	n
Erythrocytes				
Plasmalogens	↓/n	↓↓	↓↓	n
Platelets				
DHAP-AT activity	↓↓	↓	↓↓	n
Fibroblasts/amniocytes				
VLCFAs	↑↑	n	n	↑
DHAP-AT activity	↓	↓	↓↓	n
De novo plasmalogen synthesis	↓↓	↓↓	↓↓	n
Phytanic acid oxidase activity	↓↓	↓	n	n
Peroxisomal thiolast protein (kDa)	absent	44	41	41

n = normal; * = phytanic acid concentration in plasma is diet/age dependent; † = di/trihydroxycholestanoic acid; ‡ = docosahexaenoic acid; ↑ = elevated in comparison to controls; ↑↑ = highly elevated; ↓ = decreased; ↓↓ = greatly decreased; RCDP = rhizomelic chondrodysplasia punctata; NALD = neonatal adrenoleucodystrophy; DHAP-AT = dihydroxyacetonephosphate acyltransferase.

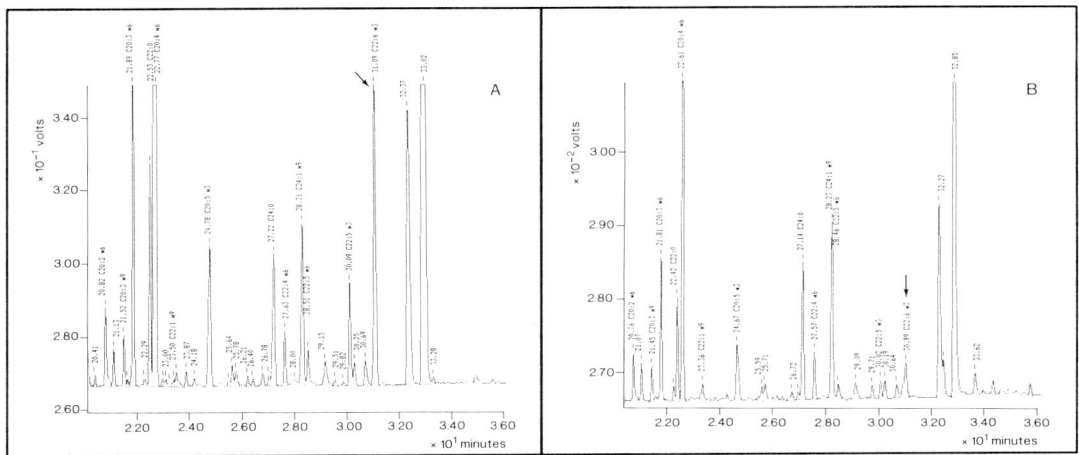

Fig. 1. Gas chromatography profiles of methyl-ester derivatives of fatty acids in plasma from a control (A) and a Zellweger's patient (B). Note the differences in sensitivity between A and B and differences in $C_{22:0}$ and $C_{22:6w3}$ (DHA) concentrations. Methyl-esters were fractionated on a Hewlett Packard 5890 gaschromatograph equipped with a capillary column (SP-2330, Supelco) with a splitless injection system, a temperature gradient from 50–250 °C and an FID detector.

However, other specific metabolites are deficient in patients including $C_{16:0}$– and $C_{18:0}$– plasmalogens and the unsaturated fatty acid docosahexaenoic acid ($C_{22:6w3}$; DHA) (Fig. 1.)

Normally, DHA is found at high levels in human grey matter and the retinal photoreceptor cells. (Anderson & Maude, 1971; Pullarkat & Reha, 1978). The possibility cannot be excluded that DHA deficiency as found in patients with Zellweger's syndrome (Martinez, 1990) plays a role in the dysmyelinogenesis and the retinopathy found in this disorder.

All peroxisomal proteins are coded by nuclear genes, synthesized on free ribosomes in the cytosol and incorporated into pre-existing intact peroxisomes.

Schram et al. (1986) found that peroxisomal β-oxidation enzyme proteins are normally synthesized in fibroblasts of patients with Zellweger's syndrome, but that these newly synthesized proteins are unstable and are rapidly degraded, probably due to the absence of intact peroxisomes. It is assumed that this mechanism is responsible for the deficiencies found for many peroxisomal enzymes. A few peroxisomal proteins like the 69-, 53-, 35- and 22-kDa (integral) peroxisomal membrane proteins (IMPs or PMPs) (Santos et al., 1988), catalase and alanine glyoxylate aminotransferase escape degradation and can be detected in normal amounts in the cytoplasm of liver and fibroblasts in Zellweger's syndrome. The finding of these IMPs in unusual large membrane structures in Zellweger's syndrome fibroblasts and liver indicates that these peroxisomes are not entirely absent in Zellweger's syndrome, but rather consist of (nearly) empty membrane ghosts. This phenomenon suggests that the primary defect(s) that causes Zellweger's syndrome involves the machinery for the post-translational import of peroxisomal proteins. Complementation studies indicate that disorders of peroxisome deficiency involve at least eleven distinct genetic defects (Brul et al., 1988; McGuiness et al., 1990; Shimozawa et al., 1993; Moser et al., 1995).

Mutation analyses in two patients with Zellweger's syndrome identified the genetic defect in these patients at the level of the gene coding for the peroxisomal assembly factor-1 (PAF-1). The nucleotide sequence of this gene encodes a protein with two highly conserved, putative membrane-spanning segments that may be responsible for localization of PAF-1 as an integral membrane protein in peroxisomes (Shimozawa et al., 1992).

There is a great homology between PAF-1 and the 35 kDa IMP (PMP). Gaertner et al. (1992) cloned and sequenced cDNA's for human PMP70 and mapped the gene to chromosome 1. Among patients with Zellweger's syndrome they found two mutant PMP70 alleles in single probands from the same complementation group.

Recently, Dodt et al. (1995) identified a mutation in the PST, (peroxisome targetting signal 1) receptor gene PXR1 in a Zellweger patient.

In RCDP, four distinct biochemical abnormalities have been found, including deficient activities of DHAP-AT, alkyl DHAP synthase and phytanic acid oxidase (Heymans et al., 1985; Schutgens et al., 1988) (Table 4). Furthermore, peroxisomal thiolase occurs in an abnormal molecular precursor form (44 kDa) instead of the mature form (41 kDa) as found in the controls (Hoefler et al., 1988). The typical biochemical features of classic RCDP allow the early prenatal and postnatal diagnosis of this disorder (Table 4). Prenatal detection in chorionic villi (CV) cells is based on the finding in Western blotting experiments of precursor peroxisomal thiolase protein (44 kDa) with anti-peroxisomal thiolase and the finding of deficient plasmalogen levels. (Schutgens et al., 1993). Prenatal diagnosis of DHAP-AT deficiency (pseudo-Zellweger's syndrome), however, is based on the finding of deficient DHAP-AT activity and of decreased plasmalogens in CV cells. Western blotting experiments with anti-peroxisomal thiolase are not informative in this disorder. This underlines that detailed biochemical analyses must be performed in the index patient before prenatal diagnostic studies can be initiated. It is assumed that the primary defect in classic RCDP is at the level of a specific receptor or carrier-protein at the peroxisomal membrane (see Heikoop, 1992). This receptor- or carrier-protein is essential for the import into the peroxisome of a specific group of proteins such as phytanic acid oxidase, DHAP-AT, alkyl-DHAP synthase and peroxisomal thiolase.

In X-ALD patients, peroxisomal VLCFA-CoA synthetase that specifically activates the VLCFAs at the peroxisomal membrane, prior to the actual peroxisomal α-oxidation, is deficient. This defect results in an accumulation of VLCFAs, but no other peroxisomal metabolites, in tissues, cultured cells and in plasma (Table 4).

Recently an elevation in the level of tumor necrosis factor in childhood ALD has been reported (Moser, 1993). The actual meaning of this finding is still unclear.

All males affected by X-ALD can be diagnosed by the demonstration of elevated VLCFAs in blood and cultured cells and/or by the finding of a deficient β-oxidation of $C_{26:0}$ fatty acid in fibroblasts. About 80 per cent of obligate heterozygotes show abnormal plasma VLCFAs. This percentage is higher (95 per cent) if also VLCFAs in fibroblasts are considered.

However, the finding of a deficient peroxisomal VLCFA-CoA synthetase activity in X-ALD does not necessarily mean that the mutation in this disease involves the gene encoding this enzyme. The primary defect may well be at the level of another gene, on the X-chromosome, the product of which is essential for the correct expression and (or) anchoring of peroxisomal VLCFA-CoA synthase in the peroxisomal membrane. Indeed, recently Mosser et al. (1993) and others (Neumann et al., 1993) identified a gene partially deleted in several independent patients with ALD. In familial cases, the deletion segregated with the disease. The deduced protein sequence shows significant sequence identity to a peroxisomal membrane protein of $M_r = 70\,000$ that is involved in peroxisome biogenesis and belongs to the 'ATP-binding cassette' superfamily of transmembrane transporters. PCR primers were developed to scan each of the 10 exons of this likely candidate gene (ALDP) and the resulting PCR amplification products screened for single-strand polymorphism to identify possible mutations. A large number of variants were identified among X-ALD patients, but none in up 60 X-chromosomes from controls. The variants were clustered primarily in exon 1, that encodes part of the transmembrane domain of the ALD-protein and in exon 5, that encodes the linker region between the transmembrane and ATP-binding domains. A large number of separate point-mutations and deletions were identified among the variants, but no correlation between the position of the mutation along the gene and the phenotypic expression of the disease could be identified (Neumann et al., 1993).

A very recent development in prenatal diagnosis for X-ALD and other X-linked inherited diseases is preimplantation female embryo selection in couples at risk. PCR analysis of sex chromosome specific sequences or fluorescence *in situ* hybridization (FISH) with sex chromosome-specific probes allows selective intrauterine transfer of female embryos. Selection is done by *in vitro* fertilization, blastomere biopsy of the 6–8-cell embryo and single cell analysis (Grifo et al., 1992).

A further step will be the preimplantation single-cell analysis of the specific gene defect, allowing selective intrauterine transfer of embryos without the gene defect (Kristjansson et al., 1994).

Patients with a defect at the level of acyl-CoA oxidase, bi(multi)-functional protein or peroxisomal thiolase respectively exhibit elevated VLCFA levels in tissues, plasma and cultured cells. Moreover, except for acyl-CoA oxidase deficiency, plasma DHCA and THCA levels are highly elevated.

Treatment

The potential for effective treatment in group I and group II disorders is limited by the multiple malformations and defects that originate in fetal life. In patients with Zellweger's syndrome the therapeutic effect of different dietary regimens has been evaluated in a limited number of patients. This includes dietary supplementation with bile acids (Setchell et al., 1992), DHA (Martinez, 1993) and/or plasmalogen precursors (Holmes et al., 1987) and a diet free of phytanic acid and precursors of phytanic acid. The outcome in patients with classic Zellweger's syndrome is doubtful.

In patients with X-ALD plasma VLCFA's can be normalized in several weeks by a dietary regimen essentially based on fat restriction and supplementation with daily doses of glycerol trioleate oil (1.7 g/kg) and glycerol trierucate oil (0.3 g/kg) (Moser et al., 1987). Asymptomatic thrombocytopenia was noted in about 15 per cent of the patients during prolonged dietary treatment. Studies with patient groups in several countries so far have found no significant evidence of a clinically relevant benefit from this treatment in patients with AMN (Aubourg et al., 1993; Moser et al., 1993, 1994; Assies et al., 1994) or in symptomatic childhood ALD patients (Moser et al., 1993; Uziel et al., 1991). The efficacy of the dietary regimen in neurologically asymptomatic boys remains to be determined.

Another approach in more than 30 boys affected by childhood ALD has been bone marrow transplantation. Normal bone marrow-derived cells contain the enzyme that is lacking in X-ALD. The striking perivascular lymphocyte accumulation in childhood ALD patients suggests that bone marrow-derived cells will enter the central nervous system of ALD patients and generate beneficial effects. There is a narrow window for transplant as there has to be unequivocal evidence of neuropsychiatric deterioration and the development of childhood ALD, but still an ability to perform IQ testing and other tests used in evaluating the effect of treatment. Bone marrow transplantation has to be performed before the cerebral demyelination has caused irreversible neurological symptoms. Some patients do remarkably well following transplantation, but in most patients it is still too early to decide whether the treatment is beneficial for the patients.

Other therapies have been tried, such as immunosuppression, intravenous administration of gammaglobulin, administration of gangliosides or carnitine and clofibrate but these therapies did not alter the course of childhood ALD (see Moser et al., 1994). Currently pentoxifylline therapy is being evaluated.

Conclusion

Substantial progress has been made in the last decade in the clinical and biochemical recognition of the different peroxisomal disorders. Prenatal diagnosis is possible in all diseases in which this is relevant. Currently several groups have successfully localized the relevant genes in the different disorders. This is followed by mutation analyses and study of the genetic and phenotypic relationships. In most disorders much still has to learned about the relationship between the biochemical defect and the pathology observed in patients.

Possibilities for effective treatment are still rather limited in peroxisomal disorders. So far the outcome of dietary treatment in X-ALD and variants in a relatively small number of patients has been disappointing. Bone marrow transplantation in childhood ALD has been beneficial in a limited number of patients, but final conclusions about its effectiveness will only be known in several years.

References

Adamo, A.M., Aloise, P.A. & Pasquini, J.M. (1986): A possible relationship between concentration of microperoxisomes and myelination. *Int. J. Med. Neurosci.* **4**, 513–517.

Anderson, R.E. & Maude, M.B. (1971): Lipids in ocular tissues – VIII. The effects of essential fatty acid deficiency on the phospholipids of the photoreceptor membranes of rat retina. *Arch. Biochem. Biophys.* **151**, 270–276.

Assies, J., van Geel, B.M., Weverling, G.J., Haverkort, E.B. & Barth, P.G. (1994): Endocrine evaluation during dietary therapy for adrenomyeloneuropathy. In: *Thomas Addison and his diseases, 200 years on*. eds. H.R. Bhatt, V.H.T. James, G.M. Besser, G.F. Botazzo and H. Keen, pp. 191–198. Bristol: Journal of Endocrinology Ltd.

Aubourg, P. & Chaussain, J.-L. (1990): Adrenoleucodystrophy presenting as Addison's disease in children and adults. *Trends Endocrinol. Metab.* **2**, 49–52.

Aubourg, P., Adamsbaum, C., Lavallard-Rousseau, M-C., Rocchiccioli F. *et al.* (1993): A two-year trial of oleic and erucic acids ('Lorenzo's oil') as treatment for adrenomyeloneuropathy. *N. Engl. J. Med.* **329**, 745–752.

Barr, D.G.D., Al Howasi, M., Kirk, J.M., Wanders, R.J.A. & Schutgens, R.B.H. (1993): Rhizomelic chondrodysplasia punctata with isolated deficiency of acyl-CoA: dihydroxyacetone phosphate acyltransferase. *Arch. Dis. Child.* **68**, 415–417.

Barth, P.G., Schutgens, R.B.H. & Wanders, R.J.A. *et al.* (1987): A sibship with a mild variant of Zellweger's syndrome. *J. Inherit. Metab. Dis.* **10**, 253–259.

Brul, S., Westerveld, A., Strijland, A., Wanders, R.J.A., Schram, A.W. *et al.* (1988): Genetic heterogeneity in the cerebro-hepato-renal (Zellweger) syndrome and other inherited disorders functions. A study using complementation. *J. Clin. Invest.* **81**, 1710–1715.

Budka, H., Sluga, E. & Heiss, W.D. (1976): Spastic paraplegia associated with Addison's disease: adult variant of adreno-leucodystrophy. *J. Neurol.* **213**, 237–250.

Caruso, U., Schutgens, R.B.H., Wanders, R.J.A. & Romano, C. (1993): Rhizomelic chondrodysplasia punctata (RCDP): heterogeneity in four patients. *Abstracts 31st SSIEM Symposium*. Abstr. W29, Manchester, UK.

Christensen, E., Van Eldere, J., Brandt, N.J., Schutgens, R.B.H., Wanders, R.J.A. & Eyssen, H.J. (1990): A new peroxisomal disorder: di- and trihydroxycholestanoyl-CoA oxidase deficiency. *J. Inherit. Metab. Dis.* **13**, 363–366.

Clayton, P.T., Eckhardt, S., Wilson, J., Hall, C.M., Youssuf, M., Wanders, R.J.A. & Schutgens, R.B.H. (1994): Isolated dihydroxyacetone phosphate acyltransferase deficiency presenting with developmental delay. *J. Inherit. Metab. Dis.* **17**, 533–540.

De Craemer, D., Kerkaert, I. & Roels, F. (1991): Hepatocellular peroxisomes in alcoholic and drug-induced hepatitis: a quantitative study. *Hepatology* **14**, 811–817.

Dimmick, J.E. & Applegarth, D.E. (1993): Pathology of peroxisomal disorders. In: *Genetic metabolic diseases*, eds. B.H. Landing, J. Bernstein & J. Rosenberg, pp. 45–98. Basel: Karger.

Dodt, G., Braverman, N., Wong, C. *et al.* (1995): Mutations in the PTS1 receptor gene, PXR1, define complementation group 2 of the peroxisome biogenesis disorders. *Nature Genet.* **9**, 115–125.

Gaertner, J., Moser, H. & Valle, D. (1992): Mutations in the 70K peroxisomal membrane protein gene in Zellweger's syndrome. *Nature Genet.* **1**, 16–22.

Grifo, J.A., Tang, Y.X., Cohen, J., Gilbert, F., Sanyal, M.K. & Rosenwaks, Z. (1992): Pregnancy after embryo biopsy and co-amplification of DNA from X and Y chromosomes. *J. Am. Med. Assoc.* **268**, 727–729.

Heikoop, J. (1992): Defects in the assembly of peroxisomes in rhizomelic chondrodysplasia punctata, the Zellweger's syndrome and related disorders. Thesis, University of Amsterdam.

Heymans, H.S.A., Oorthuys, J.W.E., Nelck, G., Wanders, R.J.A. & Schutgens, R.B.H. (1985): Rhizomelic chondrodysplasia punctata: another peroxisomal disorder. *N. Engl. J. Med.* **313**, 187–189.

Hoefler, G., Hoefler, S., Watkins, P.A., Chen, W.W., Moser, A.B. *et al.* (1988): Biochemical abnormalities in rhizomelic chondrodysplasia punctata. *J. Pediatr.* **112**, 726–733.

Holmes, R.D., Wilson, G.N. & Hajra, A.K. (1987): Oral ether lipid therapy in patients with peroxisomal disorders. *J. Inherit. Metab. Dis.* **10(Suppl. 2)**, 239–241.

Holtzman, E. (1982): Peroxisomes in nervous tissue. *Ann. NY Acad. Sci.* **386**, 523–525.

Hughes, J.L., Poulos, A., Crane, D.I., Chow, C.W., Sheffield, L.J. & Sillence, D. (1992): Ultrastructure and immunocytochemistry of hepatic peroxisomes in rhizomelic chondrodysplasia punctata. *Eur. J. Pediatr.* **151**, 829–836.

Kamei, A., Houdou, S., Takashima, S., Suzuki, Y., Becker, L.E. & Armstrong, D.L. (1993): Peroxisomal disorders in children: immunohistochemistry and neuropathology. *J. Pediatr.* **122**, 573–579.

Kelley, R.I., Datta, N.S., Dobyns, W.S., Hajra, A.K. *et al.* (1988): Neonatal adrenoleucodystrophy: new cases, biochemical studies and differentiation from Zellweger and related peroxisomal polydystrophy syndromes. *Am. J. Med. Genet.* **23**, 869–901.

Kristjansson, K., Chong, S.S., van den Veyver, I.B., Subramanian, S., Snabes, M.D. & Hughes, M.R. (1994): Preimplantation single cells analyses of dystrophin gene deletions using whole genome amplification. *Nature Genet.* **6**, 19–23.

Lazarow, P.B. & Moser, H.W. (1995): Disorders of peroxisome biogenesis. In: *The metabolic and molecular bases of inherited disease*, 7th ed., eds. C.R. Scriver, A.L. Beaudet, W.S. Sly & D. Valle, pp. 2287–2324. New York: McGraw-Hill.

Martinez, M. (1990): Polyunsaturated fatty acid changes suggesting a new enzymic defect in Zellweger's syndrome. *Lipids* **24**, 261–265.

Martinez, M. (1995): Polyunsaturated fatty acid abnormalities in patients with peroxisomal disorders: therapeutical implications. Colloquium on peroxisomal disorders, *Abstracts Royal Netherlands Academy of Arts and Sciences Colloquium*, Amsterdam, The Netherlands, in press.

McGuinness, M.C., Moser, A.B., Moser, H.W. & Watkins, P.A. (1990): Peroxisomal disorders: complementation analysis using beta-oxidation of very-long-chain fatty acids. *Biochem. Biophys. Res. Commun.* **172**, 364–369.

Moser, A.B., Borel, J., Odone, A., Naidu, S., Cornblath, D., Sanders, D.B. & Moser, H.W. (1987): A new dietary therapy for adrenoleucodystrophy. Biochemical and preliminary clinical results in 36 patients. *Ann. Neurol.* **21**, 240–249.

Moser, H.W., Moser, A.B., Smith, K.D., Bergin, A., Borel, J. *et al.* (1993): Adrenoleucodystrophy: phenotypic variability and implications for therapy. *J. Inherit. Met. Dis.* **15**, 645–664.

Moser, H.W., Kok, F., Neumann, S. *et al.* (1994): Adrenoleukodystrophy update: genetics and effect of Lorenzo's Oil therapy in asymptomatic patients. *Intern. Pediatr.* **9**, 196–205.

Moser, H.W., Rasmussen, M., Naidu, S. *et al.* (1995): Phenotype of patients with peroxisomal disorders subdivided in sixteen complementation groups. *J. Pediatr.* **127**, 13–22.

Mosser, J., Douar, A.-M., Sarde, C.-O., Koschis, P., Feil, R., Moser, H.W., Poustka, A.-M., Mandel, J-L. & Aubourg, P. (1993): Putative X-linked adrenoleucodystrophy gene shares unexpected homology with ABC transporters. *Nature* **361**, 726–730.

Neumann, S., Kok, S., Sarde C.-D., Mandel, J.L., Aubourg, P., Moser, H.W. & Smith, K.D. (1993): Mutational analysis of the ALD gene. *Abstracts 4th International Symposium.* Miami: Miami Children's Hospital Research Institute.

Poll-Thé, B.T., Saudubray, J.M., Ogier, H.A.M., Odievre, M., Scotto, J.M. *et al.* (1987): Infantile Refsum disease: an inherited peroxisomal disorder. Comparison with Zellweger's syndrome and neonatal adrenoleucodystrophy. *Eur. J. Pediatr.* **146**, 477–483.

Powers, J.M. & Tummons, R.C. (1989): Structural and chemical alterations in the cerebral maldevelopment of fetal cerebro-hepato-renal (Zellweger) syndrome. *J. Neuropathol. Exp. Neurol.* **48**, 270–289.

Pzryrembel, H., Wanders, R.J.A., van Roermund, C.W.T., Schutgens, R.B.H., Mannaerts, G.P. & Casteels, M. (1990): Di- and trihydroxycholestanoic acidaemia with hepatic failure. *J. Inherit. Metab. Dis.* **13**, 367–370.

Pullarkat, R.K. & Reha, H. (1978): Acyl and alk-1^1- enyl group composition of ethanolamine phosphoglycerides of human brain. *J. Neurochem.* **31**, 707–711.

Santos, M.J., Imanaka, T., Shio, H. & Lazarow, P.B. (1988): Peroxisomal integral membrane proteins in control and Zellweger fibroblasts. *J. Biol. Chem.* **263**, 11502–11509.

Schram, A.W., Strijland, A., Hashimoto, T., Wanders, R.J.A., Schutgens, R.B.H., van den Bosch, H. & Tager, J.M. (1986): Biosynthesis and maturation of peroxisomal β-oxidation enzymes in fibroblasts in relation to the Zellweger's syndrome and infantile Refsum disease. *Proc. Natl. Acad. Sci. USA* 6156–6158.

Schutgens, R.B.H., Heymans, H.S.A., Wanders, R.J.A., Oorthuys, J.W.E., Tager, J.M. et al. (1988): Multiple peroxisomal enzyme deficiencies in rhizomelic chondrodysplasia punctata. *Adv. Clin. Enzymol.* **6,** 57–65.

Schutgens, R.B.H., Wanders, R.J.A., Nijenhuis, A.A., Purvis, R. & Dekker, C. (1993): Rhizomelic chondrodysplasia punctata: prenatal diagnosis by biochemical analyses. *Int. Pediatr.* **8,** 45–51.

Schutgens, R.B.H. & Wanders, R.J.A. (1994): Peroxisomal disorders. In: *The inherited metabolic diseases*, 2nd edn, ed. J.B. Holton, pp. 243–263. Edinburgh: Churchill Livingstone.

Setchell, K.D.R., Bragetti, P., Zimmer-Nechemias, L. et al. (1992): Oral bile acid treatment and the patient with Zellweger's syndrome. *Hepatology* **15,** 198–207.

Shimozawa, N., Tsukamoto, T., Suzuki, Y., Orii, T., Shirayoshi, Y., Mori, T., & Fujiki, Y. (1992): A human gene responsible for Zellweger's syndrome that affects peroxisome assembly. *Science* **255,** 1132–1134.

Shimozawa, N., Suzuki, Y., Orii, T., Moser, A., Moser, H.W. & Wanders, R.J.A. (1993): Standardization of complementation grouping of peroxisome-deficient disorders and the second Zellweger patient with peroxisomal assembly Factor-1 (PAF-1) defect. *Human Genet.* **92,** 843–844.

Uziel, G., Bertini, E., Bardelli, P., Rimoldi, M. & Gambetti, M. (1991): Experience on therapy of adrenoleucodystrophy and adrenomyeloneuropathy. *Dev. Neurosci.* **13,** 274–279.

Van den Bosch, H., Schutgens, R.B.H., Wanders, R.J.A. & Tager, J.M. (1992): Biochemistry of peroxisomes. *Ann. Rev. Biochem.* **61,** 157–197.

Wanders, R.J.A., Heymans, H.S.A., Schutgens, R.B.H., Barth, P.G., van den Bosch, H. & Tager, J.M. (1989): Peroxisomal disorders in neurology. *J. Neurol. Sci.* **88,** 1–39.

Wanders, R.J.A., Casteels, M., Mannaerts, G.P., van Roermund, C.W.T., Schutgens, R.B.H., Kozich, V., Zeman, J. & Hyaneck, J. (1991): Accumulation and impaired *in vivo* metabolism of di- and trihydroxycholestanoic acids in two patients. *Clin. Chim. Acta* **202,** 123–132.

Wanders, R.J.A., Schumacher, H., Heikoop, J., Schutgens, R.B.H. & Tager, J.M. (1992): Human dihydroxyacetone-phosphate acyltransferase deficiency: a new peroxisomal disorder. *J. Inherit. Metab. Dis.* **15,** 389–391.

Wanders, R.J.A., Dekker, C., Horvath, A., Schutgens, R.B.H., Tager, J.M., van Laer, P. & Lecoutere, D. (1994): Human alkyldihydroxyacetone phosphate synthase deficiency: a new peroxisomal disorder. *J. Inherit. Metab. Dis.* **17,** 315–318.

Zoeller, R.A., Morand, O.H. & Raetz, C.H.R. (1988): A possible role for plasmalogens in protecting animal cells against photosensitized killing. *J. Biol. Chem.* **263,** 11590–11596.

Chapter 14

Four cases of rhizomelic chondrodysplasia punctata: heterogeneity and variability

Ubaldo Caruso

Laboratory for the Study of Inborn Errors of Metabolism, University Department of Pediatrics I, Giannina Gaslini Institute, Genoa, Italy

Summary

Rhizomelic chondrodysplasia punctata (RCDP) is an autosomal recessive disorder with a peculiar clinical phenotype, mainly characterized by symmetrical severe shortening of the proximal part of the humeri and femora, disturbed endochondral bone formation, punctate calcifications at joints, spine and other cartilages, atypical facial appearance, severe mental and growth delay and cataracts. Four peroxisomal functions are impaired in these patients, leading to three biochemical alterations: accumulation of phytanic acid in plasma, defect of plasmalogens in erythrocytes and other cells and the presence of peroxisomal protein 3-ketoacyl-CoA thiolase as an immature form.

This paper presents the investigations of four patients showing the classic RCDP clinical phenotype. Profound biochemical investigations have revealed that, among these four patients, three are affected by an isolated defect of acyl-CoA:dihydroxyacetone phosphate acyltransferase (DHAP-AT). The biochemical heterogeneity and the variability of the clinical expression of the disease in our patient group are here reported and discussed.

Introduction

Rhizomelic chondrodysplasia punctata (RCDP) is a rare disorder presenting with a peculiar clinical phenotype: epiphysial and extraepiphysial punctate calcifications, symmetrical severe shortening of the proximal part of humeri and femora, disturbed endochondral bone formation, atypical facial appearance, severe growth delay, mental retardation and cataracts. To date, the biochemical abnormalities found in RCDP patients are: (1) defects in phytanic acid oxidase; (2) defects in DHAP-AT and in alkyl-dihydroxyacetone phosphate synthase, two enzymes involved in plasmalogen biosynthesis; (3) defects in maturation of 3-ketoacyl-CoA thiolase, that is present in the immature form of 44 kDa. RCDP, then, belongs to the group of peroxisomal disorders characterized by a multiple loss of peroxisomal functions (Heymans *et al.*, 1985). Recently a few patients, presenting with RCDP clinical phenotype, have been reported as having an isolated defect of DHAP-AT (Wanders *et al.*, 1992; Barr *et al.*, 1993). Another patient (Poll-Thé *et al.*, 1991) presents all the biochemical alterations typical of RCDP, but not rhizomelia nor calcifications. Finally, Borochowitz, in 1991, described one patient with rhizomelic shortening of the limbs, punctate calcifications, normal growth and mental development without any recognizable defect in peroxisomal functions.

Patients

In the last four years we have studied, in our laboratory, four patients all presenting with the typical RCDP clinical phenotype.

Patient 1, R.C., a 10-year-old boy, first child of unrelated parents. Shortness of humeri was observed at birth; spontaneous movements of upper limbs were reduced and painful. Skeletal X-ray examination revealed symmetrical shortening of long bones, with abnormal epiphysial enlargements and calcified stippling located at joint cartilages of the limbs. During his first years of life, he grew very slowly, with a worsening of the morphological alterations and several severe bone fractures; bilateral cataract and repeated episodes of pulmonar, urinary and gastro-enteric infections were also reported. Currently, he is severely mentally delayed, his speech is limited to a few conventional words, and his movements are limited by joint contractures, mainly in the upper limbs. However, he is able to walk alone and to feed himself, and he attends school, showing attention and interest.

Patient 2, T.G., an 11-year-old girl, is the first child of unrelated parents. The clinical abnormalities of RCDP are strongly expressed in her. Punctate calcifications were present at joint cartilages, along the spine and at the laryngeal–tracheal cartilage. Other relevant changes were also observed: severe clefts of the vertebral bodies, cataracts, marked hypertricosis, hypoplasia of labia majora. The worsening of her bone malformations, the defect in ossification and her severe joint contractures have led to a dramatic clinical condition: the girl is immobile in bed, unable to feed or move herself. Her mental development is severely delayed and she is unable to speak.

Patient 3, A.G., is a 1-year-old boy, born to healthy unrelated parents. Three older brothers and one twin sister are in good health. At birth typical facial dysmorphysms and skeletal abnormalities like rhizomelic shortening of the limbs, metaphysial enlargement of the humeri and femora, kyphosis of the spine and calcific stipplings were evident. Cataracts and feeding difficulties were also present. Growth is delayed: at diagnosis his height was 65 cm and weight 6.5 kg (both under 3rd centile).

Patient 4, G.S., a boy was 4y 10m at diagnosis. Beyond all clinical alterations characteristic of RCDP, he presented at birth, coccyx dislocation and bilateral cryptorchidism. The latter, the cataracts and the contractures present in the lower limb joints were resolved by surgery. At the age of diagnosis he was 91 cm tall (lower segment 46 cm) and his head circumference was 49 cm. The patient is able to walk alone and attends play school.

Methods

Very-long-chain fatty acids (VLCFA), phytanic and pristanic acids were measured in plasma essentially as previously described (Caruso et al., 1991) with a slight personal modification to allow all the results in one analysis. Fractionation of plasmalogens in erythrocytes, immunoblotting studies in cultured fibroblasts, measure of de novo plasmalogen biosynthesis, DHAP-AT and phytanic acid oxidase activity in cultured fibroblasts were performed by R.B.H. Schutgens and R.J.A. Wanders (Amsterdam), by using methods reported elsewere (Bjorkhem et al., 1986; Schutgens et al., 1986; Schrakamp et al., 1988; Wanders et al., 1991).

Results

Following the protocol in use in our laboratory for the study of peroxisomal disorders, the first analytic step was to measure VLCFA, phytanic and pristanic acid, in the plasma of the patients.

As expected, VLCFA profile and pristanic acid concentrations were normal in all patients, being the peroxisomal β-oxidation not impaired in RCDP. Surprisingly, phytanic acid concentration was high only in plasma of the patient A.G. rising to 115 µmol/l (controls < 4 µmol/l), while it was 1.8 µmol/l in G.S. and under detection limit (0.2 µmol/l) in the others. Plasmalogens were then fractionated in erythrocytes, with abnormal results in all four patients: $C_{16:0}$ plasmalogens ranged between 0.9 and 37.4 per cent and $C_{18:0}$ plasmalogens ranged between 1.4 and 21 per cent of the controls. More profound biochemical investigations were carried out in cultured fibroblasts: *de novo* plasmalogen biosynthesis was impaired in all the cell lines, in agreement with the low plasmalogen levels in erythrocytes; phytanic acid oxidase activity was normal in patients T.G. and G.S., not assayed in R.C. and A.G.; Western blotting of peroxisomal proteins (3-oxoacyl-CoA thiolase and acyl-CoA oxidase) was normal in T.G., R.C., G.S., showing the abnormal band of 44 kDa in A.G. only; the activity of DHAP-AT was 0.9 nmol/2 h/mg proteins (controls: 7 ± 2 nm/2 h/mg proteins) in A.G. and less than 0.2 nmol/2 h/mg proteins in the three other patients.

Discussion

As a result of the profound biochemical investigations carried out on these patients to define precisely the biochemical alterations responsible for the clinical phenotype, we concluded that only one out of the four patients presenting with RCDP clinical phenotype showed all the biochemical alterations characteristic of the *classic* RCDP, while the other three showed an isolated defect of DHAP-AT.

Based on these results and on previous observations reported in literature (Wanders *et al.*, 1992; Barr *et al.*, 1993) we can affirm that the clinical phenotype RCDP is the expression of at least two different peroxisomal disorders having in common only the impairement of plasmalogen biosynthesis. Furthermore, the severity of the clinical appearance, in this disease is strongly variable, as demonstrated by the course of the illness in the first two patients (R.C. and T.G.) who had the same biochemical defect and were almost the same age, but showed extremely different clinical conditions. Since, to our knowledgement, there is no genetic relation between the families of the four patients, the high incidence of the isolated defect of DHAP-AT in our patient group should be underlined.

Acknowledgements

The author thanks P. Bianchi, Seriate; C. Borrone, Genova; P. Buttitta, Palermo; and L. Zelante, S.G. Rotondo, who submitted materials from their patients to our laboratory for diagnostic purposes and R. Gatti, Genova for cultures of the cells. Part of this work was presented at the Workshop on Peroxisomal Disorders, 31st Annual SSIEM Symposium, Manchester, September 1993.

References

Barr, D.G.D., Al Howasi, M., Kirk, J.M., Wanders, R.J.A. & Schutgens, R.B.H. (1993): Rhizomelic chondrodysplasia punctata with isolated deficiency of acyl-CoA dihydroxyacetone-phosphate acyltransferase. *Arch. Dis. Child.* **68**, 415–417.

Bjorkem, I., Sisfontes, L., Bostrom, B., Kase, B.F. & Bolmstrand, R. (1986): Simple diagnosis of the Zellweger's syndrome by gas–liquid chromatography of dimethylacetals. *J. Lipid Res.* **27**, 786–791.

Borochowitz, Z. (1991): Generalized chondrodysplasia punctata with shortness of humeri and brachymetacarpy: humero-mercaptal (HM) type: variation or heterogeneity? *Am. J. Med. Genet.* **41**, 417–422.

Caruso, U., Fowler, B., Erceg, M. & Romano, C. (1991): Determination of very-long-chain fatty acids in plasma by a simplified gas chromatographic–mass spectrometric procedure. *J. Chromatr.* **562**, 147–152.

Heymans, H.S.A., Orthus, J.W.E., Nick, G., Wanders, R.J.A. & Schutgens, R.B.H. (1985): Rhizomelic chondrodysplasia punctata: another peroxisomal disorder. *N. Engl. J. Med.* **313**, 187–188.

Poll-Thé, B.T., Maroteaux, P., Narcy, C., Quetin, P., Guesnu, M., Wanders, R.J.A, Schutgens, R.B.H. & Saudubray, J.M. (1991): A new type of chondrodysplasia punctata associated with peroxisomal dysfunction. *J. Inherit. Metab. Dis.* **14**, 361–363.

Schrakamp, G., Schalkwijk, C.G., Schutgens, R.B.H., Wanders, R.J.A., Tager, J.M. & van den Bosch, H. (1988): Plasmalogen biosynthesis in peroxisomal disorders: fatty alcohol versus alkyl-glycerol. *J. Lipid Res.* **29**, 325–354.

Schutgens, R.B.H., Ofman, R., Van den Bosch, H., Tager, J.M. & Wanders, R.J.A. (1986): Acyl-CoA:dihydroxyacetone phosphate acyltransferase in human skin fibroblasts. Study of its properties using a new assay method. *Biochim. Biophys. Acta* **879**, 286–291.

Wanders, R.J.A., van Roermund, C.W.T., Griffioen, P. & Cohen, L. (1991): Peroxisomal enzyme activities in the hepatoblastoma cell line Hep G2 as compared to human liver. *Biochim. Biophys. Acta* **1115**, 54–59.

Wanders, R.J.A., Schumacher, H., Hikoop, J., Schutgens, R.B.H. & Tager, J.M. (1992): Human dihydroxyacetonephosphate acyltransferase deficiency: a new peroxisomal disorder. *J. Inherit. Metab. Dis.* **15**, 389–91.

Chapter 15

Neuroradiological findings in metabolic diseases of the central nervous system

Mario Savoiardo, Ludovico D'Incerti and Elisa Ciceri

Department of Neuroradiology, Istituto Nazionale Neurologico Carlo Besta, via Celoria 11, 20133 Milan, Italy

Summary

Many metabolic disorders may affect the central nervous system, sometimes directly and selectively, and sometimes with a non-specific mechanism through a general metabolic imbalance. In some of these diseases, neuroradiological studies may be crucial for the diagnosis and the follow-up. In leucodystrophies, the distribution of the CT or MRI abnormalities, the preferential involvement of some areas or pathways, the sparing of the subcortical arcuate fibres, and the presence of megalencephaly or atrophy may be of great importance in establishing the diagnosis or in restricting the differential diagnosis. For the diagnosis of organic acidurias, the association of involvement of the peripheral, subcortical white matter and of the basal ganglia should alert the neuroradiologist. Selective involvement of some nuclei in the basal ganglia may also be seen, both in organic acidurias and in mitochondrial encephalopathies. In mitochondrial disorders, preferential involvement of the brainstem and basal ganglia is observed in Leigh's disease. In MELAS, the posterior cortical areas are usually first affected; cortical cerebellar lesions, cerebellar atrophy and calcifications in the basal ganglia are often present. In Kearns–Sayre syndrome, slight signal abnormalities in the brainstem, thalami, basal ganglia and subcortical white matter are usually present. In metabolic diseases, co-ordination between neuroradiologists, clinicians and other neuroscientists may improve the diagnostic capabilities and possibly lead to earlier treatment.

Introduction

The central nervous system may be affected by a great number of metabolic disorders, sometimes directly and selectively, sometimes as a part of a multiple organ involvement. The central nervous system may be affected in one or more of its components: grey matter, cortex or deep nuclei or systems, the whole white matter or certain regions or pathways.

In this chapter, we shall limit ourselves to the description of the neuroradiological findings observed in some of the most common or interesting metabolic disorders that may affect the central nervous system, i.e. leucodystrophies, organic acidurias and mitochondrial encephalopathies.

The leucodystrophies are among the disorders that can be best demonstrated by magnetic resonance imaging (MRI), because of its sensitivity to changes in the white matter water content. In leucodystrophies there is abnormal formation or an abnormal metabolism of myelin, which becomes progressively altered after an initially normal formation. Although the enzymatic defect which causes the leucodystrophic process, or any other metabolic disorder, is congenital, the symptoms and signs

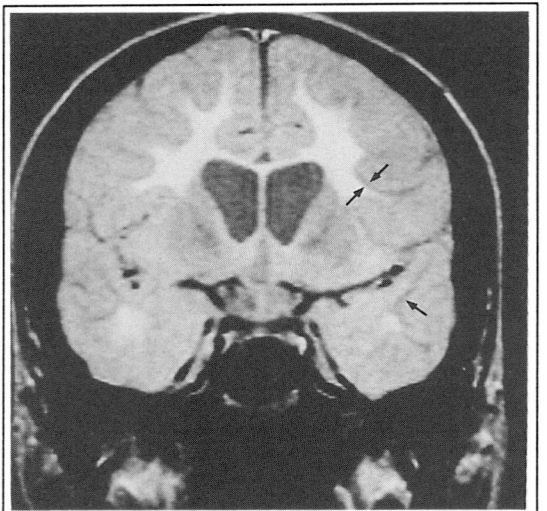

Fig. 1. Metachromatic leucodystrophy. Coronal proton density SE image shows abnormal signal intensity in the white matter with sparing of the U fibres (arrows). (From Savoiardo et al., 1991a, with permission).

of the disease and the abnormalities on imaging studies may appear at different ages, depending on several factors, such as the level of the enzymatic activity that may be completely absent or only reduced to a certain percentage of the normal activity. Moreover, the abnormal metabolites may require considerable time to accumulate and reach the level that may cause symptoms and signs and signal abnormalities on MRI. To further complicate the problem, the most frequent abnormality in leucodystrophies, that is, an increased signal intensity in T_2-weighted images, may be difficult to distinguish from the normal white matter in early infancy, because at this age the white matter is normally hyperintense owing to incomplete myelination; the early recognition of a leucodystrophic process is therefore difficult, and the neuroradiological diagnosis may be delayed to the age in which the myelination should be completed or well advanced.

The classification of the genetically determined encephalopathies is based on the enzymatic deficiency from which they originate. Classes are made according to the location of the enzyme, in the cytoplasm or in organelles. Therefore, we recognize diseases due to deficiencies of enzymes diffusely found in the cytoplasm (amino acidopathies and organic acidurias), or enzymes located in lysosomes, peroxisomes and mitochondria.

Among the lysosomal diseases, the most common leucodystrophic disorders are metachromatic leucodystrophy and Krabbe's disease. Among the peroxisomal disorders, the disease that we observe most frequently is adrenoleucodystrophy. In other leucodystrophies, such as Alexander's disease, the metabolic defect is still unknown. In Pelizaeus–Merzbacher and in Canavan's diseases, biochemical insights have recently been reached.

We shall describe the most common neuroradiological findings observed in the leucodystrophies we mentioned, in some of the organic acidurias and in mitochondrial disorders.

Leucodystrophies

In metachromatic leucodystrophy the white matter of the cerebral hemispheres is affected and appears with low attenuation values on CT scan and with high signal intensity in T_2-weighted images on MRI. MRI obviously shows greater details; the corpus callosum is involved, while the internal capsule may be affected to a lesser extent. The abnormalities may also involve the corticospinal tracts in the brainstem and the white matter of the cerebellum (van der Knaap et al., 1991). A characteristic finding in metachromatic leucodystrophy is the lack of involvement of the arcuate fibres or subcortical U fibres (Savoiardo et al., 1991a). In the initial cases, in fact, the regions first affected are the periventricular areas; the signal abnormalities then gradually extend toward the periphery in a centrifugal pattern. In advanced cases, the U fibres may also be partially involved, but their recognizability in at least a few areas indicates the centrifugal pattern of diffusion of the disease (Fig. 1).

In Krabbe's disease or globoid cell leucodystrophy, a similar distribution of pathological changes

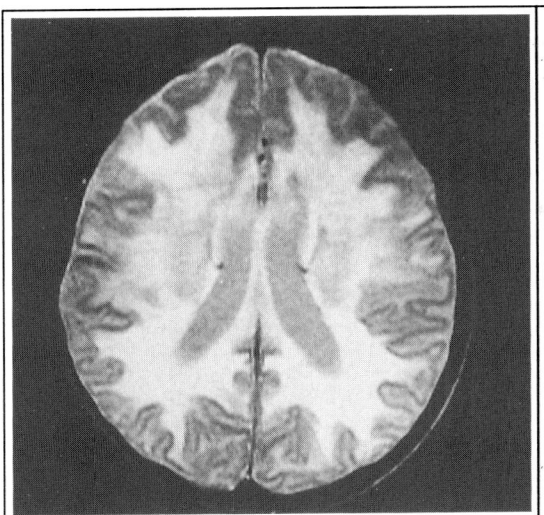 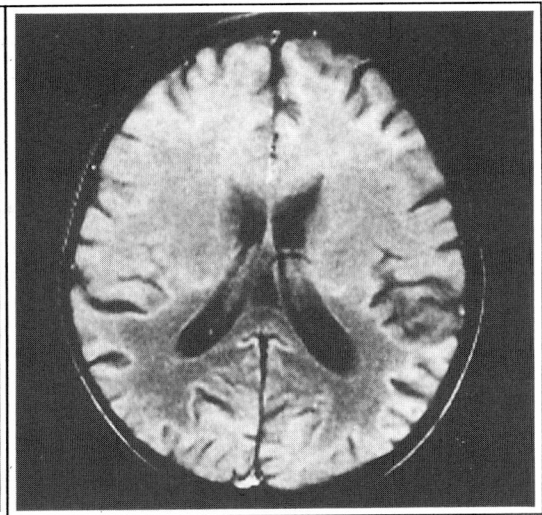

Fig. 2. Adrenoleucodystrophy. In a 7-year-old boy with a 1-year history of disease, the T_2-weighted image (a) shows extension of signal abnormalities also to the frontal lobes; the T_1-weighted image (b) better demonstrates the more severe involvement of the posterior regions, where the abnormalities have started. (From Savoiardo & D'Incerti, 1990, with permission).

and signal abnormalities is found. However, it is often difficult to demonstrate the signal abnormalities because of the earlier age of presentation. In Krabbe's disease, CT scans may be more helpful for the diagnosis; in addition to atrophy and less hypodensity that one would expect in a leucodystrophic disease, high-density areas are found in the thalami and in the posterior periventricular white matter (Kwan et al., 1984). These high-density areas are probably due to the accumulation of galactocerebroside in clusters of globoid cells, histiocytes or modified astrocytes, that give the name to the disease.

X-linked adrenoleucodystrophy is, among the leucodystrophies, the disease that can be diagnosed most easily by neuroimaging studies. In a young boy, the presence of low density on CT scan, and of low intensity in T_1- and high intensity in T_2-weighted images on MRI in the posterior periventricular areas with involvement of the splenium of the corpus callosum is characteristic of adrenoleucodystrophy. With progression of the disease, the abnormalities extend anteriorly to involve the whole temporal and parietal lobes and then the frontal lobes (Fig. 2). The subcortical arcuate fibres, initially spared, may be involved in advanced cases at least in the most affected areas of the occipital lobes. The abnormalities may variably extend to the long tracts of the brainstem; the cerebellar white matter may also be affected. In advanced cases, when the white matter of all the cerebral lobes is hyperintense in T_2-weighted images, T_1-weighted images may still show only posterior hypointensities, thus indicating the initial and more profoundly affected regions (Savoiardo & D'Incerti, 1990). Since the extension of the disease is accompanied by an active demyelination with an abnormal blood–brain barrier at the periphery, the posterior lesions present fairly well-defined margins with enhancement after contrast medium administration both on CT and MRI. In about 10 per cent of the cases, a reverse pattern of distribution of the abnormalities is observed, with initial involvement of the frontal white matter and of the genu of the corpus callosum and backward progression.

A different pattern of the white matter involvement is seen in Canavan's disease, which has been found to be associated with a profound deficiency of the enzyme aspartoacylase, resulting in an increased amount of N-acetylaspartic acid in urine and plasma. The ability of ^{1}H MR spectroscopy

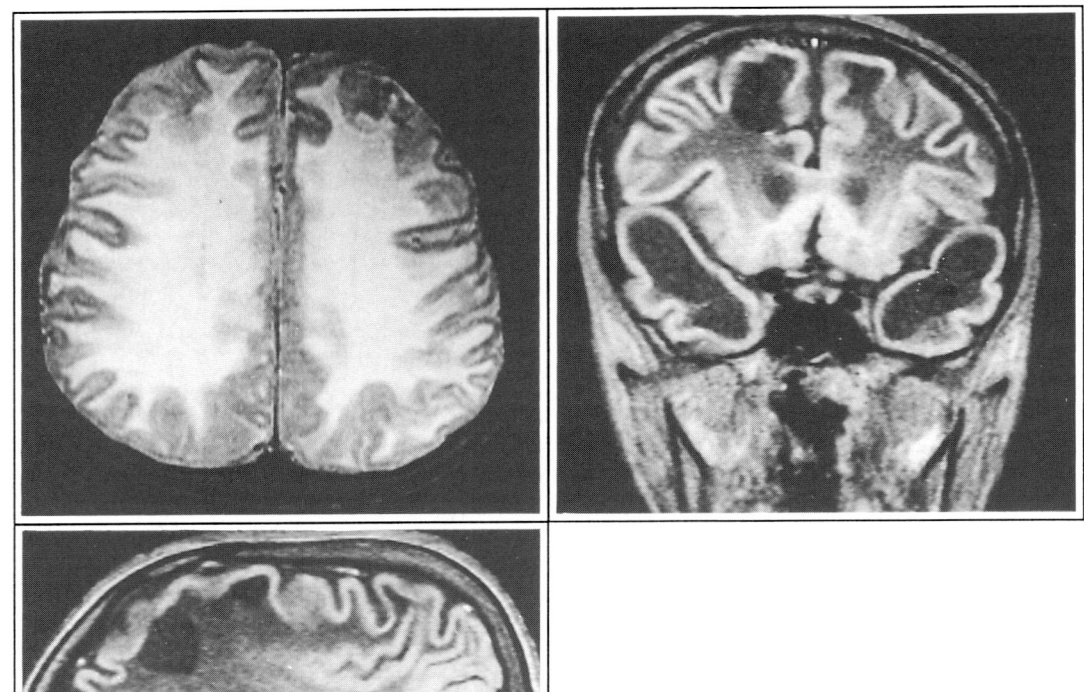

Fig. 3. Alexander's disease. Axial T_2-weighted image (a) shows diffuse abnormalities in the whole white matter of the cerebral hemispheres. Coronal (b) and sagittal (c) T_1-weighted images also show cavitations in the frontal and anterior temporal regions. Megalencephaly is present.

to demonstrate excessive concentrations of N-acetylaspartate in the brain of children with Canavan's disease (as well as a few other metabolites in other metabolic disorders), has added this MR technique to the diagnostic tools used in the metabolic diseases of the central nervous system (Grodd et al., 1991; Tzika et al., 1993; Zimmerman et al., 1993). In Canavan's disease, MRI demonstrates diffuse white matter abnormalities in the cerebral hemispheres, almost always primarily involving the subcortical white matter. This finding correlates well with a spongy state observed in pathological studies just beneath the cortex in the region of the arcuate fibres. The internal and external capsules and the corpus callosum are sometimes spared. White matter changes may sometimes occur in the brainstem and cerebellum. Macrocephaly is often present; slight atrophy may rarely develop in advanced cases (Brismar et al., 1990). In a series of nine patients, Brismar et al. (1990) noted that there was no correlation between the severity of white matter disease and the clinical symptomatology, nor with age or aspartoacylase level. A similar discrepancy has been observed by us in six cases of metachromatic leucodystrophy (Savoiardo et al., 1987).

Alexander's disease is one of the few leucodystrophies still without a known biochemical defect; therefore, diagnosis must be made by brain biopsy or may be attempted on the basis of clinical and neuroradiological findings, and by exclusion of other diseases. In Alexander's disease profound white matter abnormalities with very low attenuation values on CT scans and hypointensity in T_1- and high-signal intensity in T_2-weighted images on MRI are seen in addition to megalencephaly. Contrast enhancement may be present in the early stages around the frontal horns. The white matter abnormalities are more marked in the frontal regions where they initiate; the disease involves the subcortical white matter with a marked contrast with the overlying normal or slightly thinned cortex; as the disease progresses, cavitations may occur initially in the frontal subcortical regions but may extend posteriorly with destruction of most of the white matter (Fig. 3).

Pelizaeus–Merzbacher disease also remains without biochemical proof; however, it is caused by a defective biosynthesis of a central nervous system myelin-specific proteolipid protein for which a DNA probe has been found (Brismar et al., 1990). MRI demonstrates very little or no myelin, suggesting a very early arrest of myelination, perhaps before birth. A decrease of the bulk of white matter with marked atrophy is usually present (van der Knaap et al., 1991).

A specific diagnosis of a leucodystrophy requires biochemical studies, or a biopsy or molecular genetic studies. However, the observation on MRI of the distribution of the abnormalities, of the involvement or sparing of the subcortical arcuate fibres, of megalencephaly or atrophy, or, rarely, characteristic CT changes may give important clues to accelerate the diagnosis (Table 1).

Table 1. Characteristic abnormalities in leucodystrophies

	Megalencephaly	Atrophy	Initial distribution	U fibre involvement
MLD	–	+	Periventricular	–
Krabbe	–	+	CT high density	–
ALD	–	–	Posterior	–
Alexander	+	–	Anterior	+
Canavan	+	–	Diffuse	+
Pel. Merzb.	–	+	Diffuse	+

+ = present; – = absent; for CT in Krabbe's disease see text; MLD = metachromatic leucodystrophy; ALD = adrenoleucodystrophy; Pel.Merzb. = Pelizaeus–Merzbacher disease

Table 2. Mitochondrial encephalomyopathies studied with MRI and CT of the brain at the Istituto Nazionale Neurologico Carlo Besta.

	No. of cases	Mean age (years)
β-oxidation deficiency	1	2
Leigh's disease	11	2.5
MELAS	3	8.5
Kearns–Sayre syndrome	3	17
MERRF	2	23.5
Leber's hereditary optic neuropathy	3	28
CPEO	9	47
CPEO-plus	6	27
Others	7	15

Organic acidopathies

The various organic acidurias may present different neuroradiological findings. However, the areas or structures most commonly involved are the basal ganglia and the cerebral white matter, particularly in the subcortical areas (Uziel et al., 1988; Savoiardo et al., 1991a; van der Knaap et al., 1991).

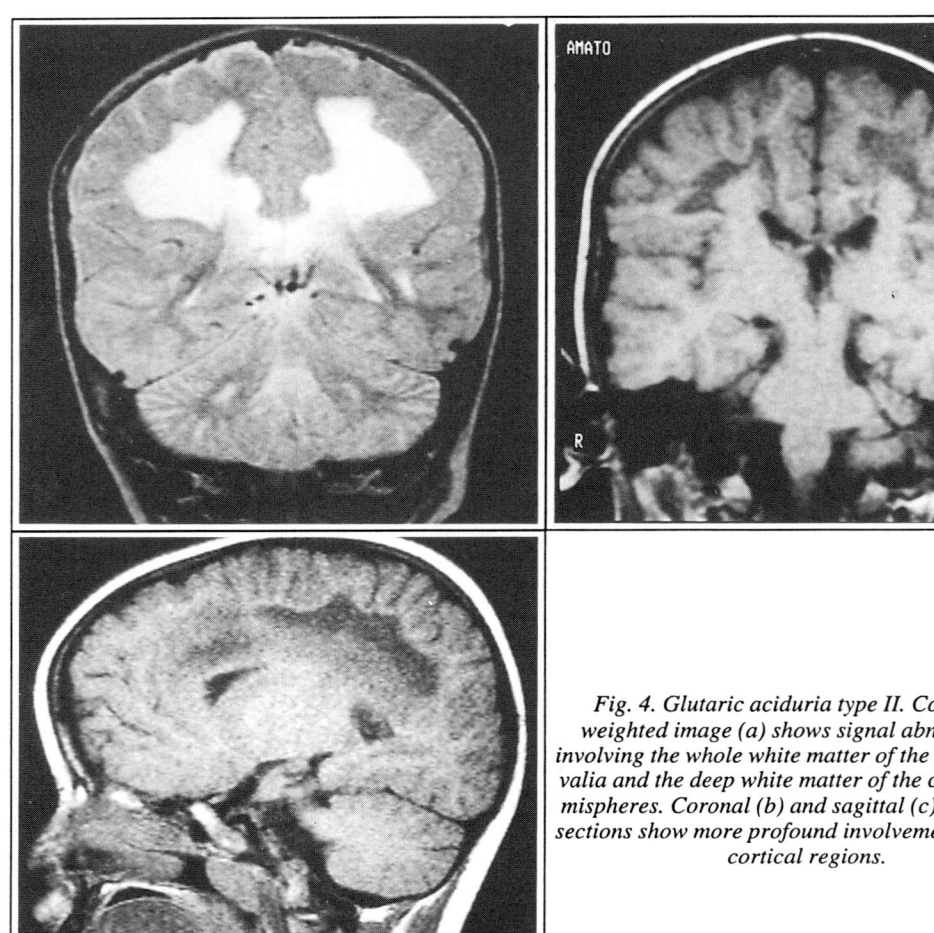

Fig. 4. Glutaric aciduria type II. Coronal T_2-weighted image (a) shows signal abnormalities involving the whole white matter of the centra semiovalia and the deep white matter of the cerebellar hemispheres. Coronal (b) and sagittal (c) T_1-weighted sections show more profound involvement of the subcortical regions.

We recently reviewed the MRI findings of 11 cases of biochemically proved organic acidurias. The biochemical diagnosis was: glutaric aciduria type II in two brothers of 2 and 4 years of age; glutaric aciduria type I in one child aged 3; 2-hydroxyglutaric aciduria in three cases ranging from 11 to 17 years of age; methylmalonic aciduria in three patients (aged 6 months–4 years), one of whom was without proved enzymatic deficiency; 3-methyl-glutaconic aciduria in one boy aged 6; 4-hydroxybutyric aciduria in a girl aged 7. These patients had a total of 20 MRI studies.

The two brothers with glutaric aciduria type II presented marked signal hyperintensity in T_2-weighted images in the centra semiovalia of the cerebral hemispheres and in small areas of the cerebellar white matter. T_1-weighted images demonstrated a more severe involvement of the peripheral, subcortical white matter of the cerebral hemispheres with, however, partial sparing of the U fibres (Fig. 4). The youngest boy also had diffuse atrophy.

The girl with glutaric aciduria type I had only minimal abnormalities of the peripheral white matter, but more evident signal abnormalities in the basal ganglia (Fig. 5), and tiny, isolated, symmetrical

Chapter 15 Neuroradiological findings in metabolic diseases of the central nervous system

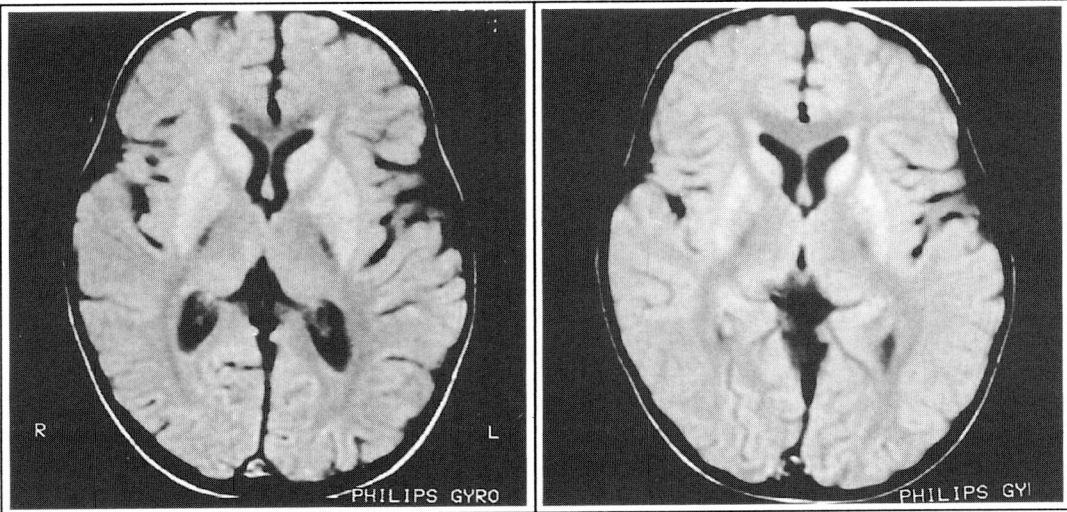

Fig. 5. Glutaric aciduria type I. MRI proton density images. First examination (a) shows increased signal intensity in the whole lenticular nucleus and in the head of caudate nucleus. Follow-up examination 4 months later (b) shows regression of signal abnormalities in the pallidum; the neostriatum has slightly shrunk and the ventricles have enlarged. Minimal white matter abnormalities are also present.

areas of high-signal intensity in the pontine tegmentum. She did not present the bilateral middle fossa arachnoid cysts nor the marked widening of the sylvian fissures reported in other cases (Hald et al., 1991; Mandel et al., 1991); the sylvian fissures were only slightly enlarged.

The three patients with 2-hydroxyglutaric aciduria all presented severe abnormalities in the subcortical white matter with involvement of the U fibres (Fig. 6), and slight signal alterations in the basal

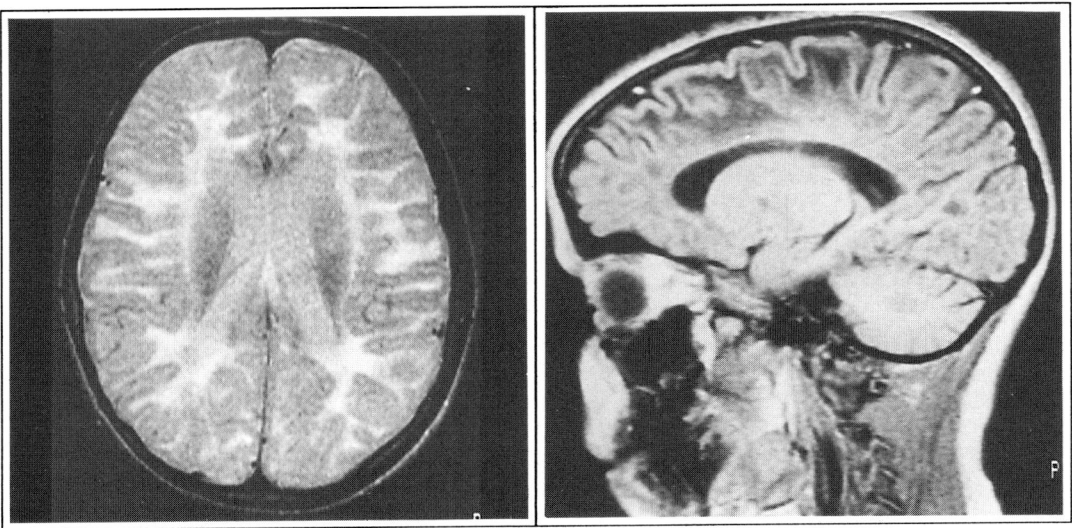

Fig. 6. 2-hydroxyglutaric aciduria. An axial T_2-weighted image (a) shows diffuse white matter abnormalities, with involvement of subcortical U fibres. A sagittal T_1-weighted image (b) better demonstrates the involvement of the peripheral white matter.

ganglia; in addition, one patient presented an increase in signal intensity in the deep cerebellar white matter and questionable abnormalities in the pontine tegmentum, while another presented mild cerebellar atrophy.

Of the three cases with methylmalonic aciduria, two presented signal abnormalities in the basal ganglia, but the pallidum, which is usually selectively involved as reported by Andreula et al. (1991) and observed by us in other cases, was relatively spared; in these two cases the abnormalities were more severe in the neostriatum, and more so in the putamen than in the caudate nucleus. Mild abnormalities were also present in the pontine tegmentum and were questionable in the peripheral white matter. The 6-month-old child without proved enzymatic deficiency only had a borderline increase in signal intensity in the pallidum, which on repeat MRI scan was considered normal.

The patient with 3-methylglutaconic aciduria presented slight abnormalities of the posterior, mostly periventricular, white matter, and mild cerebellar atrophy.

The girl with 4-hydroxybutyric aciduria had small, distinct areas of increased signal intensity in T_2-weighted images in the pallidum and in the most peripheral white matter in the axis of a few convolutions near the vertex (Savoiardo et al., 1991a).

From these data and from other cases reported in the literature (van der Knaap et al., 1991) we can conclude that the areas of white matter more frequently involved in patients with organic aciduria are the subcortical ones, sometimes with remarkable contrast and neat outline vs the overlying normal cortex. When the signal hyperintensity in T_2-weighted images also extend to the periventricular white matter, T_1-weighted images still demonstrate a greater involvement with a more marked hypointensity in the subcortical areas. These areas, together with the paraventricular white matter superior to the trigones, are the last to myelinate; as Barkovich et al. (1993) noted, diseases like Canavan's and Kearns–Sayre syndrome (and organic acidurias), in which a spongy state of the white matter is observed in pathological studies, show abnormalities mostly in the areas of 'new' or more recent myelination. It is not known whether the new myelin is more vulnerable to spongiotic disorders, or whether any disorder of the white matter affecting the areas of more recent myelination results in a spongy degeneration (Barkovich et al., 1993). The other structures most commonly involved in organic acidurias are the basal ganglia, often the pallidum, which in metabolic or degenerative disorders seems in general to be less vulnerable than the neostriatum. In spite of the cases here described, an isolated involvement of the pallidum in the appropriate clinical condition should raise the suspicion of methylmalonic aciduria (Naidu & Moser, 1991).

In organic acidurias, other areas such as pontine tegmentum and cerebellum may be variably involved. A combination of these findings, particularly abnormalities of basal ganglia and subcortical white matter, however, are not pathognomic of organic aciduria as may be seen in other metabolic disorders, particularly in Kearns–Sayre syndrome.

Mitochondrial encephalopathies

Imaging studies are becoming more and more important in the definition and in the clinical follow-up of some mitochondrial disorders (Barkovich et al., 1993); however, their relevance and reliability in the diagnosis of mitochondrial encephalopathies have not yet been fully assessed. To help define the role of imaging studies, we recently reviewed all the neuroradiological examinations performed in a series of 45 patients, well-defined from the genetic and biochemical standpoints, observed at our Institute (Savoiardo & Ciceri, 1994). Many of these patients had had more than one study; 44 had had at least one MRI scan of the brain. The diagnoses of these 45 patients are given in Table 2. We shall describe and discuss only the cases presenting in childhood and adolescence.

A few mitochondrial disorders, such as fatty acids β-oxidation deficiencies, may cause severe metabolic disorders with hypoglycaemia and coma, that non-specifically affect the central nervous system, causing diffuse brain lesions. In this group we usually find young children or infants, in whom the episodes of severe hypoglycaemia, frequently precipitated by fasting, may cause brain

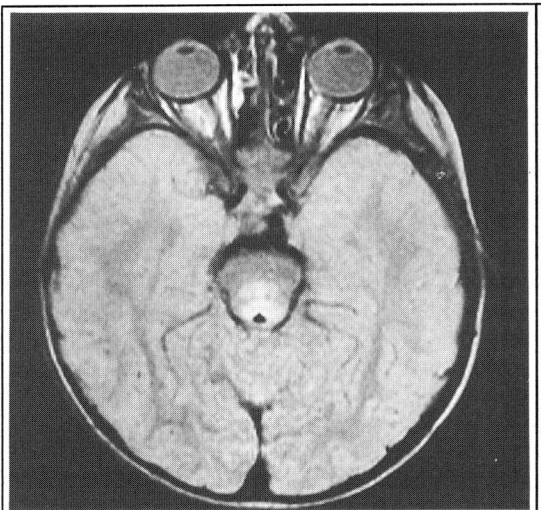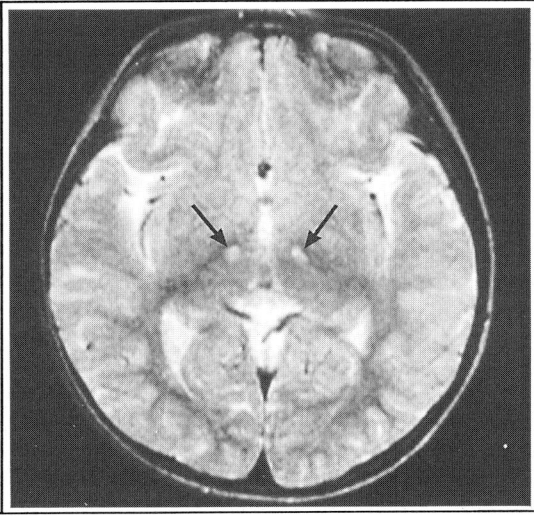

Fig. 7. Leigh's disease with cytochrome-c-oxidase deficiency. Proton density image (a) demonstrates signal abnormalities in the ponto-mesencephalic tegmentum. A more cranial T_2-weighted image (b) shows well-defined abnormalities in the subthalamic nuclei (arrows).

lesions and lead to death. In a 2-year-old boy, in acute hypoglycaemic coma caused by carnitine-palmitoyl-transferase deficiency, CT scans showed diffuse cortical and subcortical low attenuation values of the cerebral hemispheres, with oedema and compression of the ventricles and cisterns, sparing posterior fossa structures and basal ganglia. After correction of the acute metabolic imbalance, the CT abnormalities partially regressed with disappearance of the oedema, but persistence of diffuse cortical and subcortical abnormalities, from necrosis or spongiosis, and the development of diffuse cerebral atrophy and ventricular dilatation (Savoiardo *et al.*, 1992).

Other mitochondrial diseases cause more specific and characteristic damage on the central nervous system. In the paediatric age, the most common disorder is Leigh disease; in adolescence or young adulthood, MELAS and Kearns–Sayre syndrome may have their onset.

Leigh's disease, or subacute necrotizing encephalopathy, presented various neuroradiological aspects in our series. On CT scans, the most frequent finding in Leigh's disease was considered to be hypodensity in the neostriatum. In our MRI series, the most common abnormalities were in the brainstem, particularly in the pontine tegmentum and in the midbrain periaqueductal area. Signal abnormalities with symmetrical hyperintensities in T_2-weighted images may also occur in the medulla oblongata, in the inferior cerebellar peduncles, in the deep white matter of the cerebellum, in the subthalamic nuclei, in the neostriatum and in the white matter of the cerebral hemispheres, rarely with a diffuse leucodystrophic pattern (Fig. 7). The putamen is probably the second most common location after the brainstem. The location in the subthalamic nuclei is quite interesting; we have seen it only in mitochondrial disorders, and all but one case were Leigh's disease with cytochrome-*c*-oxidase deficiency (Savoiardo *et al.*, 1991b). An attempt at correlating the neuroradiologic distribution of abnormal findings with the enzymatic deficiency was unsuccessful. A few cases with diffuse abnormalities of the white matter in a leucodystrophic pattern and with clinical presentation similar to that of other cases of Leigh's disease and an identical biochemical defect (cytochrome-*c*-oxidase deficiency) had a different clinical course and are listed in our series in the 'others' group.

Mitochondrial encephalomyopathy with lactic acidosis and stroke-like syndrome (MELAS), may present neuroradiological abnormalities of various severities according to the stage of the disease.

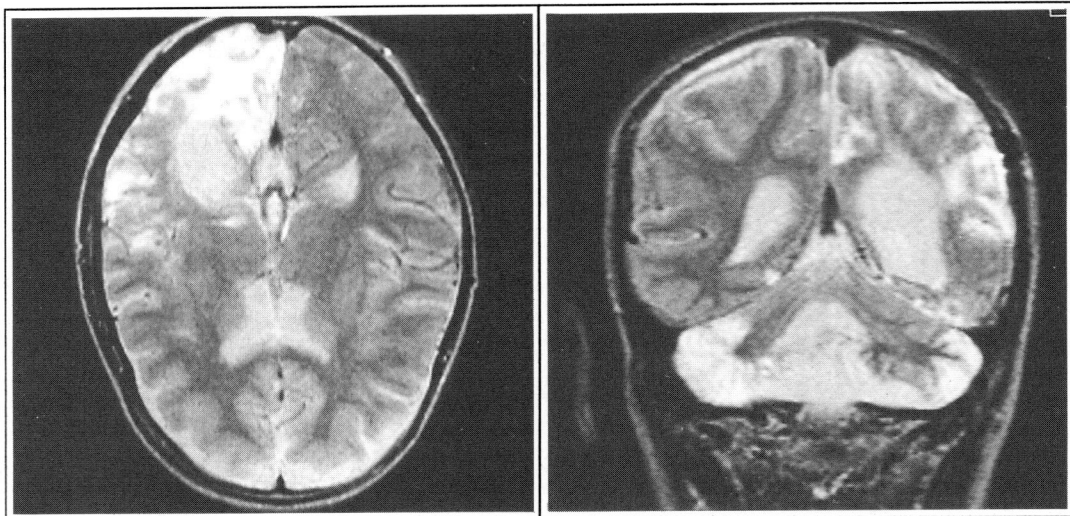

Fig. 8. MELAS. Axial T2-weighted image (a), after the first stroke-like episode, shows signal abnormalities in the posterior regions of the left cerebral hemisphere and in the left thalamus. Coronal T2-weighted image (b) also demonstrates signal hyperintensity in the cerebellar cortex. The cerebellum is atrophic.

Generally, the first acute stroke-like episode that marks the disease involves the posterior regions of the cerebral hemispheres, often on one side only. CT scans or MRI demonstrate involvement both of the cortex and of the underlying white matter with a distribution that does not correspond exactly to vascular territories. Approximately half of the patients are found to have calcifications in the basal ganglia, more visible on a CT scan; slight or moderate cerebellar atrophy is also often present. These findings obviously pre-exist, and their association with an acute cerebral lesion in a young patient may lead to the diagnosis. With correction of the metabolic imbalance and clinical improvement, the acute lesions may sometimes fade or even disappear, thus confirming that they did not represent ischaemic areas leading to necrosis. Most of the time some abnormality persists; other acute episodes occur, and the brain and cerebellum show multiple cortical areas of low density on CT and high signal intensity in T_2-weighted images on MRI. The lesions may involve all the cerebral lobes, basal ganglia, and thalami; in the cerebellum the posterior and lateral cortex of the hemispheres is affected (Fig. 8); so far, we are not aware of cases with lesions in the brainstem. Even if the distribution of the lesions does not represent vascular territories, it seems that the areas involved are the distal areas of the vessels, the lesions often being centred on the watershed areas (Savoiardo *et al.*, 1992). The distribution usually observed in the cerebellum may in fact represent the distal territories of the superior, anterior inferior and posterior inferior cerebellar arteries. With the development of these lesions, diffuse severe atrophy ensues.

Cerebellar atrophy and calcifications in the basal ganglia in a young patient should suggest a mitochondrial disease. These findings are often also present in Kearns–Sayre syndrome.

Kearns–Sayre syndrome, clinically characterized by chronic external ophthalmoplegia, retinal degeneration, heart block, high protein content in the CSF, ataxia, weakness, sensorineural hearing loss and onset before age 20, may also show faint hypodensity of the subcortical white matter on CT scans. On MRI, the white matter abnormalities are more evident as hyperintensities in T_2-weighted images. MRI may also reveal signal abnormalities in the supratrigonal white matter, an area of late myelination like the subcortical region (Barkovich *et al.*, 1993). In addition, MRI may show signal abnormalities in the brainstem, mostly in the pontine and midbrain tegmentum, in the red nuclei, in the thalami and in the pallida. Often a diffuse, slight atrophy is present.

Not all cases of proved mitochondrial disease fit into the best clinically characterized syndromes. Overlapping or various combinations exist. We have already mentioned the cases with leucodystrophic pattern in cytochrome-*c*-oxidase deficiency, not fitting in with Leigh's disease. We also observed a girl with cerebellar atrophy and cerebellar cortex abnormalities identical to those observed in MELAS, without any episode of 'stroke' and with complex I and IV deficiencies of the respiratory chain (Savoiardo *et al.*, 1992).

Another recent case not included in this series is worth mentioning. This was a female infant referred to our Institute at the age of 10 months for a stereotactic midbrain biopsy. She had poor growth, generalized muscle hypotonia and brainstem signs for the previous 3 months; metabolic acidosis with elevated blood lactate and pyruvate were also present. MRI showed an asymmetric swelling of the midbrain, consistent with a glioma. On reviewing the MRI, tiny, symmetrical areas of increased signal intensity in T_2-weighted images were also noted in the pontine tegmentum and in the inferior cerebellar peduncles. These findings were considered compatible only with a metabolic disorder and a possible diagnosis of Leigh's disease or other mitochondrial encephalopathy was entertained in spite of the pseudotumoral appearance of the brainstem. A muscle rather than brain biopsy was then performed; biochemical assays of the respiratory chain complexes revealed a marked deficiency of NADH-Co-Q reductase (complex I). In the follow-up, a transient signal abnormality appeared in the subthalamic nuclei; the midbrain enlargement disappeared in the following months.

From these data, we can conclude that mitochondrial disorders may present different aspects in the different syndromes, but that even in the same disease a strict uniformity of findings is rarely seen. However, in a child, prevalence of abnormalities in the brainstem and in the basal ganglia with some characteristic distribution should raise the suspicion of Leigh's disease. In older children, adolescents, or young adults, calcifications in the basal ganglia associated with some degree of cerebellar atrophy should raise the suspicion of other mitochondrial encephalopathies: MELAS when a stroke-like episode occurs, Kearns–Sayre syndrome when abnormalities in the subcortical white matter are also present, obviously in the appropriate clinical setting.

Conclusions

In establishing a diagnosis of metabolic disease, the essential neuroradiological data usually are the symmetry of the abnormalities, the selective involvement of some structures or areas, with sparing of adjacent structures. Rarely is the distribution of the abnormalities not symmetrical, as in MELAS; other times, as in adrenoleucodystrophy, the areas most commonly involved may be spared and a different, reverse pattern of distribution may be observed.

Many metabolic disorders are rare, and the number of the cases reported is insufficient to establish the characteristic neuroradiological features of a disease. Neuroradiological–pathological correlations are rarely obtained, and one has to attempt to correlate the neuroradiological findings with the reported pathological findings of other cases; however, the pathological reports of cases of metabolic diseases are rare and often it is difficult to extract from these reports what MRI features should be expected.

In the most common metabolic disorders, however, MRI may suggest the specific diagnosis; in many instances, the neuroradiological features may at least restrict the possible diagnosis to a group of disorders. Nevertheless, in metabolic disorders the diagnosis always requires a biochemical confirmation. A close collaboration between the neuroradiologist and the clinician, with the support of the biochemist and of the molecular geneticist, is necessary for a specific diagnosis, which is the first step before treatment can possibly be attempted.

References

Andreula, C.F., De Blasi, R. & Carella, A. (1991): CT and MR studies of methylmalonic acidemia. *AJNR* **12**, 410–412.

Barkovich, A.J., Good, W.V., Koch, T.K. & Berg, B.O. (1993): Mitochondrial disorders: analysis of their clinical and imaging characteristics. *AJNR* **14**, 1119–1137.

Brismar, J., Brismar, G., Gascon, G. & Ozand, P. (1990): Canavan's disease: CT and MR imaging of the brain. *AJNR* **11**, 805–810.

Grodd, W., Krägeloh-Mann, I., Klose, U. & Sauter, R. (1991): Metabolic and destructive brain disorders in children: findings with localized proton MR spectroscopy. *Radiology* **181**, 173–181.

Hald, J.K., Nakstad, P.H., Skjeldal, O.H. & Stromme, P. (1991): Bilateral arachnoid cysts of the temporal fossa in four children with glutaric aciduria type I. *AJNR* **12**, 407–409.

Kwan, E., Drace, J. & Enzmann, D. (1984): Specific CT findings in Krabbe disease. *AJNR* **5**, 453–458.

Mandel, H., Braun, J., El-Peleg, O., Christensen, E. & Berant, M. (1991): Glutaric aciduria type I. Brain CT features and a diagnostic pitfall. *Neuroradiology* **33**, 75–78.

Naidu, S.B. & Moser, H.W. (1991): Value of neuroimaging in metabolic diseases affecting the CNS. *AJNR* **12**, 413–416.

Savoiardo, M., Bracchi, M., Visciani, A., Milanese, C. & Uziel, G. (1987): Radiology of demyelinating diseases and other disorders of the white matter. In: *Clinical neuroimmunology*, eds. J.A. Aarli, W.M.H. Behan & P.O. Behan, pp. 467–481. Oxford: Blackwell Scientific Publications.

Savoiardo, M. & D'Incerti, L. (1990): Multiple sclerosis, dysmyelinating and degenerative diseases. *Riv. Neuroradiol.* **3 (Suppl. 2)**, 101–107.

Savoiardo, M., D'Incerti, L. & Strada, L. (1991a): La RM nella patologia infiammatoria e degenerativa encefalica. *Riv. Neuroradiol.* **4 (Suppl. 3)**, 57–63.

Savoiardo, M., Uziel, G., Strada, L., Visciani, A., Grisoli, M. & Wang, G. (1991b): MRI findings in Leigh's disease with cytochrome-*c*-oxidase deficiency. *Neuroradiology* **33 (Suppl.)**, 507–508.

Savoiardo, M., Strada, L., Uziel, G., Ciceri, E., Antozzi, C. & Zeviani, M. (1992): La risonanza magnetica nelle encefalomiopatie mitocondriali. *Riv. Neuroradiol.* **5 (Suppl. 1)**, 25–32.

Savoiardo, M. & Ciceri, E. (1994): La neuroradiologia delle malattie mitocondriali. *Riv. Neurobiol.* **40**, 237–242.

Tzika, A.A., Ball, W.S.Jr, Vigneron, D.B., Dunn, R.S. & Kirks, D.R. (1993): Clinical proton MR spectroscopy of neurodegenerative disease in childhood. *AJNR* **14**, 1267–1281.

Uziel, G., Savoiardo, M. & Nardocci, N. (1988): CT and MRI in maple syrup urine disease. *Neurology* **38**, 486–488.

van der Knaap, M.S., Valk, J., de Neeling, N. & Nauta, J.J.P. (1991): Pattern recognition in magnetic resonance imaging of white matter disorders in children and young adults. *Neuroradiology* **33**, 478–493.

Zimmerman, R.A., Valk, J. & Wang, Z. (1993): Clinical proton MR spectroscopy of neurodegenerative disease in childhood. *AJNR* **14**, 1282–1284.

Chapter 16

Neuropsychological development of children with metabolic diseases

Roberto Militerni, Antonella Gritti, Monica Ghezzi and Giancarlo Parenti

Department of Paediatrics, Università di Napoli, Via Pansini 5, 80131 Naples, Italy

Summary

We discuss some general points related to the results of a multicentre study (Milano–Napoli–Padova) on neuropsychological development of children with metabolic diseases. The simplest level of analysis that can be performed is based on the prevalence of neuromotor, sensory and cognitive impairment. However, a more accurate analysis should take into account many other variables possibly affecting the outcome of patients with inborn errors of metabolism. The current knowledge of neuroanatomy, and possible effects of metabolic diseases on different stages of brain development, is reviewed. These findings are also discussed in relation to parental attitudes and child emotional aspects.

Introduction

The neuropsychological development of infants with metabolic diseases is a very complex field that has not received adequate attention by various researchers. Actually, there are many studies on *long-term evaluation* of such diseases (Saudubray et al., 1982; Matsui et al., 1983; Leonard et al., 1984; Msall et al., 1984; Rousson & Guibaud, 1984; Rinaldo et al., 1987; Berry et al., 1988; Chalmers, 1989; Gatti et al., 1990; Willems et al., 1990; Kaplan et al., 1991; Surtees et al., 1992; Widhalm et al., 1992). However, a study on the neurological or intellectual outcome of a specific disease is something different from a study on the *assessment of the neuropsychological profile* of a child with this disease.

This is not just a semantic issue, but a substantial point, as these studies employ different methodologies. In fact, in studies of long-term evolution only two variables are considered (Fig. 1). The first is the disease; the second is the patient's outcome, expressed as a nosographical label on a nominal scale. This type of study is complicated to the utmost by adding, as a third variable, the effects of therapy (Fig. 2). In other words, these studies underestimate a series of incident variables that can considerably influence the dependent variable chosen as the target.

For example, the intelligence quotient (IQ), on which the diagnosis of mental retardation is commonly based, provides a measure of the cognitive level; however, the IQ is necessarily conditioned by extra-cognitive factors, namely motivation, interest and attention, and is strongly influenced by the current level of language development (Fig. 3). In the absence of other indicators, therefore, we may risk labelling as mentally retarded a child who suffers from completely different problems.

By contrast, studies aimed at evaluating the neuropsychological development of a child affected by

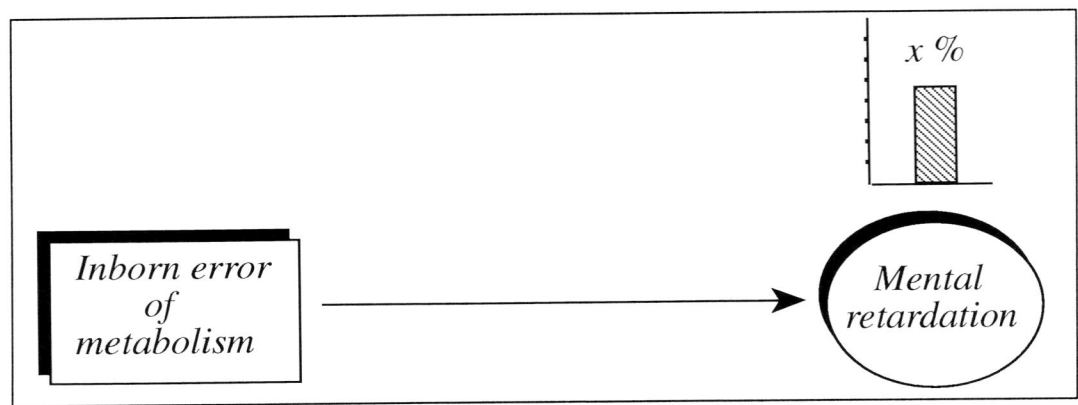

Fig. 1. The simplest model of study.

a certain illness do not use pre-defined diagnostic labels, and try to gather more information about each child over time. This methodology allows us to answer some crucial questions:

– does a developmental profile exist, that can be considered typical of a certain disease?

– is it possible to identify in the neurological or psychological examination single features that could be considered specific?

– and if so, is such a feature specific for a certain metabolic disease or can it be the result of different metabolic diseases?

The goal of the Milano–Napoli–Padova multicentric study for the evaluation of the neuropsychological development of children with metabolic diseases was to provide answers to these questions. The research is still in progress. Here we discuss some of the data obtained.

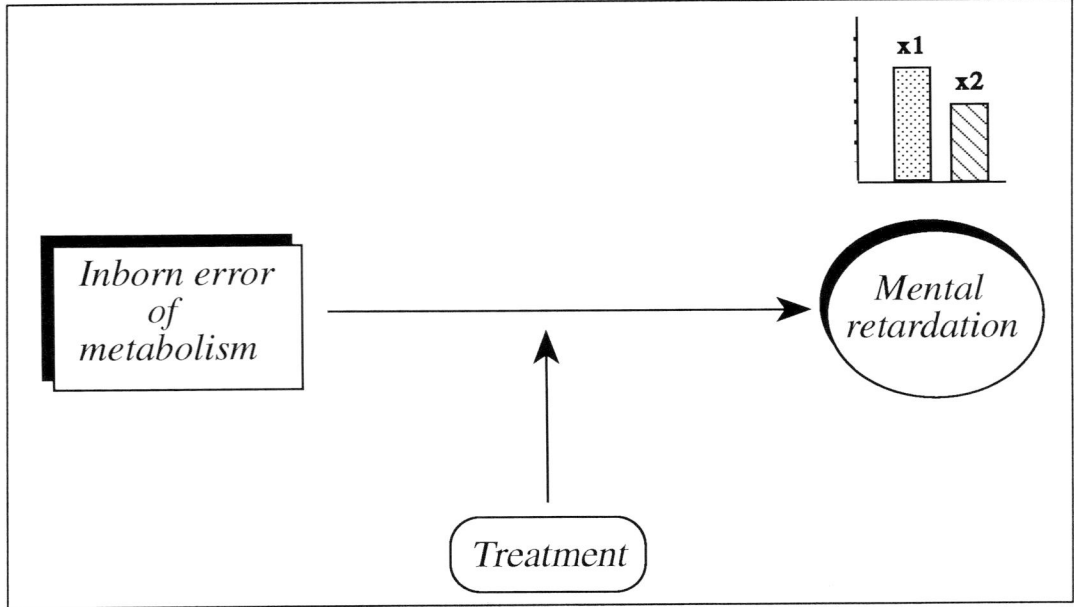

Fig. 2. Introduction of a new variable: the treatment.

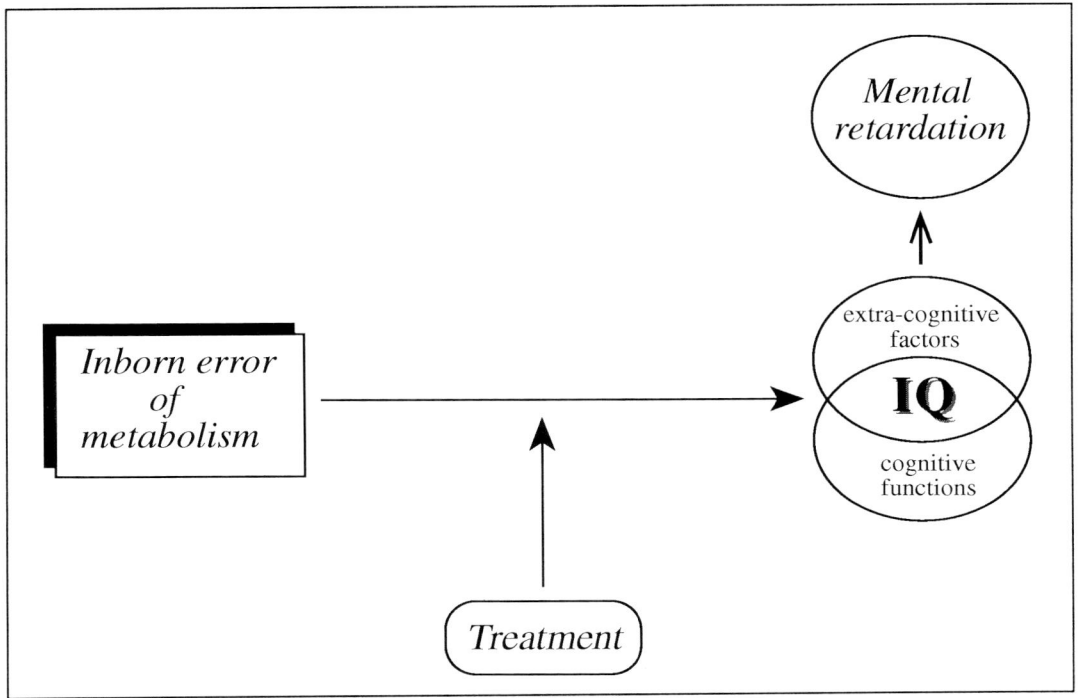

Fig. 3. The IQ as a measure composed cognitive and extra-cognitive factors.

Developmental profile of patients with metabolic diseases

Nyhan et al. (1989) studied five patients with inborn errors of metabolism: two of them were affected by maple syrup urine disease (MSUD) and three by methylmalonic acidaemia (MMA). The authors tried to define the areas of cognition and learning damaged by these disorders. The neuropsychological findings demonstrated deficits in the cognitive/language areas, with interesting individual differences. Furthermore, all the children exhibited very short attention spans.

Nord et al. (1991) described the development of nine children with MSUD. Measures and variables examined included: full IQ, verbal IQ, performance IQ, neurological involvement, speech/oral motor difficulties, school progress and family IQ. One of the most interesting findings was that the verbal IQ was higher than the performance IQ: this difference ranged from 5 to 25 points, with a mean difference of 15 ($P < 0.001$). To understand this finding, one should consider the items that are included in the performance scale of the WISC-R. 'Picture completion', 'picture arrangement', 'block design', 'object assembly', 'coding': all these items reflect some basic abilities represented by visual–spatial perception, visual–spatial and motor integration, fine motor co-ordination, verbal and visual–spatial memory span, etc. A specific fall in the performance scale means a specific difficulty in one or more of these functions (Fig. 4).

These results reflect a trend that we also noticed in our sample. In our patients, the scores on the performance scale of the WISC-R were considerably lower than those in the verbal scale. However, we would like to emphasize that this major involvement was observed not only in two patients affected by MSUD, but in the whole sample, which includes patients with other organic acidurias, glycogenosis and urea cycle disorders.

Moreover, we found that the performance IQ was highly correlated with a number of neurological disorders referred to as soft neurological signs (Tupper, 1987), such as associated movements,

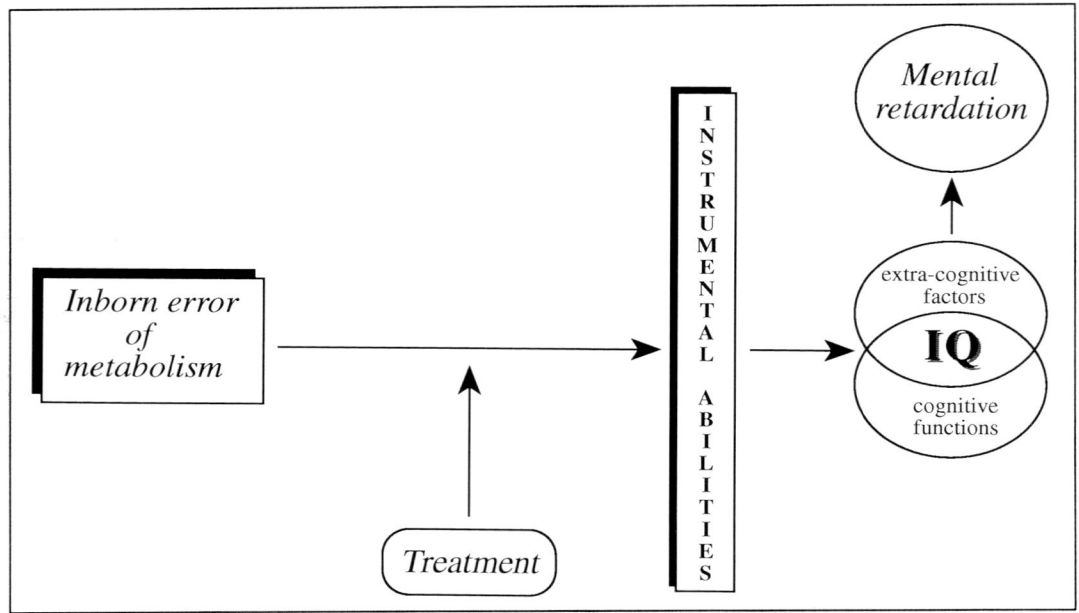

Fig. 4. Introduction of a further variable: instrumental abilities.

immature grasp of a pencil, inability to catch a ball, motor awkwardness, motor instability, dysdiadochokinesis, speech articulation problems, word-finding difficulty, slowness of gait, hand movements, opposing the fingers to the thumb and tapping. In our sample we found a cluster of children with similar patterns of skills and deficits that we would rather define as minor developmental disabilities (Militerni, 1990). These were more frequent than 'major' disabilities, such as mental retardation, psychosis or cerebral palsy.

This finding presents two interesting questions: one concerning pathogenesis, the other prognostic value.

Mechanisms of central nervous system involvement

For the pathogenesis, it looks as if the sequelae were shifted from a major injury towards a minor one. It is possible that early diagnosis and the availability of new therapeutic approaches succeeded in preventing major sequelae, but are not sufficient to protect the anatomic–functional integrity of the central nervous system. In this respect, the concept of minimal brain dysfunction (Wender, 1971) is recalled. However, if one does not want to refer to this diagnostic label for its controversial implications (Rutter, 1977), the idea of a subtle neurobiological impairment appears particularly suggestive, considering the period when the metabolic disease seems to exert its pathogenetic effects (Fig. 5).

Actually, we refer to metabolic errors whose clinical manifestations appear early in development with acute and often recurring crises. The disease represents a 'metabolic storm' that affects the central nervous system in a period of crucial importance for its general development.

In fact, a significant correlation between the age of onset of symptoms and the severity of prognosis has been frequently found in the natural history of different metabolic diseases (Matsui et al., 1983; Msall et al., 1984; Rousson & Guibaud, 1984; Kaplan et al., 1991; Nord et al., 1991; Bellini et al., 1992; Surtees et al., 1992). This finding should be analysed in view of the complex events that take place in the first months of central nervous system development. In gross anatomical terms this

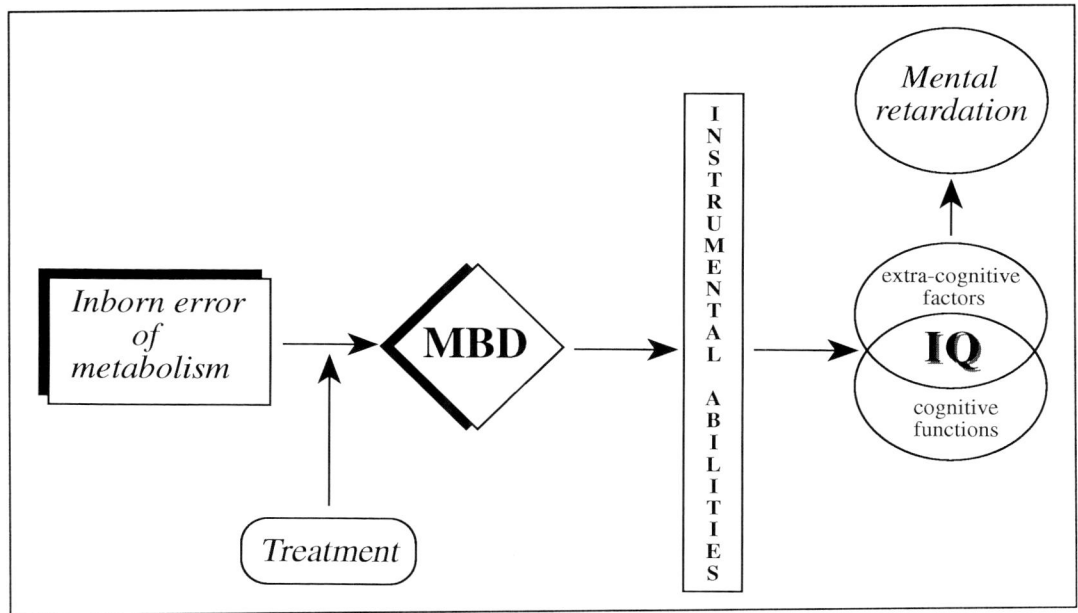

Fig. 5. The minimal brain dysfunction as a neuropathological basis of impairment in ability.

period coincides with the growth spurt (Dobbing & Sands, 1973). It begins at about mid-gestation, when the adult neuronal cell number has already been largely achieved, except for some cerebellar neurons, and ends at the 18th month of life, with a peak in the first months. During this period the central nervous system is highly vulnerable. The sequence of developmental events underlying the brain growth spurt is complex and poorly defined. Glial multiplication, growth in cell size, dendritic branching, synaptic proliferation, and myelination are likely to be involved.

This is the period of the overrepresentation of neuronal cells with exuberant projections, followed by a pre-defined programme of cell differentiation, selective stabilization of synapses and neuronal cell death (Cowan et al., 1984). These latter processes are regulated by a fine balancing of growth factors and cytolytic mediators that eliminate the functionally redundant neurons or those whose axons grow to the wrong target area. A rapidly growing body of evidence suggests that, in the developing brain, the excitatory amino acids (EAA), in addition to their role in neurotransmission, play a critical role both in physiological brain development and in the occurrence of brain injury (Pearce et al., 1987; Hattori & Wasterlain, 1990). Recent evidence has suggested that the post-synaptic receptor activity of the EAA system is more active early in life than in adulthood (Represa et al., 1989).

Clinical indicators of these complex events are the increase of brain weight and the degree of myelination (Dobbing & Sands, 1973). Currently, magnetic resonance imaging (MRI) has established that the normal pattern of myelination follows a predictable sequence, starting in the brainstem and cerebellum and extending superiorly and anteriorly to the cerebrum (Barkovich et al., 1988; Harbord et al., 1990; van der Knaap et al., 1991). Consequently, a 'delayed' myelination (Nowell et al., 1987) represents the expression of a neuronal disorder (Harbord et al., 1990; Fujii et al., 1993).

Therefore, it would be conceivable that an acute metabolic imbalance may adversely affect the cellular functions, initiating a cascade of potentially harmful events. Apart from the gross neuropathological damage (Heidenreich et al., 1988; Andreula et al., 1991; de Sousa et al., 1989;

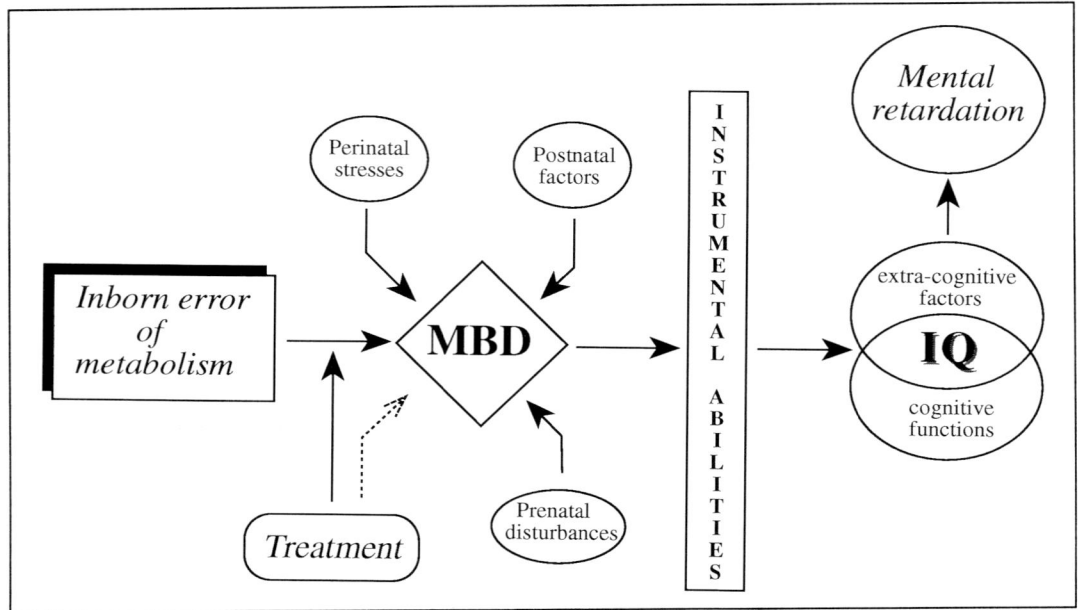

Fig. 6. Associated factors in determining brain damage.

Thompson et al., 1989; Hald et al., 1991; Naidu & Moser, 1991; Kamei et al., 1992; Stockler et al., 1992; Treacy et al., 1992; Agamanolis et al., 1993), evidence from MRI studies suggests that the *transitory* disturbance of the myelination process often found in the first months of life (Amir et al., 1989; Nyhan et al., 1989; Surtees et al., 1992) may be the result of more subtle damages following metabolic insults.

In view of all this, our model is further complicated (Fig. 6).

In fact, the concept of a minimal neurobiological dysfunction implies that possible interactions of many other factors, such as prenatal stresses, perinatal disturbances or postnatal factors, not necessarily correlated with the metabolic disease, are to be taken into account (Farquharson et al., 1992; Gluckman & Williams, 1992; Vannucci & Yager, 1992).

Psychosocial considerations

It has become clear that factors other than the metabolic ones may contribute to the genesis of a basic neurobiological impairment. However, in researching behavioural, psychiatric, or learning disorders, which often have a varied aetiological basis, the need for truly multifactorial methodology becomes obvious.

The risk is that, whatever this child does or does not do, this is *sic et simpliciter* attributed to even a minimal organic defect of which he is likely to be a carrier.

Such a view worries neuropsychiatrists: it is a short-sighted determinism that does not take into account a series of affective–relational factors which play a critical role both in the interpretation of some falls in the level of performance and, particularly, in guaranteeing the future well-being of the person.

In this respect, we would like to emphasize that in a high percentage of the patients examined we found behavioural disturbances such as oppositivity, impulsivity, anxiety, distractability; these

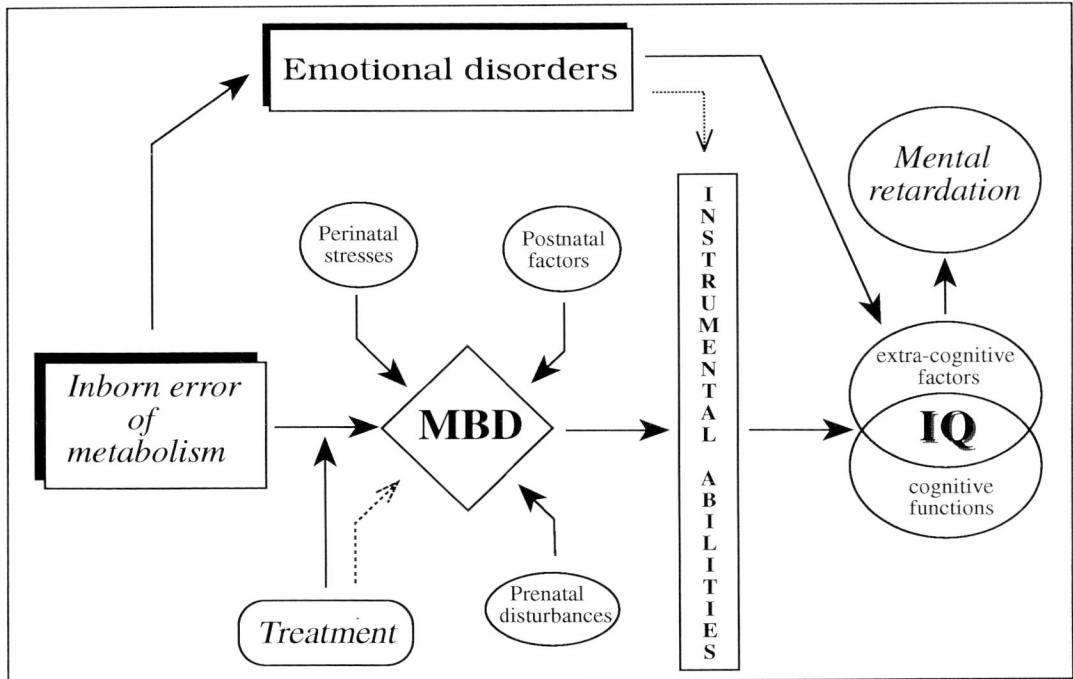

Fig. 7. Introduction of 'emotional disorders' affecting the performance even beyond the level of neuropathological damage.

disturbances were not easily classified into a definite nosographic category (psychosis, neurosis, etc.), but were the result of a generic affective immaturity of a reactive nature.

Our initial scheme, therefore, becomes more and more complicated (Fig. 7).

It would be possible to speculate that the disabilities observed in children with metabolic diseases are not due to a basic neuroanatomical impairment, but are related to these emotional aspects. In fact, it would not be difficult to say that the limitations intrinsically related with the therapeutic protocols, life style and low initiative of the subject are responsible for a reduction of his experiences. The reduced experiences lead in turn to scarce exercising of developing functions, which are hardly transformed into competencies.

For the genesis of these emotional disorders it is necessary to complicate our scheme further by inserting another variable, viz, the quality of parental attitudes (Fig. 8).

In fact, psychodiagnostic examinations based on interviews extended to the parents allowed us to notice the presence of widespread uneasiness in the whole family. Particularly, parents perceive their child's disease as a 'rare' disease, a 'hereditary' disease, a disease 'the cause of which is poorly understood and the evolution is unknown'. This generates fantasies that condition the spontaneity, and quality of the affective–pedagogic attitudes towards the child. Intrafamilial relationships are complicated by a series of contents which impair the child's emotional development. All paediatricians know the importance of the parents complying with therapy.

Moreover, our interest for these affective–relational aspects cannot be limited to an instrumental prospective. Their significance is of a much more general nature. It is necessary to point out that good social adjustment of the patients depends exclusively on their personality structure and then on the quality of their emotional and relational experiences. This is true either if a somatic and

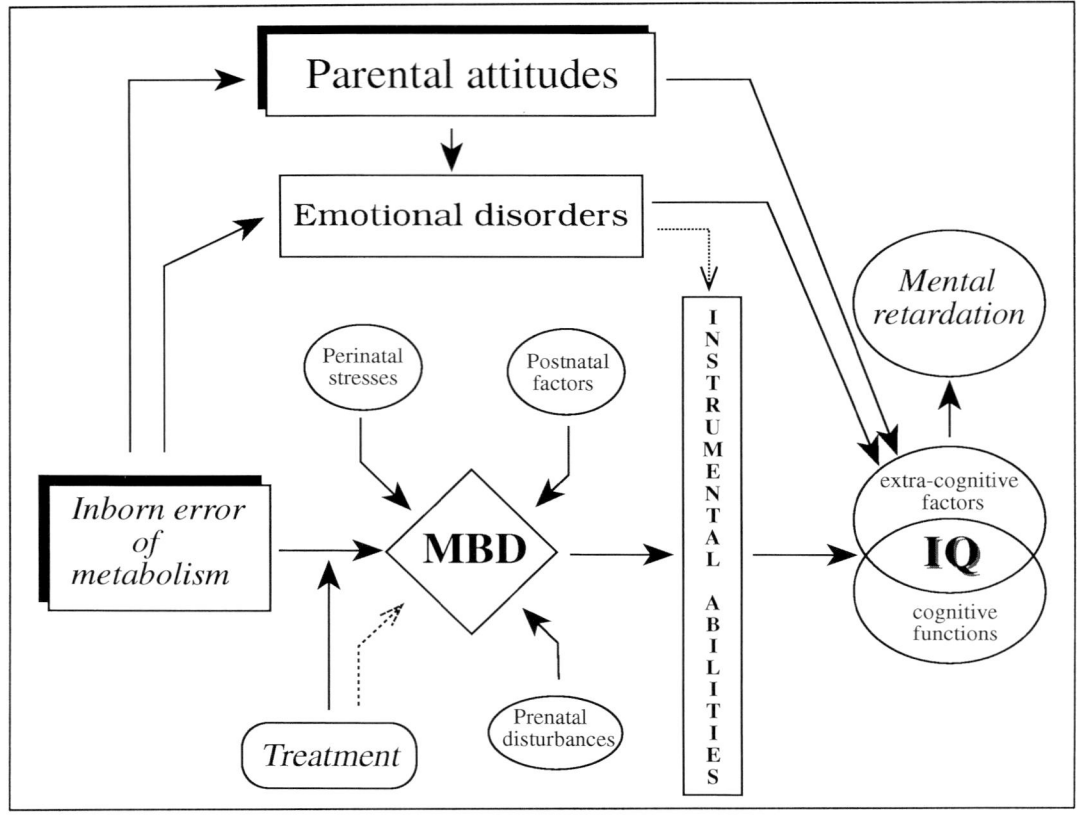

Fig. 8. The crucial role of parental attitudes.

neurological development of the patient is achieved or if, in spite of all our efforts, a disability results from the disease.

Acknowledgements

This study was supported by a grant from the Fondazione Pierfranco e Luisa Mariani, Milan, Italy.

References

Agamanolis, D.P., Potter, J.L. & Lundgren, D.W (1993): Neonatal glycine encephalopathy: biochemical and neuropathologic findings. *Pediatr. Neurol.* **9**, 140–143.

Amir, N., Elpeleg, O.N., Shalev, R.S. & Christensen, E. (1989): Glutaric aciduria type I: enzymatic and neuroradiologic investigations of two kindreds. *J. Pediatr.* **114**, 983–989.

Andreula, C.F., De Blasi, R. & Carella, A. (1991): CT and MR studies of methylmalonic acidemia. *AJNR* **12**, 410–412.

Barkovich, A.J., Kjos, B.O., Jackson, D.E. & Norman, D. (1988): Normal maturation of the neonatal and infant brain: MR imaging at 1.5 T. *Radiology* **166**, 173–180.

Bellini, C., Cerone, R., Boanacci, W., Caruso, U., Magliano, C.P., Serra, G., Flower, B. & Romano, C. (1992): Biochemical diagnosis and outcome of 2 years treatment in a patient with combined methylmalonic aciduria and homocystinuria. *Eur. J. Pediatr.* **151**, 818–820.

Berry, G.T., Yudkoff, M. & Segal, S. (1988): Isovaleric acidemia: medical and neurodevelopmental effects of long-term therapy. *J. Pediatr.* **113**, 58–64.

Chalmers, R.A. (1989): Current research in the organic acidurias. *J. Inherit. Metab. Dis.* **12,** 225–239.

Cowan, W.M., Fawcett, J.W., O'Leary, D.D.M. & Stanfield, B.B. (1984): Regressive events in neurogenesis. *Science* **225,** 1258–1265.

de Sousa, C., Piesowicz, A.T., Brett, E.M. & Leonard, J.V. (1989): Focal changes in the globi pallidi associated with neurological dysfunction in methylmalonic acidaemia. *Neuropediatrics* **20,** 199–201.

Dobbing, J. & Sands, J. (1973): Quantitative growth and development of human brain. *Arch. Dis. Child.* **48,** 757–767.

Farquharson, J., Cockburn, F., Patrick, W.A., Jamieson, E.C. & Logan, R.W. (1992): Infant cerebral cortex phospholipid fatty-acid composition and diet. *Lancet* **340,** 810–813.

Fujii, Y., Konishi, Y., Kuriyama, M., Maeda, M., Saito, M., Ishii, Y. & Sudo, M. (1993): MRI assessment of myelination patterns in high-risk infants. *Pediatr. Neurol.* **9,** 194–197.

Gatti, R., Di Rocco, M., Barabino, A., Pesce, F., Canini, S. & Borrone, C. (1990): Diagnostic and therapeutic approach to hepatic glycogenosis. Report of 36 patients. *Riv. Ital. Pediatr.* **16,** 549–558.

Gluckman, P.D. & Williams, C.E. (1992): When and why do brain cells die? *Dev. Med. Child Neurol.* **34,** 1010–1021.

Hald, J.K., Nakstad, P.H., Skjeldal, O.H. & Stromme, P. (1991): Bilateral arachnoid cysts of the temporal fossa in four children with glutaric aciduria type I. *AJNR* **12,** 407–409.

Harbord, M.G., Finn, J.P., Hall-Craggs, M.A., Robb, S.A., Kendall, B.E. & Boyd, S.G. (1990): Myelination patterns on magnetic resonance of children with developmental delay. *Dev. Med. Child Neurol.* **32,** 295–303.

Hattori, H. & Wasterlain, C.G. (1990): Excitatory amino acids in the developing brain: ontogeny, plasticity, and excitotoxicity. *Pediatr. Neurol.* **6,** 219–228.

Heidenreich, R., Natowicz, M., Hainline, B.E., Berman, P., Kelley, R.I., Hillman, R.E. & Berry, G.T. (1988): Acute extrapyramidal syndrome in methylmalonic acidemia: 'metabolic stroke' involving the globus pallidus. *J. Pediatr.* **113,** 1022–1027.

Kamei, A., Takashima, S., Chan, F. & Becker, L.E. (1992): Abnormal dendritic development in maple syrup urine disease. *Pediatr. Neurol.* **8,** 145–147.

Kaplan, P., Mazur, A., Field, M., Berlin, J.A., Berry, G.T., Heidenreich, R., Yudkoff, M. & Segal, S. (1991): Intellectual outcome in children with maple syrup urine disease. *J. Pediatr.* **119,** 46–50.

Leonard, J.V., Daish, P., Naughten, E.R. & Bartlett, K. (1984): The management and long-term outcome of organic acidaemias. *J. Inherit. Met. Dis.* **7(Suppl. 1),** 13–17.

Matsui, S.M., Mahoney, M.J. & Rosemberg, L.E. (1983): The natural history of the inherited methylmalonic acidemias. *N. Engl. J. Med.* **308,** 857–861.

Militerni, R. (1990): *La diagnosi neuroevolutiva*. Naples: Idelson.

Msall, M., Batshaw, M.L., Suss, R., Brusilow, S.W. & Mellits, E.D. (1984): Neurologic outcome in children with inborn errors of urea synthesis. *N. Engl. J. Med.* **310,** 1500–1505.

Naidu, S. & Moser, H.W. (1991): Value of neuroimaging in metabolic diseases affecting the CNS. *AJNR* **12,** 413–416.

Nord, A., Van Doorninck, W.J. & Greene, C. (1991): Developmental profile of patients with maple syrup urine disease. *J. Inherit. Metab. Dis.* **14,** 881–889.

Nowell, M.A., Hackney, D.B., Zimmerman, R.A., Bilaniuk, L.T., Grossaman, R.I. & Goldberg, H.I. (1987): Immature brain: spin-echo pulse sequence parameters for high-contrast MR imaging. *Radiology* **162,** 272–273.

Nyhan, W.L., Wulfeck, B.B., Tallal, P. & Mardsen, D. (1989): Metabolic correlates of learning disabilities. *Birth Defects* **25,** 153–169.

Pearce, I.A., Cambray-Deakin, M.A. & Burgoyne, R.D. (1987): Glutamate acting on NMDA receptors stimulates neurite outgrowth from cerebellar granule cells. *FEBS Lett.* **223,** 143–147.

Represa, A., Tremblay, E. & Ben-Ari, Y. (1989): Transient increase of NMDA-binding sites in human hippocampus during development. *Neurosci. Lett.* **99,** 61–66.

Rinaldo, P., Zacchello, G., Chiandetti, L. & Zacchello, F. (1987): Follow-up of seven patients affected by methylmalonic acidosis. *Riv. Ital. Ped.* **13,** 66–73.

Rousson, R. & Guibaud, P. (1984): Long term outcome of organic acidurias: survey of 105 french cases (1967-1983). *J. Inherit. Metab. Dis.* **7 (Suppl.),** 10–12.

Rutter, M. (1977): Brain damage syndromes in childhood: concepts and findings. *J. Child Psychol. Psychiatry* **18,** 1–21.

Saudubray, J.M., Ogier, H., Charpentier, C., Manesme, A.O., Coudé, F.X. & Frézal, J. (1982): Acute and long-term management of infants with amino-acidopathies and organic acidurias. In: *Human genetics. Part B: Medical aspects*, ed. B. Bonne-Tamir, pp. 589–596. New York: Alan R. Liss.

Stockler, S., Slavc, I., Ebner, F. & Baumgartner, R. (1992): Asymptomatic lesions of the basal ganglia in a patient with methylmalonic aciduria. *Eur. J. Pediatr.* **12**, 920.

Surtees, R.A.H., Matthews, E.E & Leonard, J.V. (1992): Neurologic outcome of propionic acidemia. *Pediatr. Neurol.* **8**, 333–337.

Thompson, G.N., Christodoulou, J. & Danks, D.M. (1989): Metabolic stroke in methylmalonic acidemia. *J. Pediatr.* **115**, 499.

Treacy, E., Clow, C.L., Reade, T.R., Chitayat, D., Mamer, O.A. & Scriver, C.R. (1992): Maple syrup urine disease: interrelations between branched-chain amino-, oxo- and hydroxyacids; implications for treatment; associations with CNS dysmyelination. *J. Inherit. Metab. Dis.* **15**, 121–135.

Tupper, D.E. (1987): *Soft neurological signs*. Orlando: Grune & Stratton.

van der Knaap, M.S., Valk, J., Bakker, C.J., Schooneveld, M., Faber, J.A.J., Willmse, J. & Gooskens, R.H.J.M. (1991): Myelination as an expression of the functional maturity of the brain. *Dev. Med. Child Neurol.* **33**, 849–857.

Vannucci, R.C. & Yager, J.Y. (1992): Glucose, lactic acid, and perinatal hypoxic–ischemic brain damage. *Pediatr. Neurol.* **8**, 3–12.

Wender, P.H. (1971): *Minimal brain dysfunction in children*. New York: Wiley.

Widhalm, K., Koch, S., Scheibenreiter, S., Knoll, E., Colombo, J.P., Bachmann, C. & Thalhammer, O. (1992): Long-term follow-up of 12 patients with the late-onset variant of argininosuccinic acid lyase deficiency: no impairment of intellectual and psychomotor development during therapy. *Pediatrics* **89**, 1182–1184.

Willems, P.J., Gerver, W.J.M., Berger, R. & Fernandes, J. (1990): The natural history of liver glycogenosis due to phosphorylase kinase deficiency: a longitudinal study of 41 patients. *Eur. J. Pediatr.* **149**, 268–271.

Chapter 17

Multicentric study of a group of Italian patients with metabolic diseases

Paola Vizziello[†], Roberto Militerni[*], Olimpia Caropreso[*], Andrea Pasqui[‡] and Ermellina Fedrizzi[§]

[†]USSL 75/I SIMEE 1, Milan, Italy, [*]Cattedra di Neuropsichiatria Infantile, Facoltà di Medicina, Seconda Università di Napoli, Italy; [†]; [‡]Dipartimento di Pediatria, Università di Padova, Italy; [§]Divisione Neuropsichiatria Infantile, Istituto Neurologico Carlo Besta, Milan, Italy

Summary

We report the preliminary results of a multicentric study on the neuropsychological development of children with metabolic diseases. Fifty-eight patients were divided into four subgroups according to biochemical characterization of the disorder. We have investigated four functional areas: neurological, behavioural, linguistic, and cognitive areas. In our experience, the overall prognosis was disappointing, because more than 50 per cent of patients showed an impairment in one or more of the functional areas investigated. However, these impairments were often *minor*, because they did not assume the features of a definite clinical condition. We conclude that a more extensive follow-up is necessary. Moreover, each particular child must be evaluated from as many viewpoints as possible for the development of appropriate strategies of intervention.

Introduction

Inborn errors of metabolism, certainly rare as single entities, are quite frequent when considered as a group. Over the past decade much progress has been made in defining the biochemical and genetic bases of these disorders. Despite these advances, little is known about the neuropsychiatric aspects. This is surprising if we consider that there is often neuropsychiatric involvement. The few reports on long-term outcome are limited by methodological weaknesses, such as a small number of affected children, the absence of control subjects, and the lack of standardization of assessment protocols. However, these studies suggest the importance of three specific fields of investigation concerning neuropsychological, neuroradiological and emotional aspects.

For the neuropsychological aspects, several patients seem to show deficits in perceptual/conceptual development, with delays in visual–spatial–motor integration, fine motor coordination, and verbal and visual–spatial memory span (Nyhan *et al.*, 1989). Attention deficit disorders are also reported (Berry *et al.*, 1988; Nyhan *et al.*, 1989; Nord *et al.*, 1991). Finally, severe dysfunctions in speech and language development, often unrelated to cognitive or behavioural disorders, seem to be very frequent (Berry *et al.*, 1988; Nyhan *et al.*, 1989; Kaplan *et al.*, 1991; Nord *et al.*, 1991).

Magnetic resonance imaging (MRI) has become an important tool in the study of these diseases (Naidu & Moser, 1991). In glutaric acidaemia type I, MRI has revealed significant frontotemporal atrophy in both symptomatic and asymptomatic patients with white matter abnormalities that are considered pathognomonic of this disorder (Yager *et al.*, 1988; Amir *et al.*, 1989). Specific lesions of the basal ganglia have been demonstrated in patients with methylmalonic aciduria and propionic aciduria (Heidenreich *et al.*, 1988; de Sousa *et al.*, 1989; Thompson *et al.*, 1989; Andreula *et al.*, 1991; Stockler *et al.*, 1992). Some authors suggest that MRI should be performed in all patients even if there are no signs of neurological involvement (Stockler *et al.*, 1992).

Finally, the importance of the emotional aspects is widely emphasized (Fava Vizziello *et al.*, 1991 and chapter 18 in this volume). Nevertheless, an intervention programme for these aspects does not exist.

A multicentric study has been carried out since 1990. It is still in progress. Here, we give the preliminary results for the following factors:

1. assessing the overall prognosis of patients with different metabolic diseases;
2. finding the factors that could interfere with the prognosis;
3. looking for similarities in developmental patterns.

Methods

The Centres participating in the study were the following:

Milan   Division of Child Neuropsychiatry of the National Neurological Institiute 'Carlo Besta'
Pediatric Department of the University of Milan

Naples   Chair of Chil Neuropsychiatry of the II University
Pediatric Department of the University 'Federico II'

Padua   Pediatric Department of the University of Padova
Neuropsychiatry Clinic of the University

For the data reported in this chapter we have selected a sample according to the following criteria:
(1) age at last examination over 2 years;
(2) the availability of complete clinical and metabolic documentation.

A total of 58 patients was studied. The age ranged from 2 to 24 years (mean age 8 years).

The sample was divided into four subgroups, according to the type of metabolic disorder:

Subgroup I = Urea cycle disorders (UCD), 16 patients;

Subgroup II = Organic acidurias (OA), 20 patients;

Subgroup III = Carbohydrate metabolism disorders (CMD), 13 patients;

Subgroup IV = other disorders (Other), nine patients.

Table 1 shows the distribution of the patients according to the type of metabolic disorder and the Centre from which they came.

Table 1. Distribution of the patients by Centre of origin and metabolic disorder

	Milan	Naples	Padua	Total
Urea cycle disorders	13	3	–	16
Organic acidurias	11	7	2	20
Carbohydrate metabolism disorders	2	7	4	13
Other	6	–	3	8
Total	32	17	9	58

We then evaluated the frequency distribution of neuropsychiatric impairment in the whole sample and in each subgroup.

The neurological assessment was carried out with a standardized examination (Touwen, 1979). In addition to the classical examination, well-standardized tests were used to assess general intelligence and abilities in different fields of cognition. The Griffiths Scales and Wechsler Preschool and Primary Scale of Intelligence (WPPSI) or revised Wechsler Intelligence Scale for Children (WISC-R) were administered, according to age. Behavioural assessment was based on observations of child and parent–child relationships, with interviews extended to the parental couple.

We have, therefore, considered four functional areas: i.e. neurological, behavioural, linguistic, and cognitive areas. For each area we have described the following diagnostic categories:

Neurological area

Normal (Norm) absence of any impairment; minor neurological impairment (minNI): isolated impairments such as asymmetry of passive tone, mild hypotonia, clumsiness, poor visual–motor integration which did not cause disability; major neurological impairment (majNI): impairments which interfered with mobility and caused disability.

Behavioural area

Normal (Norm): absence of any abnormality; minor behavioural disorder (minBD): presence of abnormalities, such as anxiety, hyperactivity, inhibition, which do not interfere with a normal style of life; major behavioural disorder (majBD): presence of abnormalities, which cause disability.

Linguistic area

Normal (Norm): normal language development; abnormal (Abnorm): includes abnormalities ranging from speech difficulties to impairments of more complex expressive functions.

Cognitive area

Normal (Norm): IQ score of 80 or above;
Mild mental retardation (Mild): IQ score between 50 and 79;
Marked mental retardation (Marked): IQ score below 50.

Finally, we looked for factors in the clinical history which could interfere with the outcome. After a preliminary study of significance by a stepwise regression analysis we selected five factors, coded in the following manner:

Quality of the delivery

1: normal
2: abnormal

Age at onset of the symptomatology, expressed in days

Furthermore, we have also considered three categories:
Early: with onset below 30 days;
Medium: with onset between 31 and 160 days;
Late: with onset above 161 days.

Age at diagnosis, expressed in days

Severity of the clinical course before the diagnosis

This was evaluated according to various factors such as number and length of hospitalizations, severity of clinical variables, and rates of growth. By these criteria three categories could be considered:

Mild

Moderate
Severe

Quality of the clinical course after the diagnosis

This was assessed referring to the same factors expressed above. The following categories were recognized:

Good
Satisfactory
Poor
Bad

We also evaluated the frequency of seizures, but the assessment of this aspect is still in progress.

Statistical analysis

StatView 512+™ (release 1.01, 1986) was used, and statistics included the t-test, χ^2 testing, one-way analysis of variance, and multiple stepwise regression analysis.

Results

Frequency distribution of the diagnostic categories (Fig. 1)

Neurological area

Twenty-one of 58 patients had a neurological abnormality: 13 had a minNI and eight had a majNI. The subgroup II (OA) presented the most serious involvement: out of 20 patients, nine had a neurological abnormality (six with a minNI and three with a majNI). The subgroup I (UCD) showed the highest frequency of majNI: five of 16 patients had a major impairment. The distribution of the diagnostic categories was not, however, significantly different in the four subgroups ($\chi^2 = 9.96$, ns).

Behavioural area

Only 25 of 58 patients were normal. The other 33 had a behavioural disorder: 20 patients had a minBD and 13 had a majBD. The differences between the subgroups were significant ($\chi^2 = 12.97$, $P < 0.05$). Subgroup II (OA) contained a higher frequency of abnormalities. This subgroup also had the highest proportion of majBD. In subgroup III (CMD) no patient showed any majBD.

Linguistic area

Twenty-four of 58 patients had language disorders. Subgroups II (OA) and IV (Other) showed higher proportions of abnormalities; whilst subgroup III (CMD) had relatively fewer. The distribution of the diagnostic categories, however, was not significantly different in the four subgroups ($\chi^2 = 2.69$, ns).

Cognitive area

Twenty-seven of 58 patients had a global IQ of less than 80: 22 had mild mental retardation and five had marked mental retardation. Subgroup II (OA) showed higher proportions of mental retardation. Subgroup III (CMD) had the lowest frequency of retardation, and none of the patients showed any marked retardation. The differences between the four subgroups were not significant ($\chi^2 = 4.37$, ns).

QIV vs QIP

In 32 patients whose IQ scores were assessed with the Wechsler Intelligence Scales the mean values of verbal–performance IQ scores were compared. Most of these patients showed higher verbal than performance IQ scores, and the mean difference was 5.7 ($P < 0.05$).

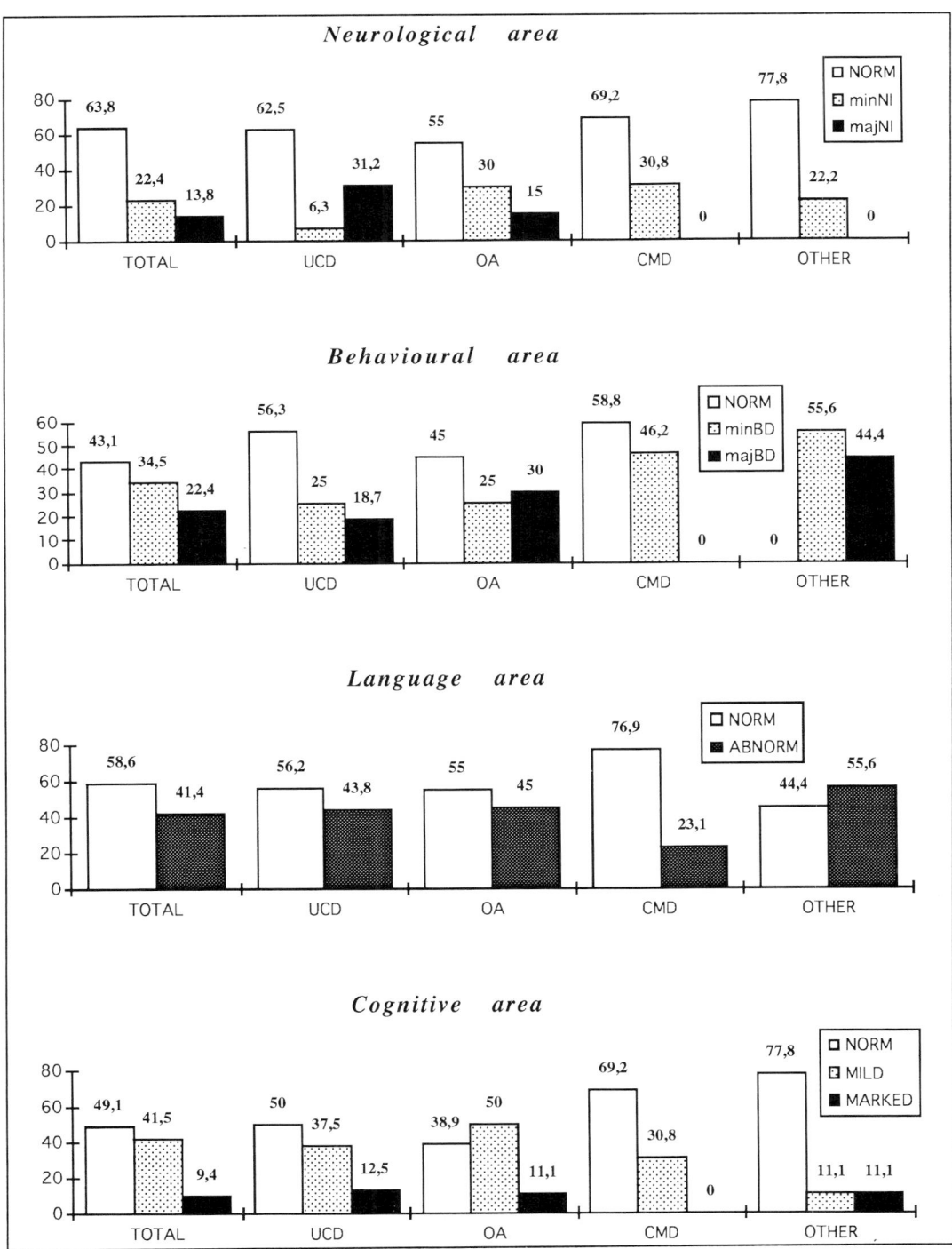

Fig. 1. Comparison of diagnostic categories in the functional areas considered.

Correlations between the functional areas

Table 2 shows the correlation matrix for the functional areas investigated.

Table 2. Correlations between the functional areas examined

Areas	Neurological	Behavioural	Linguistic	Cognitive
Neurological	1.00			
Behavioural	0.53	1.00		
Linguistic	0.61	0.41	1.00	
Cognitive	0.66	0.60	0.62	1.00

The correlation coefficients indicated a high degree of association between all the variables.

Factors related to the outcome

The factors chosen by the stepwise regression analysis were the following: quality of the delivery, age at onset of symptomatology, severity of the clinical course before the diagnosis, age at diagnosis, and severity of the clinical course after the diagnosis.

Table 3 shows the multiple regression output for such variables predicting the outcome of the functional areas investigated.

Table 3. Multiple regression analysis output for variables predicting the outcome

	Neurological T	Behavioural T	Linguistic T	Cognitive T
Delivery	2.22*	1.48	1.86	1.33
Age at onset	1.30	1.82	1.91	2.89†
Age at diagnosis	0.46	1.80	0.54	2.19*
Severity before	2.47*	2.98†	3.16†	2.86†
Severity after	1.31	4.14†	1.81	2.10*
F-ratio	3.70†	6.84†	5.56†	4.68†

* $P < 0.05$; † $P < 0.01$.

The variable 'severity of clinical course before diagnosis' was the most significant: it was related to all the areas. Among the functional areas, the cognitive area was significantly related to many factors.

The 'age at onset' variable was significantly related only to the cognitive outcome. But it had a high degree of association with the severity of the clinical course before the diagnosis: when multiple regression analysis was performed only on those patients with medium and late onset, the importance of the severity of clinical course before the diagnosis was no longer significant.

Frequency distribution of the factors related to the outcome

Figure 2 shows the frequencies of the various factors in the sample.

The variables 'age at onset of the symptomatology' and 'severity of clinical course before diagnosis' showed the highest differences between the subgroups. An early onset was present in 13 of 20 patients of subgroup II (OA), in six of 16 patients of subgroup I (UCD), in seven of 13 patients of subgroup III (CMD), and in none of the patients of subgroup IV (Other). The differences were significant ($\chi^2 = 13.58$, $P < 0.05$).

A severe clinical course before the diagnosis was present in three of 16 patients of subgroup I (UCD), in nine of 20 patients in subgroup II (OA), in one of nine patients in subgroup IV (Other), and in none of the patients in subgroup III (CMD). The distribution was significantly different ($\chi^2 = 20.38$, $P < 0.01$).

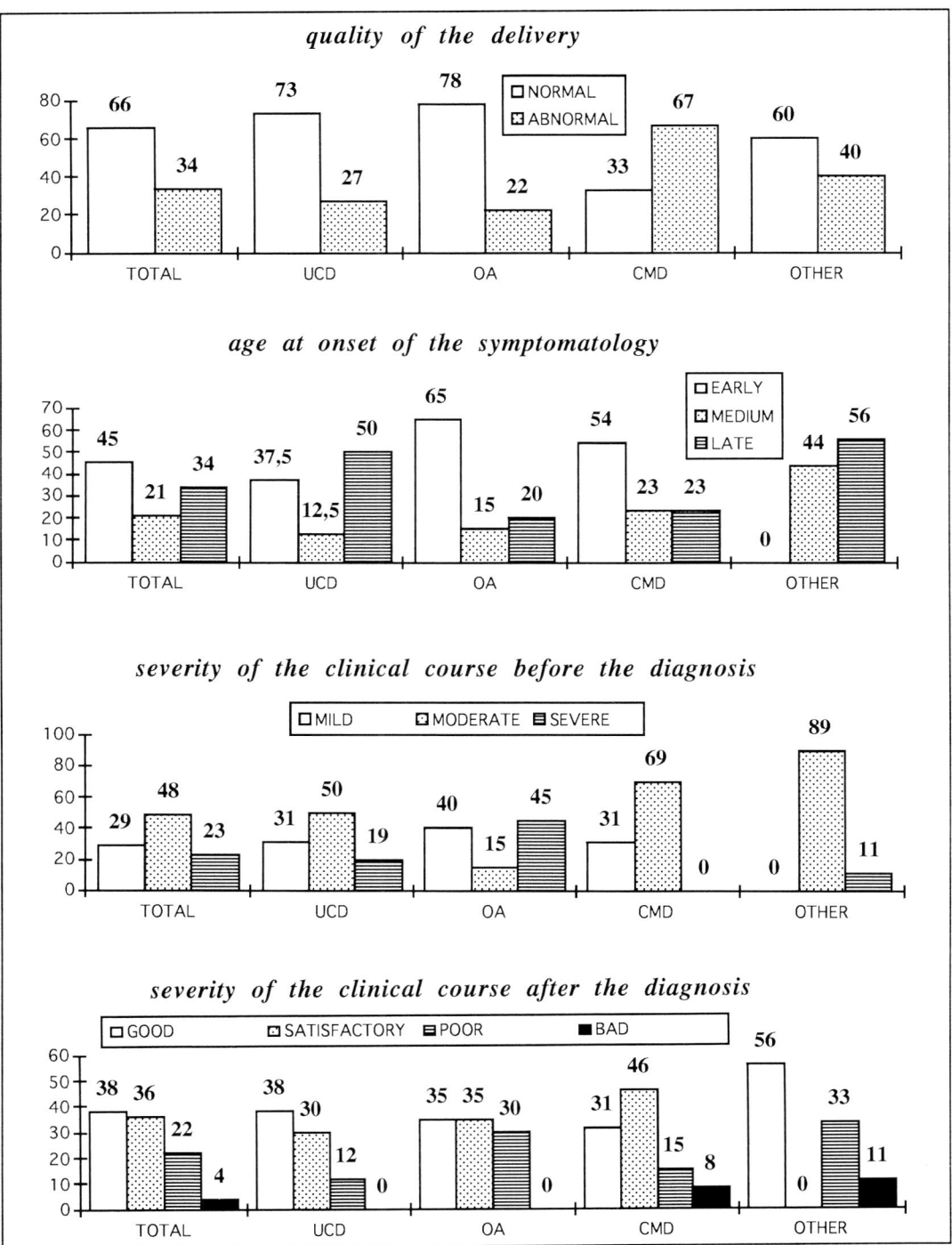

Fig. 2. Frequency distribution of the factors related to the outcome.

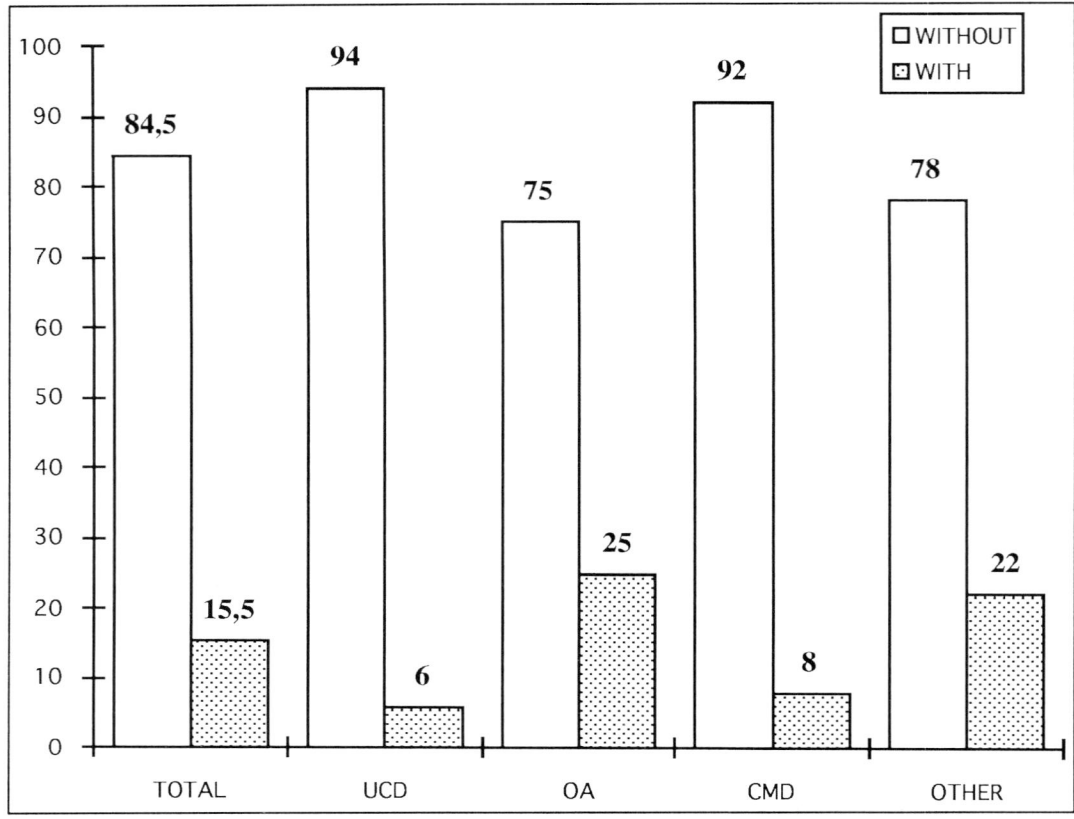

Fig. 3. Distribution of seizures in the different subgroups.

The differences of the other factors were not significant. The mean values of the age at diagnosis are summarized in Table 4.

Seizures

Figure 3 shows the frequency of seizures in the sample. They were present in nine of 58 patients. Subgroups II (OA) and IV (Other) showed the highest proportions, but the differences in the four subgroups were not significant ($\chi^2 = 3.33$, ns).

Discussion

One of the purposes of our study was to assess the overall prognosis of patients with different metabolic diseases considered as a unitary sample or, at the most, divided into four main subgroups. We have found that the outcome was disappointing, because more than 50 per cent of the patients had an impairment in one or more of the functional areas investigated. The behavioural and cognitive areas showed the most severe involvement. In subgroups II (OA) and IV (Other) the outcome was much worse. In these subgroups the neurological area was also very involved. In subgroup III (CMD) subgroup the overall prognosis was much better.

These findings are consistent with other reports (Leonard et al., 1984; Rousson & Guibaud, 1984; Rinaldo et al., 1987; Gatti et al., 1990; Willems et al., 1990; Levy, 1991; Maestri et al., 1991; Andria, 1992; Parini, 1992; Hilliges et al., 1993), but they cannot be used to assess the efficacy of

Table 4. Mean values of the age at diagnosis (in days)

	Total	UCD	OA	CMD	Other
Mean	943	1990	311	576	1016
SD	2028	3475	446	1166	855

dietary treatment. One should not forget that these samples are very heterogeneous not only for clinical and biochemical aspects but also for treatment protocols. Moreover, the inclusion of patients with a wide range of ages results in different treatments related to the changes of therapeutic approaches over time.

A second aim of our study was to find the factors which could interfere with the outcome. Special attention was addressed to the age at diagnosis, because it coincides with the onset of the treatment.

A significant association between the age at diagnosis/treatment and the outcome was emphasized in patients with isovaleric acidaemias (Berry et al., 1988), partial ASL deficiency (Widhalm et al., 1992), and MSUD (Leonard et al., 1984; Kaplan et al., 1991; Hilliges et al., 1993).

Some authors (Levy, 1991; Maestri et al., 1991; Bellini et al., 1992; Hilliges et al., 1993), however, suggested that the metabolic improvement following the therapeutic interventions did not always assure a good cognitive prognosis.

Many other authors drew attention to the age at the onset of the symptomatology and to its severity. A significant association between precocity/severity of the symptomatology at onset and the outcome was emphasized mainly for methylmalonic aciduria and propionic aciduria (Matsui et al., 1983; Leonard et al., 1984; Rousson et al., 1984; Surtees et al., 1992), but also for UCD and MSUD. Msall et al. (1984), in patients with UCD, showed that the length of the neonatal coma was a crucial factor for the outcome. Nord et al. (1991), in patients with MSUD, observed that the variable 'severity of clinical course at onset' was significantly related to the outcome, while the age at diagnosis was not.

In our experience, 'severity of clinical course before diagnosis' was the most important variable: it was significantly related to the outcome of all the functional areas. The 'age at diagnosis' variable showed a significant association only with the cognitive outcome.

The age at the onset of the symptomatology was of little importance to the prognosis, but it showed a significant negative linear correlation with the severity of the clinical course before the diagnosis. In particular, in considering only those patients whose symptomatology began after the age of 6 months, the severity of the clinical course before the diagnosis had a lesser influence on the outcome of all the functional areas.

This close relationship between precocity/severity of the symptomatology and the overall prognosis in such a heterogeneous sample suggests some considerations about the pathogenesis of brain damage. On the basis of such findings one can hypothesize that brain damage is not only a metabolic-dependent effect but also an age-dependent effect. In other words, the immaturity of SNC, that is directly correlated with age, results in a marked vulnerability. Therefore a metabolic disorder produces greater consequences the earlier it appears, initiating cascades of events that often have no other association with the initial metabolic disorder (Gluckman & Williams, 1992). Msall et al. (1984), in patients with UCD, showed that the length of neonatal coma was significantly related to the intellectual outcome, whereas the peak ammonia levels were not. Naughten et al. (1982) and Nord et al. (1991) noted that the severity of the neonatal course of patients with MSUD appeared to be associated with subsequent IQ scores, whereas initial levels of BCAA (branched chain amino acids) and the time necessary to achieve leucine levels 1000 mmol/l did not show a clear relation to outcome measures of IQ. Surtees et al. (1992), reported that the late-onset group of PA showed a better prognosis than the early-onset group, even if the levels of plasma ammonia at presentation did not differ significantly between the two groups.

Moreover, MRI highlights specific findings, such as the abnormalities of the basal ganglia and the white matter changes in several metabolic diseases (Amir et al., 1989; Nyhan et al., 1989; Andreula et al., 1991; Naidu & Moser, 1991; Surtees et al., 1992; Treacy et al., 1992). As Naidu et al. (1991) suggested, the energy depletion brought about by mitochondrial involvement in these conditions could result in neuronal injury from a relative excess of or an increased sensitivity to endogenous excitatory amino acid (EEA). Recent evidence has suggested that post-synaptic receptor activity of the EEA system is more active early in life than in adulthood (Represa et al., 1989; McDonald & Johnstone, 1990). This transient hypersensitivity renders the immature brain vulnerable to pathological excitation of the EEA. The preferential involvement of brain regions, such as striatum, hippocampus, and Golgi cells of the cerebellum, is related to the different distribution of the receptor sites (Barks et al., 1988; Hattori & Hasterlain, 1990).

Therefore, brain damage can be linked to several factors. In our sample, for example, neurological outcome shows a significant association with the severity of the clinical course before the diagnosis, but also with the quality of the delivery. The seizures are strongly related to the quality of the delivery and the perinatal period, but not to the variables associated with the metabolic diseases. It is apparent that additional factors will profoundly influence the final outcome.

The last purpose of our study was to look for similarities in developmental patterns. In this respect, we considered those patients without any major syndrome, such as mental retardation, psychosis or cerebral palsy. Many of such patients showed soft neurological signs and/or language disorders and/or difference in verbal and performance IQ scores of 20 or more points on the WISC (with total score >80) and/or minor behavioural disorders. The frequent association between two or more of such findings suggests the diagnosis of minimal brain dysfunction (MBD). The label 'MBD' has been applied to 'children of near average, average, or above average general intelligence with certain learning or behavioural disabilities ranging from mild to severe, which are associated with deviations of function of the central nervous system. These deviations may manifest themselves by various combinations of impairment in perception, conceptualization, language, memory, and control of attention, impulse, or motor function' (Clements, 1966). But the concept of MBD as a unitary diagnostic entity has been highly criticized, particularly from a psychiatric viewpoint. As Rutter (1977) pointed out 'to put all the different syndromes into the same ragbag is to lose valuable information'. The behavioural aspect is the most controversial, because the existence of a specific 'organic' syndrome associated to 'brain damage' is still in doubt.

In our sample comparable behavioural problems existed with and without neurological symptomatology. This fact emphasizes that soft neurological signs may merely reflect a certain vulnerability of the nervous system, so that the child's ability to cope with his environment in the broadest sense becomes endangered (Touwen, 1987). Although increased vulnerability may well play a role in the pathogenesis of psychiatric disorders in general, specific symptoms come to be defined in the course of the interaction between a particular child and his familial environment. In fact, the psychodiagnostic examination based on interviews extended to the parental couple allowed us to notice the presence of widespread uneasiness in the whole family. Particularly, parents perceived their child's disease as a 'rare' disease, a 'hereditary' disease, a disease 'the cause of which is poorly understood and the evolution is unknown'. This generated fantasies that conditioned the spontaneity and quality of the affective–pedagogic attitudes towards the child. From this viewpoint we must take into account the significant association found between the severity of the clinical course after the diagnosis and behavioural outcome. We can hypothesize that the severity of the clinical course after the diagnosis can interfere with the 'emotional metabolism' of fears, doubts, and distress.

In conclusion, we prefer to avoid any diagnostic label and assess the strengths and weaknesses of each particular child from as many viewpoints as is possible for the development of appropriate strategies of intervention.

Acknowledgements

This study was supported by a grant from the Fondazione Pierfranco e Luisa Mariani, Milan, Italy.

References

Amir, N., Elpeleg, O.N., Shalev, R.S. & Christensen, E. (1989): Glutaric aciduria type I: enzymatic and neuroradiologic investigations of two kindreds. *J. Pediatr.* **114**, 983–989.

Andreula, C.F., De Blasi, R. & Carella, A. (1991): CT and MR studies of methylmalonic acidemia. *AJNR* **12**, 410–412.

Andria G. (1992): Terapia degli errori congeniti del metabolismo: lo stato dell'arte in Italia. *Prospettive in Pediatria* **22**, 191–195.

Barks, J.D., Silverstein, F.S., Greenamyre, J.T. & Johnston, M.V. (1988): Glutamate recognition sites in human fetal brain. *Neurosci. Lett.* **84**, 131–136.

Bellini, C., Cerone, R., Boanacci, W., Caruso, U., Magliano, C.P., Serra, G., Flower, B. & Romano, C. (1992): Biochemical diagnosis and outcome of 2 years treatment in a patient with combined methylmalonic aciduria and homocystinuria. *Eur. J. Pediatr.* **151**, 818–820.

Berry, G.T., Yudkoff, M. & Segal, S. (1988): Isovaleric acidemia: medical and neurodevelopmental effects of long-term therapy. *J. Pediatr.* **113**, 58–64.

Clements, S.D. (1966): *Minimal brain dysfunction in children. NINDB Monograph No. 3*, pp. 9–10. Washington DC: U.S. Department of Health, Education and Welfare.

de Sousa, C., Piesowicz, A.T., Brett, E.M. & Leonard, J.V. (1989): Focal changes in the globi pallidi associated with neurological dysfunction in methylmalonic acidaemia. *Neuropediatrics* **20**, 199–201.

Fava Vizziello, M.G., Bricca, P., Cassiba, R., De Rocco, G. & Zingarello, C. (1991): Disturbi psicosomatici e funzionamento psichico di bambini ad alto rischio neuropsichico ricoverati alla nascita. *G. Neuropsich. Età Evol.* **11**, 231–246.

Gatti, R., Di Rocco, M., Barabino, A., Pesce, F., Canini, S. & Borrone, C. (1990): Diagnostic and therapeutic approach to hepatic glycogenosis. Report of 36 patients. *Riv. Ital. Pediatr.* **16**, 549–558.

Gluckman, P.D. & Williams, C.E. (1992): When and why do brain cells die? *Dev. Med. Child Neurol.* **34**, 1010–1021.

Hattori, H. & Hasterlain, C.G. (1990): Excitatory amino acids in the developing brain: ontogeny, plasticity, and excitotoxicity. *Pediatr. Neurol.* **6**, 219–228.

Heidenreich, R., Natowicz, M., Hainline, B.E., Berman, P., Kelley, R.I., Hillman, R.E. & Berry, G.T. (1988): Acute extrapyramidal syndrome in methylmalonic acidemia: 'metabolic stroke' involving the globus pallidus. *J. Pediatr.* **113**, 1022–1027.

Hilliges, C., Awiszus, D. & Wendel, U. (1993): Intellectual performance of children with maple syrup urine disease. *Eur. J. Pediatr.* **152**, 144–147.

Kaplan, P., Mazur, A., Field, M., Berlin, J.A., Berry, G.T., Heidenreich, R., Yudkoff, M. & Segal, S. (1991): Intellectual outcome in children with maple syrup urine disease. *J. Pediatr.* **119**, 46–50.

Leonard, J.V., Daish, P., Naughten, E.R. & Bartlett, K. (1984): The management and long-term outcome of organic acidaemias. *J. Inherit. Met. Dis.* **7**(Suppl. 1), 13–17.

Levy, H.L. (1991): Nutritional therapy in inborn errors of metabolism. In: *Treatment of genetic diseases*, ed. R.J. Desnick, pp. 3–22. New York: Churchill-Livingstone.

Maestri, N.E., Hauser, E.R., Bartholomew, D. & Brusilow, S.W. (1991): Prospective treatment of urea cycle disorders. *J. Pediatr.* **119**, 923–928.

Matsui, S.M., Mahoney, M.J. & Rosemberg, L.E. (1983): The natural history of the inherited methylmalonic acidemias. *N. Engl. J. Med.* **308**, 857–861.

McDonald, J.W. & Johnston, M.V. (1990): Physiological and pathophysiological roles of excitatory amino acids during central nervous system development. *Brain Res. Rev.* **15**, 41–70.

Msall, M., Batshaw, M.L., Suss, R., Brusilow, S.W. & Mellits, E.D. (1984): Neurologic outcome in children with inborn errors of urea synthesis. *N. Engl. J. Med.* **310**, 1500–1505.

Naidu, S. & Moser, H.W. (1991): Value of neuroimaging in metabolic diseases affecting the CNS. *AJNR* **12**, 413–416.

Naughten, E.R., Jenkins, J., Francis, D.E.M. & Leonard, J.V. (1982): Outcome of maple syrup urine disease. *Arch. Dis. Child.* **57**, 918–921.

Nord, A., Van Doorninck, W.J. & Greene, C. (1991): Developmental profile of patients with maple syrup urine disease. *J. Inherit. Metab. Dis.* **14**, 881–889.

Nyhan, W.L., Wulfeck, B.B., Tallal, P. & Mardsen, D. (1989): Metabolic correlates of learning disabilities. *Birth Defects* **25**, 153–169.

Parini, R. (1992): Il trattamento delle malattie metaboliche ad esordio acuto. *Prospettive in Pediatria* **22**, 211–219.

Represa, A., Tremblay, E. & Ben-Ari, Y. (1989): Transient increase of NMDA-binding sites in human hippocampus during development. *Neurosci. Lett.* **99**, 61–66.

Rinaldo, P., Zacchello, G., Chiandetti, L. & Zacchello, F. (1987): Follow-up of seven patients affected by methylmalonic acidosis. *Riv. Ital. Ped.* **13**, 66–73.

Rousson, R. & Guibaud, P. (1984): Long term outcome of organic acidurias: survey of 105 French cases (1967–1983). *J. Inherit. Metab. Dis.* **7(Suppl.)**, 10–12.

Rutter, M. (1977): Brain damage syndromes in childhood: concepts and findings. *J. Child Psychol. Psychiatry* **18**, 1–21.

Saudubray, J.M. & Ogier, H. (1990): Clinical approach to inherited metabolic disorders. In: *Inborn metabolic diseases*, eds. J. Fernandes, J.M. Saudubray, K. Tada, pp. 3–39. Berlin: Springer.

Stockler, S., Slavc, I., Ebner, F. & Baumgartner, R. (1992): Asymptomatic lesions of the basal ganglia in a patient with methylmalonic aciduria. *Eur. J. Pediatr.* **12**, 920.

Surtees, R.A.H., Matthews, E.E & Leonard, J.V. (1992): Neurologic outcome of propionic acidemia. *Pediatr. Neurol.* **8**, 333–337.

Thompson, G.N., Christodoulou, J. & Danks, D.M. (1989): Metabolic stroke in methylmalonic acidemia. *J. Pediatr.* **115**, 499.

Touwen, B.C.L. (1979): Examination of the child with minor neurological dysfunction. 2nd edn. *Clinics in Developmental Medicine, No. 71.* London: SIMP.

Touwen B.C.L. (1987): The meaning and value of soft signs in neurology. In *Soft neurological signs*, ed. D.E. Tupper, pp. 281–295. Orlando: Grune & Stratton.

Treacy, E., Clow, C.L., Reade, T.R., Chitayat, D., Mamer, O.A. & Scriver, C.R. (1992): Maple syrup urine disease: interrelations between branched-chain amino-, oxo- and hydroxyacids; implications for treatment; associations with CNS dysmyelination. *J. Inherit. Metab. Dis.* **15**, 121–135.

Widhalm, K., Koch, S., Scheibenreiter, S., Knoll, E., Colombo, J.P., Bachmann, C. & Thalhammer, O. (1992): Long-term follow-up of 12 patients with the late-onset variant of argininosuccinic acid lyase deficiency: no impairment of intellectual and psychomotor development during therapy. *Pediatrics* **89**, 1182–1184.

Willems, P.J., Gerver, W.J.M., Berger, R. & Fernandes, J. (1990): The natural history of liver glycogenosis due to phosphorylase kinase deficiency: a longitudinal study of 41 patients. *Eur. J. Pediatr.* **149**, 268–271.

Yager, J.Y., McClarty, B.M. & Seshia, S.S. (1988): CT-scan findings in an infant with glutaric aciduria type I. *Dev. Med. Child Neurol.* **30**, 808–820.

Chapter 18

From communicating to the family to communicating with the family: the process and its discontinuity

Graziella Fava Vizziello

University of Padua, Department of Developmental and Socialization Psychology, Via Beato Pellegrino 26, 35100 Padova, Italy

Summary

This chapter considers the common factors which determine intervention methods for chronic pathologies, such as metabolic disorders, regarded as pathologies of the real and fantasmatic family system, and more precisely: (1) each intervention at each point of the system modifies both representations and relations, and the family offers or chooses a privileged entry point, or forces the members of the team into it; (2) each organic impairment has different values in the child and family: it is therefore worked through at different levels; (3) the family's positive transference is maintained on account of interpretation and decoding of non-compliance and aggressiveness; (4) interventions are determined by the family system, which must be decoded moment by moment, since the quality of the child's life and his very survival depend on its functioning.

Introduction

Metabolic disorders are chronic, organic pathologies, generally of hereditary origin, whose treatment requires the cooperation of the family, which in turn is profoundly modified by the presence of the disease, both in terms of internal functioning and of communication with the outside world. The family, and later the school, is often able to identify signs and symptoms at a very early stage.

Communicating the diagnosis to the family corresponds to the traditional medical model and can only be done at a given moment. Many follow-up studies show that there is a link between the child's survival and quality of life (Manificat *et al.*, 1993) and the way the family handles the illness.

All approaches to chronic organic pathologies that occur at an early and very early age have a number of aspects in common, which we would like to summarize (Fava Vizziello & Stern, 1992).

(1) Intervention is always in a system consisting of real and fantasmatic family interactions. The

position of the operator within the team, his professional role and training will all affect the way of entering the system.

At whatever point of the system we enter (e.g. by acting on real interaction, such as by the introduction of a diet), we also modify fantasmatic interaction. Vice versa, if we intervene in the fantasmatic world (e.g. by verbally supporting the family), real interaction becomes modified too.

The point of entry into the system is not, however, neutral. Sometimes the family offers only one point of entry, as when it is unable to accept the diagnosis and to adapt to a programme, forcing the caregivers to take action and prolonging, for example, the child's stay in hospital. Often the family is the one to choose the member of staff with whom it finds it easiest to communicate.

The very diagnosis modifies the parents' representation of the child and their way of treating him. When parents modify their representation of their child, they are also forced to modify all other related ones and accompanying affects, including representations of themselves, their partner, and their own parents, leading to a change in family and affective transactions.

(2) Any organic pathology, supposing (and this is not always the case for metabolic disorders) that it remains stable over the years, has a different meaning and impact for the child and his family during the various stages of development. It must therefore be worked through at each stage or crisis situation on the basis of newly emerging functions, as shown by longitudinal studies (Fava Vizziello et al., 1991; Fava Vizziello et al., 1992).

(3) Family transference must always be kept positive, to enable the team's help to be sought as soon as a problem arises or recurs, in the certainty of finding a sympathetic ear. This implies that family symptomatology is part of the positive semiotics used by the team, enabling them to understand that non-compliance or aggressiveness may signal a need for help.

(4) The functional team serves as a source of history and memory for the child and his family, too overwhelmed by circumstances to be able to build that *continuity*, which also assures full development of various functions (language, learning, even motor skills). It is likely that many functional disorders are only partially connected with organic problems.

(5) In therapy, what the team decide to do and decide not to do are equally important. This is particularly so in the case of children with metabolic disorders, who are subject to so many interventions.

(6) In most cases, the type of intervention is not usually determined by the child's specific pathology, for which the diagnosis is known, but rather by changes brought about in real and fantasmatic interaction.

The aetiopathogenic, symptomatic and therapeutic polymorphism of the two hundred or so metabolic pathologies (Saudubray & Rapoport, 1985) known to date obliges us to select only a few of the most recurrent aspects, in particular the moments of crisis (Harris, 1990) which all families must face sooner or later:

(1) learning the diagnosis and discussing the implications;

(2) living at home with the child or taking part in specific treatment programmes;

(3) accepting and coping with the start and possibly the end of a diet (Rapoport et al., 1983a);

(4) preparing for school life and handling a wide range of associated problems (Rapoport et al., 1993b);

(5) accepting and living with the gradual loss of certain functions;

(6) eugenic planning (Horgan, 1993).

These crises obviously have different connotations according to the purpose of the considerable restrictions imposed by treatments at various levels (hospitalization, rehabilitation programmes, diets, etc.), with which the family and child must live for years, in some cases always – whether, that is, the treatments are to limit the effects of the pathology, and can therefore be considered an inconvenience which, however serious, will have a positive outcome; whether they are a way of restricting damage to a minimum; or whether they are simply a way of accompanying a child to his death with the least possible suffering or deterioration.

Even this initial differentiation implies predictive capacities which staff do not yet have for all diseases. Owing to new intensive neonatal therapies, for most pathologies we are now starting to have infants surviving acute crises and comas in their early months of life, without knowing what course their pathology will take and/or their life expectancy.

How should we communicate to and with the families?

We should distinguish at least two situations:

(a) acute pathologies which occur unexpectedly in the early months of life, with acute decompensation, leading to immediate hospitalization;

(b) the slow onset of psychic pathologies, with progressive deterioration in intellect and an increase in behavioural disorders, at times accompanied by psychotic organization of personality and/or by the establishment of devastating dysmorphia.

In the former case, having overcome the fear of the child dying, parents above all want to know what his future holds. When staff ask for time to go further into the diagnosis and assess the child's ability to recover after the acute situation, parents closely watch the caregivers' every glance and movement to try to understand what they are looking for. They find it hard to believe that staff 'don't know', or that they know the name of a pathology but not how their child with that pathology will develop. The 'great wait' for answers differs greatly according to relational functioning in the various families, and the intrapsychic functioning of that particular father or that particular mother. Studies by Saudubray & Rapoport which go back to 1983 on three groups of children (23 with typical phenylketonuria (PKU) diagnosed before 3 months of age, 10 with atypical PKU treated prior to 3 months of age, and 14 treated later) show that ability to adhere to a balanced diet during the first four years of treatment does not depend either upon parents' intelligence or on sociocultural environment; rather, it depends on disturbances in the environment, e.g. on marital conflicts and personality disorders in the parents. Reber et al. (1987), on the other hand, found a relationship between a well-controlled diet, good cognitive performance, social skills and cohesion and strong stereotypies of family adaptation. The mothers from the above group of 46 children considered their families to be more rigid and less cultured than mothers in the general population, and the fathers found their families less adaptable.

There is no right, complete way of informing families. The one thing that staff looking after these children must do (in particular, those taking care of bodily functions) is to make time available again and again so that parents can communicate what and how much they have grasped up until then and what they need to discuss differently in order to comprehend fully. In the study by McBean (1971) on how parents experience the pronouncement of the diagnosis, parents clearly describe their 'confusion' with regard to information received at the outset and the difficulties encountered in asking questions about other children. Their tiny baby being in a coma and the announcement of a serious pathology catastrophically interrupt the psychic work, which began a long time before conception in the mind of the individual parent and, later in the couple's mind, on making a home for a beautiful, healthy baby which, despite well-being and beauty, will create problems and aggressiveness by stealing space, time, autonomy and intimacy from the couple. The overwhelming sense of injustice and rebellion caused by the pathology upsets all equilibria achieved, and is coupled with the need to fend off desperation to try and rebuild a representation of the new baby. Corresponding to these early catastrophes is the mother's difficulty in modifying her own representations. This may lead to the most disparate types of behaviour: at one extreme, we have seen parents with a conflictual relationship suddenly unite and run off, leaving the child in hospital; we have seen parents make appointments at other centres to which to take the child; we have seen parents petrified by distress; the emergence in some couples of previously hidden conflict; parents who try to introduce religious rituals into the ward; others who try to talk with everyone to receive reassurance; and ones who get angry with everybody and feel persecuted. Defence mechanisms are infinite while caregivers' ability to understand all of them are not. On the other hand, doctors find it very hard to widen their skills (and often resist doing so) to treat these reactions from a psychological point of view.

A metabolic disorder, like all chronic diseases, is an illness which affects the family; the transactions of the entire family will suffer for years because of it. Often parents are referred to as 'cotherapists', although this would appear to be a contradiction in terms. Parents greatly need to be treated too, even if they lend themselves to providing very complicated care for their children. Burdening them and their actions with the role of therapist means giving them enormous responsibilities, power of life and death over their children, consequently making them even more distressed.

To enable their child to live at home, parents have to learn to take care of his diet, however it has to be administered. But the psychological problems linked with feeding involve the whole family. It is just as hard for a mother to handle a feeding tube as it is for a child to use one, and the child's level of acceptance partly depends on his mother's. Responsibility for obtaining the family's utmost compliance depends on the ability of the doctor, dietician and team to assess what can be done by that particular family at that particular time, and to reassess it at each checkup, as part of a process of accepting the disease and its consequences, which aspects are continually brought into question and which need to be helped again and again.

Cotherapists and members of staff have a duty to control their own drives, aggressiveness, dependency and fear. This is not the case for parents, who have a right to have others help them with their problems and consider them natural, without this making them less important correlates of the metabolic disorder. This is also very important from a utilitarian point of view, as it avoids actions. Aggressiveness, ambivalence and guilt towards their child are felt by parents subjected to enormous stress, though these cannot and must not be analysed or interpreted. Parents need, instead, to be supported and contained, to protect their self-esteem in spite of these feelings.

Often diagnosis of the pathology comes after weeks of stressful waiting and hits a young couple who, during this period, have already imagined very frightening and/or miraculous outcomes to the situation. Only on the child's return home do they realize that one of them will have to give up work, just when the cost of this difficult 'care' is so clear to two very tired, fraught parents, who are not getting enough sleep and feel alone. The child's illness embarrasses and perplexes parents and friends, to such a point that in the months that follow, some old friends fall by the way, radical changes come about in relations with the child's grandparents, and new acquaintances are made on account of the baby's requirements.

Chronic pathologies always bring about these types of change in the social network, with induced relational formalities, whose effects are often harder to bear and difficult to reverse, such as in partial remissions which are almost always accompanied by serious psychological difficulties.

A different group of children consists of ones in which the diagnosis is made at a later date, for example in an attempt to establish a diagnosis on the basis of different psychopathological pictures (learning, behavioural and personality difficulties) which over the years, despite all sorts of treatment, seem to worsen. The defence mechanisms which parents bring into play range from total negation and rejection of any form of intervention, to actual relief and removal of guilt feelings where the psychic pathology had previously been put down to difficult family relations – as though genetics were preferable to psychological responsibility.

The time factor is often essential as initial standpoints change and there may be an opening, with treatment of the child being reconsidered, provided that the team is able to *wait* and take account of internal times. We are in fact convinced that if development of the disease is considered as a whole, psychological factors sometimes need to be given greater importance than physical ones, with a view to enabling better integration of the child.

Diet

One of the greatest pleasures and most profitable educational experiences of the mother–child dyad (or of the father–mother–child triad, where the child is bottle-fed) is represented by feeding.

Feeding, which not only meets the need for food and affection, but also provides an opportunity for organizing a routine, a period of waiting and role alternation, becomes 'controlled', or at times is even replaced by parenteral feeding 24 h a day. The result is, in our opinion, partly to blame for a number of symptoms, which are part of the development of these forms and are attributed to organic impairment, such as language and learning disorders.

Harris (1990) and Rapoport et al. (1983a) state that diets, even when well-accepted, remind parents and child every meal time that the child is ill. The distress brought on by every change in diet is proof of this: 'What will happen if he refuses this food, seeing as there are no alternatives'?

We feel that the distress behind these questions stem from other feelings which the mother has:

(1) of being rejected in the most spontaneous, enjoyable and devoted part of her maternal functions;

(2) of having to introduce her need to give love among the complicated numbers in the diet charts, which could, moreover, be used by anyone else without making the slightest difference;

(3) of being inescapably bound to her child by that hateful diet, which will cause considerable difficulties at each step of the slow separation process which will come about over the years;

(4) of constantly running the risk of forcing the child to make rigid sacrifices which may not be necessary. All this plays a role in compliance.

We know that even the best paediatricians, psychologists or child neuropsychiatrists cannot prevent mothers and fathers from suffering like this. What they can do, however, is help rebuild a life's course in which moments of crisis and second thoughts are seen as necessary, so that they are readily recognized and discussed. Together with the parent, clinicians may also try to build a picture of him- or herself as parent including failure, but which also emphasizes the exceptional investments required of him or her. Nevertheless, it is clear that this also depends on the doctor's ability to assess the risks of an overly strict diet, and to modify it, taking into account psychological requirements, while maintaining those cardinal points which are so important in helping the family feel supported and enabling the child to survive. It is also essential that parents are not considered cotherapists and therefore errors or infringements of the diet should be seen as signals to be decoded and *not* reprehensible shortcomings to be punished.

We would like to draw attention to another problem: whenever the oral sphere is involved, there prove to be problems of identity regarding where the child's needs start and where the mother's end and consequently the meaning of the messages sent out by the dyad. At times it is amazing to see how signals made by the child, which could more aptly be called simple tantrums, are considered to be symptoms of the disease and trigger off complex chain reactions, which tend to worsen the situation.

In these situations it is often more appropriate to adopt a much more active intervention strategy than the one described thus far, with specific aids for decoding the various categories of the child's needs, thereby enabling the parent to meet at least some of them. This work, which starts from concrete interaction observed between parent and child, may also bring about a change in the parent's representation (Stern, 1985). This consequently narrows the gap between representation and the real child and reduces, on the one hand, problems of separation, which are particularly hard from a child who is still unknown, and on the other hand, projections onto him which have an important role in the formation of psychotic personality traits.

What is needed is a therapeutic attitude modulated between waiting, listening and active support. This requires a continuous review of countertransference, especially when it contains and is shaped around free aggressive instances, which all parents have in these situations, but recognition of which is prevented in every way.

The start of school

Should a mother send her child to nursery school, seeing that all other children go? Should he be given school meals? Who should be informed? How much should be explained so that the child is protected, without being considered 'special'? Besides, what is this child, who has made so much progress at home, really like, when his mother compares him with his peers?

The fear that something may happen to the child at school undoubtedly stems from a mother–child relationship orientated around the illness, but it is also a potential reality. It is as though the entire relationship had an ambiguous, confused aspect (Bleger, 1967), requiring more time for individuation, and often help, even when the outcome of the diet is a healthy child.

At as early as 3 years of age, and again at the start of primary school, middle school and high school, comparison with schoolmates often cruelly emphasizes the child's shortcomings with respect to his peers. This not uncommonly leads to varying degrees of depression in parents, who for the first time realize their problems and are forced to consider the future, something the child's succession of needs had previously allowed them to put to one side.

Particularly when the person chosen by the team to discuss the future is not himself able to project a future for the child, the most positive aspect of intervention lies in sharing the distress and experience relating to a time which seems to belong to eternity, or worse, to a time which is rapidly changing.

The child's identity through deterioration in intelligence and other functions

The evolution of some metabolic disorders leads to gradual, inescapable, very painful deterioration in which, despite all efforts, the outcome is negative. The impact of this ineluctable march towards the worst tends to make the family cling to one of the members of staff, whom it chooses as a constant, stable reference point.

At times, the unexpected death of seriously ill, but not moribund, children occurs when the paediatrician leaves the centre. There is a reduction in the parent's social network although there are incomprehensible data provided by some American studies which describe the social network of these families as being increased) and hence in the enormous investment made by the paediatrician, who is often the only remaining reference point in families stricken by misfortune after the nightmare of years of watching inescapable transformations in their children.

Genetic counselling

How and when should genetic counselling be proposed, either to find out whether any other children have problems, or to provide information about the future?

Although most of these pathologies are recessive and therefore involve both parents, their original families often blame the partner in order to shun genetic responsibility. Serious problems often arise in couples with respect to future children who may help compensate for their failure, or who may be feared because ethico-religious beliefs prohibit the use of contraceptives.

Furthermore, the decision to take a healthy child for a checkup, with the risk of having him turned into a potentially sick one after a laboratory test, is very hard to take. It requires a preparation time which is difficult to assess, since working through these complex problems differs from one parent to the next.

Conclusions

Psychological support for families and children is absolutely essential in chronic pathologies, which are in most cases hereditary, with different holding conditions, which change and demand continuous adaptation by the family, and turn all normal caregiving into complex activities that have to be monitored. Nowadays, it is clear that these parents are normal people who have to cope with a seriously abnormal situation. It is not therefore a question of providing for adaptation strategies, but rather of understanding which ones adopted by families present fewer problems in order to help those which present most problems. Sometimes it means helping families with the same problem to meet and mutually support each other, by the exchange of coping strategies and in particular by mutual identification, since they are sensitized to each other's situation.

We feel that the question of who should support the family and by whom this support will be accepted is one of the many which need to be answered moment by moment, in this type of treatment. Investments in the various members of staff (paediatrician, dietitian, rehabilitation therapist, child neuropsychiatrist, and psychologist) change according to the stage of development of the family, the individual parent, the child and his pathology, and the staff's ability to understand, explain and reassure.

That is, we feel that relevant professional qualifications and rank should be limited to professional registers and rolls and should have nothing to do with the needs of these children and their families, who simply want answers.

Hence, if the various professional figures to whom we have referred (and others, according to needs) appear on the staff, their function in communicating to the family can and must vary greatly over the years. At times they should help other members of staff to interpret and programme situations; at others they will help through targeted, focal or long-term interventions. In particular, as far as anyone from the field of psychology is concerned, we feel that psychotherapy is not advisable unless there is close, continuous communication with the other members of staff, particularly those looking after physical problems.

We would like to stress this point since, while doing field work at mental health centres, we have come into contact with children with metabolic disorders who had difficult relations with hospitals. We clearly remember psychotherapies which turned into accusations of families for their child's relentless deterioration, or caused the shelving and denial of psychic or social problems because there was 'an organic disease'. As always, where there is a long-standing illness, there is loneliness and thus a need for contact (Canevaro, 1994) between the interventions that may be needed in moments of crisis. Added to this general aspect are specific characteristics, some of which we have already hinted at.

These aspects are already included in our programme and many others will be added in the near future, with a view to developing semiotics in which the assessment of family functioning and potential communication within it form an integral part of treatment, for the fact is that this is just as responsible for the child's survival and quality of life as management of the initial organic situation.

References

Belger, J. (1967): *Simbiosis y ambiguedad*. Buenos Aires: Paidòs Editor.

Canevaro, A. (1994): Accompagnare nella vita. In: *I percorsi delle dipendenze*, eds. G. Fava Vizziello & S. Pigatto, Padua: Clup Editore.

Fava Vizziello, G., Bottos, M. & Zorzi, C. (1992): *Figli delle macchine*. Milan: Masson Editore.

Fava Vizziello, G., Colucci, R. & Disnan, G. (1991): *Genitori psicotici*. Turin: Bollati Boringhieri Editore.

Fava Vizziello, G. & Stern, D.N. (1992): *Dalle cure materne all'interpretazione*. Milan: Raffaello Cortina Editore.

Harris, J.C. (1990): Neuropsychiatric and psychosocial issues in the care of the child with an inborn error of metabolism. In: *Inborn metabolic diseases. Diagnosis and treatment*, eds. J. Fernandes, J.M. Saudubray & K. Tada, pp. 120–141. New York: Springer.

Horgan, J. (1993): L'eugenetica rivisitata. *Le Scienze* **300,** 80–88.

Manificat, S., Guillaud-Bataille, J.M. & Dazord, A. (1993): La qualité de vie chez l'enfant atteint de maladie chronique. Revue de la littérature et aspects conceptuels. *Pédiatrie* **7/8,** 519–527.

McBean, M.S. (1971): The problems of parents of children with phenylketonuria. In: *Phenylketonuria*, eds. B. Bickel, F.P. Hudson & L.I. Woolf, pp. 280–282. Stuttgart: Thieme Press.

Rapoport, D., Depondt, E. & Saudubray, J.M. (1983a): Le régime de la phénylcétonurie. Aspects psychologiques. *Arch. Fr. Pediatr.* **40,** 265–267.

Rapoport, D., Saudubray, J.M., Ogier, H., Hatt, A., Berges, J., Depondt, E., Charpentier, C. & Frézal, J. (1983b): Devenir psychologique et résultats scolaires de trente-trois enfants hyperphénylalaninémiques dépistés tôt. *Arch. Fr. Pediatr.* **40,** 273–279.

Reber, M., Kazak, A.E. & Himmelberg, P. (1987): Phenylalanine control and family functioning in early treated phenylketonuria. *J. Dev. Behav. Pediatr.* **8,** 311–317.

Saudubray, J.M. & Rapoport, D. (1985): Manifestations psychiatriques des maladies héréditaires du métébolisme. In: *Psychiatrie de l'enfant et de l'adolescent*, Vol. 1, eds. S. Lebovici, M. Soulé & G. Diatkine, pp. 537–573. Paris: Masson.

Stern, D.N. (1985): *The interpersonal world of the infant*, New York: Basic Books.

Chapter 19

Children with chronic disease and their family: a psychoanalytical point of view

Danièle Brun

Université de Paris VII, 66 Boulevard Saint Michel, 75006 Paris, France

Introduction

'I shall never forget how kind you were to me, I shall remember your smiles to all those young children who give you their lives to protect'. The young woman who thus spoke had several times delayed sending of letter to the doctor who had taken care of her when she had cancer in her childhood. 'To write to you', she said, 'means being immersed once more in a past I would so much wish to forget about; thus every time I wanted to do so, I postponed it and time passed'. Introducing my chapter with this fragment of a letter means that I will not speak in terms of optimism or pessimism. I mainly wish to stress the nature of the psychical conflict that may arise through chronic illnesses. Among those, a place should be made nowadays, owing to huge progress in medicine, for cancer as a chronic disease. Furthermore, cancer, as well as chronic and metabolic diseases, involves both parents, siblings and children in various psychical processes which are linked to the evolution of the medical treatment.

The acknowledgement of a debt which is part of the relationship between parents, doctor and child does not exclude ambivalent feelings. To evoke a past such as the story of the illness itself over the years can sometimes promote the expression of this ambivalence which will indirectly include the relationship with the doctor. Such an ambivalence, which is not necessarily aggressive, is caused by antagonistic wills directing the course of the illness. The patient's unconscious will, in which, paradoxically, his attachment to illness finds its roots, is indeed opposed to his conscious will, in the name of which he contracts therapeutic bonds, and greatly seeks recovery, even if he partly knows that it is not possible.

Referring to the Freudian idea that psychopathology is not a mere enlargement of normality but some kind of critical normality, the question of chronic illness must then be analysed in terms of a psychopathology of its processes.

Let us say first that the evolution of a chronic illness should not be summed up in terms of failure or success, nor be inscribed in a kind of secondary position that would be lateral to the compromise which the illness can sometimes represent.

When the causes of inadequacy, from which stem feelings of pain, impotence or contradicted life, are closely examined, in particular when everyday life begins to get better, one is forced to go beyond the sole effect of progress.

If it is true that in the field of mental health one rarely asks the patient to acknowledge that his symptoms have diminished or communicates one's own satisfaction or optimism, one is well aware that the prospect of recovery, however implicit it may be, is indeed present in the therapeutic relationship. In other circumstances – such as autism for example, and despite the constant development of new research on the subject – caution and silence are the rule, precisely because there is no hope of full recovery.

In the medical field the problem is quite different, all the more so when the patient's life has been threatened. Two cases may then rise: either the child is not ever going to improve, or one can hope that his condition may ameliorate even if the illness cannot be finally overcome. To begin with, let us study the second case.

When breaking through his reserve, the physician then tries to be more persuasive. He suggests to the patient that he should resume multifold activities and find a professional, emotional and family environment[1]. It is almost as if a return to health might imply a continuity and homogeneity with a former state. Nobody can actually say whether this state ever existed or whether it is the result of a construction built in the course of the illness, a construction which the physician could have been requested to share and to which he would implicitly have agreed.

Here is a conjecture whose contradictions are clearly evident in cases of recovery from cancer, which I know rather well. The medical knowledge imparted to the patient functions for him as a revelation of the fact that he had deluded himself with demands for recovery, often reiterated. His delusion derives mainly from his state of being which he finds to be unsatisfactory.

Announcing that there has been a recovery leads the doctor to talk about the illness in the past tense and to take for granted a symbolic elaboration which is far from being achieved spontaneously. For if, on a practical level, such a recovery represents the outcome of constant efforts to obtain it, the multiplicity of the reactions it induces leads to further thoughts according to the three points of view which Freud found essential: that is to say, the topical, the economic and the dynamic.

Remaining, at first, on the level of description, one should note that the reactions against the knowledge of a chronic illness can lead the relationship between the parents, the child and the physician into an unusual conflict of opposed forces. Notwithstanding their varied forms of expression, such reactions aim at opposition. It looks as if the patients and their families feel unable to take the physician at his word. In the case of children who recover from cancer, for example, one sees parents building up a mistrustful attitude towards the future. One sees them insisting on telling the physician about irrational and unjustified fears of relapse, of metastasis, or the appearance of a new stage of the illness sooner or later. And, however confident or buoyant they try to look, they cannot believe, deep down inside, that their child will have the opportunity to choose his own way of life in the future.

Such a reversal is also the expression of a crisis entailed by the differing effects of the trauma

---

1 On that topic, Maurice Tubiana writes: *'Il faudrait, dès le début de la maladie, préparer cetter reconversion vers la santé, et les trop longs arrêts de travail, quand ils ne sont pas imposés par l'état physique, favorisent un repli sur soi générateur d'anxiété [...]. De plus, ce ralentissement s'accompagne d'un besoin d'hyperactivité, d'une sorte d'hypervigilance, comme si les anciens malades voulaient constamment contrôler tout ce qui les concerne* ('One should, at the very beginning of a illness, start to prepare the patient for this readaptation to health and in this sense sick leave from work, when it is not imposed by the patient's physical state, tends rather to encourage introversion which in its turn produces anxiety [...]. Moreover, the slower pace of life brings a need for hyperactivity, a sort of excessive vigilance, as if people who have once been ill constantly wanted to control all that touches them'). Tubiana, M. (1977): Le refus du réel, p. 278. Paris: Robert Laffont.

trauma following the threat of death. But when we say this, we do not in any way solve the problem of the apparent illogicality of the reactions at stake which belong to a certain psychical functioning that is far less exceptional than it seems at first.

The surprise these reactions entail does not allow one to ignore any longer the heterogeneity existing between the demand for care and the illusory satisfaction created by the wish to recover in its very ambiguity. One is thus forced to take into account a new logic revealed by the crisis, springing from any improvement of the chronic illness itself. Parents and child are then in the situation of having to make the disabilities coming from the outside world their property. In other words, they have to cope with various forms of sequels, and none of them ever suspected the psychic processes which are here involved.

This picture does not gain from a confrontation with the criterias of the norm, of normality or of anomaly. On the contrary it stresses in a more essential way the originality of psychopathology of a chronic illness.

The paradoxes of the processes of chronic illness

Some authors have already listed the paradoxes inherent in chronic illness. These have not however been used to understand psychic life as a whole, as a psychic capital so far unexploited and in a close relationship to the life of the body. Jean Starobinski's work[1], entitled *Remedy in Evil*, enables us now to state the problem more precisely in terms of chronic illness processes and their psychopathology. The title, borrowed from Jean-Jacques Rousseau, defines a major theme in his life, thought and work. According to Starobinski, it is appropriate given the circumstances of the writer's birth, as described in his *Confessions*. Here is a short passage:

> *Je naquis infirme et malade; je coûtai la vie à ma mère, et ma naissance fut le premier de mes malheurs ... J'étais né presque mourant; on espérait peu de me conserver. J'apportai le germe d'une incommodité que les ans ont renforcée, et qui maintenant ne me donne quelquefois des relâches que pour me laisser souffrir d'une autre façon.*
>
> (I was born handicapped and sick; my birth cost my mother her life, and it was the first of my misfortunes ... I was born almost dead; there was little hope I would survive. I brought the seed for a discomfort which was strengthened through the years and which now releases me only when I am to suffer in another way.)

Starobinski adds:

> *Il importe à Rousseau de pouvoir dire dans un même souffle le sauvetage initial et le crescendo implacable du mal apporté en naissant.*
>
> (It is important for Rousseau to voice in the same breath both the initial rescue and the fatal crescendo of evil that accompanies birth.)

Moving on in his commentary on the *Confessions*, Starobinski never misses an opportunity of underlying the narcissistic advantages which Rousseau found in the feeling that he would soon die[2]. And he stresses the sadomasochistic alternatives that he believes to be inseparable from Rousseau's philosophy. Starobinski strongly insists on this point, only finding at the end of his paper the reasons for such an emphasis.

A few weeks before his death, at Easter 1778, Rousseau gave an account of one of his last day-dreams which, as he reminds us, was dominated by the presence of 'maman'. The atmosphere of this final day-dream, at last peaceful, is liable to induce perplexity. And one sees Starobinski

---

1 *Starobinski, J. (1978):* Nouvelle revue de psychanalyse, *no. 17, pp. 251–74. Paris, Gallimard.*
2 *One should note that the same causes do not always produce the same effects for such was also Goethe's case: he was thought to be dead when he was born. See Goethe J.W.,* Dichtung und Wahrheit, Goethes Werke, Hamburger Ausgabe, Christian Wegner Verlag, 1960.

linking the word '*maman*' with the 'I was born almost dead' written on the first pages of the *Confessions*, interpreting this final day-dream in terms of 'he died almost cured'. Thus he concludes with the hypothesis that the life forces are irrigated by the very source that also nourishes the opposing force that once threatened them.

Not settling for a mere obliteration of the illness, he adds, is the unquestionable economy of Rousseau's attitude, whose work bears a living stamp, all the more I might add, as this illness comes from childhood. Thus the strength and the infallible nature of the image of a mother–child couple cemented by the death threat (and which Starobinski finds constantly latent in Rousseau's work) give us here a perfect example of what neither the growing child nor his mother will probably ever want to give up. Anyway they often fail to untie the unconscious knot of representations which keep their faithfulness and bond to this fantasmatic couple. Psychotherapeutic work with children and mothers, as much as collaboration with paediatricians, find here their entire justification.

When the death threat imposes itself as a reality, one is led to believe that it introduces a split between bodily and psychic life. Thus, value judgements and the acknowledgement of the discrepancy with the norm overtake the reference to the unconscious. Ignoring the silent workings of the unconscious deprives the clinical approach, and leads it either towards anecdote or towards specific diagnosis.

Thus one should not only take into account the effects of a death threat in its psychological components, even when pondering upon what we normally call our 'relationship to death'. To be heard in its demands, and not simply in its apparent negative critical dimension, our present proposition requires, symmetrically, a brief presentation of the psychopathology of chronic illness processes.

Specifics of the psychopathology of chronic illness

Considering both its methodological and research aspects, the psychopathology of chronic illness processes cannot be reduced to psychological disorders or transient symptoms which we know are linked with some somatic illnesses and sometimes recoveries. Likewise, the specifics of this psychopathology are not to be found in demands for the newest treatments or for specific surgery which, although it can be achieved by the miracles of medicine, has unsuspected psychic costs.

As far as organic physiological shortcomings are concerned, one witnesses a growing demand for results[1]. Any reference to the subject must be accompanied by the appropriate saving gesture. Whether in the field of a disease that could be neonatal, or lethal, or involving sterility, grafts and transplants, one has to face up to the blossoming of a psychopathology of chronic illness processes against a background of deceit and dissatisfaction.

If it would indeed be superficial to consider such a psychopathology as being a neocreation ascribable to the progress of science, we should however admit that the latter does participate in the sense that such manifestations become more and more present and diversified. Yet, the dialectics of request and reply, even when analysed in terms of its internal and external dynamics, is not sufficient to define and stress the differences of opinions between the physician and the psychopathologist. For the physician illness remains a dysfunction and it is very difficult for him to admit that a return to order, that is to say remission of the illness, progress or recovery, should produce disorder.

Using the works of Goldstein & Leriche, Georges Canguilhem in *The Normal and the Pathological*[2]

---

1 Here is a theme for which I tried to retrace the numerous effects within a study entitled 'L'envie du vagin' taking into account the complexity of the processes linked with recovery from cancer. See Brun, D. (1990): La maternité et le féminin, Ch. 3. Paris: Denoël.

2 Canguilhem, G. (1972): The normal and the pathological, p. 128. Paris, PUF

stresses the link between the medical position and the Bergsonian theory of disorder. As Bergson said:

> *Il n'y a pas de désordre, il y a substitution à un ordre attendu ou aimé d'un autre ordre dont on n'a que faire ou dont on a à souffrir.*
> (Disorder does not exist; what happens is that a familiar order, to which we are attached, is replaced by another order which we do not care about at all and which only makes us suffer.)

This sentence is heavy with implications about chronic illness and the inadequacy of what it brought compared to the hopes which remain in the parents' thoughts. Such a different approach opens up new territories and fields for action: this does not in any way hinder close collaboration between medicine and psychoanalysis. What the former aims at eradicating is at the centre of the latter's quest to listen to the parents and child's own story and creation. This is the moment for a therapeutic demand that the problem be examined first in its specific aspects and then in its general dynamics. These various aspects help in the understanding of the functioning and the cohesion of all the new associations of people with diabetes, cystic fibrosis and grafts or transplants, in the midst of which these people regain a new identity.

Hence I wish to concentrate on the narcissistic aspect of the child's illness with their consequences on the parents, brothers' and sisters' minds rather than the objective aspect of the illness. Neither the presumption nor the existence of deadly and murderous maternal attitudes, nor the reference to death wishes, are able to justify, I believe, a plain causal interpretation.

When, after a handicap, a malformation or a serious illness, parents focus their attention on their child, they are unable to appreciate that their solicitude also belongs to the world of fantasy. Indeed, they are not in a position to acknowledge repressed death wishes from their own childhood which, as one knows, are the wishes which meet with the most important resistance. In order to escape censorship and avoid repression, these wishes tend to remain hidden behind the 'worry that becomes active during the day'[1]. It is obvious that the parents' reactions come in answer to unconscious motives and that it would be an error to think they are exclusively aimed at the real child. This is why I feel that those who attempt to make the mothers responsible have opted for a static approach rather than a dynamic one. In this sense, what one begins to think or feel through seeing the wounded mother's face would probably be more adequate.

Regarding the relational and transferential impact of the identification with a child in danger, major aspects of it come from the silent work of mourning a defective child.

Yet it is impossible to ascribe the long-lasting effects of such a trauma only to the reality of the event called 'illness'. Neither is it possible, unless one refers exclusively to the external reality, to assimilate the instant of the trauma to the very trauma itself. This kind of reference would wipe out the transposition of the illness within the psychic reality.

The psychotherapeutic technique, in such circumstances, does not mean using the 'representation of the child given up as dead' as a vehicle for interpretation but as a theme which may induce therapeutic instruments and enable numerous omnipresent but forbidden thoughts to escape from exile and to find a place in a specific psychotherapeutic space.

Dynamic aspects of the chronic illness situation

The dynamic aspects of the chronic illness situation deal with the characteristics of three kinds of transformations which take place in the course of the illness irrespective of its outcome. These

---

1 *Cf. Freud S. (1967):* L'interprétation des rêves (The interpretation of dreams), *p. 232. Paris, PUF. SE, IV, p.267. This passage is quoted and commented on in Brun D. (1989):* L'enfant donné pour mort (The child given up as dead), *Ch. 4. (L'interruption d'une lignée) and Ch.10. (La scène onirique de la maladie mortelle). Paris: Dunod.*

transformations can be gathered into three different categories. They refer to the relationship regarding knowledge, objects of love and a sense of time. The general impression is that they do not become conscious. It rather seems as if their influence spreads in an indirect manner. The contradictory reactions of doubt, of dissatisfaction and incredulity which I have formerly described are evidence of this influence. Nevertheless, one should not refer such paradoxes to a mere anticipating illusion – in which the physician would also be engaged – of shared satisfaction and coherence between what is expected and what is obtained.

Convinced that he has communicated to the patients and their families the information he had at hand, in terms which he chooses to be understandable, the physician believes that such a direct explanation can resist the influence of a fantasy potential. It is the same for the idea of death, though he is well aware of its tenacity because of the very recurring power of illness. Thus he neglects the 'cognitive' value of the news or of the information he may give during the illness. One should indeed use the term 'cognitive' since the information conveyed, from the outside, is knowledge clad with the weight of medical authority.

This authority ratifies, confirms and embodies an inner knowledge which is hard or impossible to impart or communicate. This inner knowledge is peculiar because close family members and patients gather it silently during the illness. And they feel that, in doing so, they, in a way, are transgressing the forbidden. Thus it is easier to understand why the medical information forces the partners to an act of ownership of their own morbid thoughts. They thought that death was close, even though they did their best for it not to be known and not to happen. Hence they try to go through with the mourning for an object they love, which they should consider as dead although still living. This interior and idealized object can no longer coincide with the real one. Thus, they feel guilty as if they had committed an offence towards the living child, towards themselves and others. Besides, the living presence of the real child leads them to discover that any previous attempts to make the real object and the fantasized one coincide is regularly bound to fail.

This point leads me to the third transformation created by long-lasting illnesses, that of the relationship to time. Many children who have been seriously ill move without any transition from childhood to adulthood without knowing or experiencing the pangs of adolescence. Isolated from their peers, they grow mature artificially. The adults also find that they have lost contact with their contemporaries, as far as time, ideas, and ideology are concerned, and they suffer from this. Despite the knowledge they acquired during the illness, they continue to widen the gap which separates them from the others because their sense of values has been altered. On the other hand, they never lose their vigilance towards the slightest sign coming from the injured body, neither are they afraid of being more learned or more pessimistic than their physician.

Others, on the contrary, such as certain children who have become adults, decide to behave as if nothing has happened, thus hoping they will convince themselves that the illness was none of their business but was their parents'. Almost as if to dismiss the disease from their thoughts they create a misleading symbolic split with their own parents. This split is all the more illusory in that the patient sometimes forgets to take care of himself and no longer thinks about his own safety. This is a proof of the enormous psychic impact of such transformations, which can also weaken everyday life.

One cannot avoid mentioning the new reshuffling of the distribution of the narcissistic economy, that is to say of defences, adaptation and mechanisms which cope more or less with the illness or with any lethal deficit. I am thinking, in particular, of procreation techniques, grafts and transplants involving either life received, or life to be kept or be given.

All things considered, the course of the illness reveals in an almost experimental way the polemical and dynamic concept of normalization which Georges Canguilhem criticized as 'negatively qualifying that sector of data which is concerned with extension rather than comprehension'. Thus, weakening or frailty, however denied it may be, cannot possibly be separated from an internal and external demand for normalization. And frequently the uncertainty concerning the future counterbalances the certainty of a diagnosis which continues, in an almost fetishistic way, to be acknowledged in its reality and at the same time denied.

Regarding the development of a multifold psychopathology, one should focus attention, among other manifestations, on the fear of change, the approach to the future and the aspect which I have called a resistance to oblivion[1]. All of them are concerned and none of them should be underestimated.

To conclude, let us refer to the question of mourning which is part of the illness and its differed action.

Let us for example mention here weaning the patient from the relationship with the physician. Whatever the words uttered to justify the less frequent appointments, patients and their relatives believe it means 'I am leaving you'. However one-sided it may seem, the motto is adequate for illustrating the difficulties one meets in psychotherapy with these patients. Whether one has to deal with patients themselves or with healthy relatives who accompanied them during the illness, the psychotherapy enhances a feeling of emptiness comparable to the breaking up of a close relationship. That is to say that psychotherapeutic work reveals the attachment to the physician as being one figure of the lost narcissistic image of the perfect child.

As far as methodology is concerned, the different phases of this study have enabled epistemological and methodological reflection on the instruments which help both paediatricians and psychoanalysts to think about their work in a close collaboration.

---

1 One may refer to the chapter dealing with this problem in Brun, D., L'enfant donné pour mort, *op. cit.*

Chapter 20

Genetic counselling and prenatal diagnosis

Faustina Lalatta

Laboratorio di Citogenetica, Istituti Clinici di Perfezionamento, via Commenda 9, 20122, Milan, Italy

'The objective of medical genetics is to help people with a genetic disadvantage to live and reproduce as normally as possible' (WHO Advisory Group 1985).

Summary

Genetic counselling involves communication following a genetic diagnosis. It refers to the occurrence and the risk of recurrence of a genetic disorder in an individual or in a family. To make or to review the diagnosis, apart from taking the medical history, the necessary physical and laboratory examinations and the calculation of risk, is an essential part of the counselling process. It is now widely recognized that the purpose of genetic counselling is not only to prevent genetic disease but to help the patient decide what to do with the information provided. In the past 20 years, with the advent of prenatal testing, the practice of medical genetics has evolved towards a more comprehensive service which includes discussion and support during pregnancies at risk. Specific knowledge of the technical aspects of prenatal procedures and the risks involved are necessary, even for clinical geneticists to help the patient in the decision-making process. An accurate diagnosis is crucial in identifying precise prenatal tests. Traditional laboratory investigations are now supported by more sophisticated methods of recognizing mutations. Molecular cytogenetics and molecular biology already play a major role in ascertaining genetic risks. An increasing number of genetic diseases can be diagnosed during pregnancy in time for the option of selective abortion, and some can be detected in early infancy in time for successful treatment. The selection of foetuses affected by serious genetic disorders through prenatal diagnosis and consequent termination of pregnancy cannot be considered a valid goal; strategies for the *in utero* treatment of these diseases must be developed. A combination of systematic checking, the maintenance of a genetic register and the offer of genetic testing to those at risk, forms the basis of a comprehensive prevention programme.

Introduction

With the increasingly successful control of environmentally caused illnesses in the developed world, diseases which are either wholly or partly genetically determined have assumed a far more prominent role in childhood illness and mortality.

Genetic diseases and congenital malformations occur in approximately 3 to 5 per cent of live births. (Table 1) (Weatherall, 1991).

Table 1. The total load of genetic disease

Type of genetic disease	Frequency per 1000 population
Single gene	
– Dominant	1.8–9.5
– Recessive	2.2–2.5
– X-linked	0.5–2.0
Chromosome abnormalities	6.8
Common disorder with significant genetic component	7–10
Congenital malformations	19–22
Total (approx)	37.3–52.8

From Weatherall (1991).

Many are associated with chronic and distressing mental or physical handicaps or both. Table 2 shows the classification of congenital anomalies and estimates of the total disability caused (Modell & Modell, 1992).

Table 2. Congenital anomalies: classification and estimate of total disability generated annually in Europe

Category of defect	Births/1000	Annual births (no.)	Early mortality		Chronic problems		Successful treatment		Main therapeutic needs
			%	n	%	n	%	n	
Congenital malformations	30	408 000	22	89 800	24	98 000	54	220 500	Paediatric surgery
Chromosomal disorders	3.2	43 500	34	14 800	64	28 000	2	900	Social support
Inherited diseases (single gene defects)	7.0	95 200	58	55 200	31	29 500	11	10 500	Medical treatment and support
Total	40	546 700	29	160 000	28	155 500	43	232 900	

Total annual births ≈ 13.6×10^6. (Calculations based on Czeizel & Sankanarayanan, 1984 and Modell, et al., 1990). Treatment is considered successful if it permits an approximately normal length and quality of life, including education, work, and the ability to have a family.

Hence genetic diseases place a considerable burden on health, social and educational services. In addition they cause immense stress and misery for the families of affected children. The demand for genetic services has therefore steadily increased over the years. This is also the consequence of greater awareness among clinicians and the public of the possibilities of preventing genetic diseases. Table 3 lists ways to avoid some of them.

Table 3. Control of genetic disease

Primary prevention
    Mutagen control
Population screening
    Prospective counselling
Retrospective counselling
Antenatal diagnosis
    Prenatal diagnosis
        Selective termination
Neonatal screening

From Weatherall (1991).

I will concentrate on genetic counselling and prenatal diagnosis, the two fields where the recent advances in molecular technologies have had a major impact on defining the aetiology of numerous disorders and on detecting carriers.

Genetic counselling

One definition of the role and the scope of genetic counselling has been given very effectively by Harper (1993). 'Genetic counselling is the process by which patients or relatives at risk of a disorder that may be hereditary are advised of the consequences of the disorder, the probability of developing or transmitting it and the ways in which this may be prevented, avoided or ameliorated'. In this definition three main aspects are mentioned: the diagnosis, the actual estimation of risks and the supportive role of genetic counselling in ensuring that people who ask for advice actually benefit from it and get to know the various forms of management and the preventive measures that may be available for their own problems.

Genetic counselling requires specific knowledge, adequate time and the ability to communicate, and should be inspired by at least three key ethical principles: the autonomy of the individual or couple, their right to complete and accurate information, and the highest level of confidentiality (Fletcher, 1985). It is widely accepted that genetic counselling should be 'non-directive' but this does not mean simply giving people the facts and leaving them to make up their own minds. It involves actively helping them to reach the decision that they feel is right for themselves in the light of their own unique social and moral situation.

The practice of genetic counselling has undergone profound changes in the past 30 years, during which time options available to patients at risk have gone from being very limited (remain childless or take the risk of having an affected child), to a few more (use prenatal diagnosis, prenatal treatment or use AID or another form of 'assisted reproduction').

By looking at the most common causes of referral for genetic counselling, as listed in Table 4, we will notice that, despite recent developments, most of the problems and concerns of the affected families have not changed over the years. While parental needs are frequently expressed in terms of the risk of occurrence and recurrence, the unstated and frequently much deeper concerns centre around the affected child itself and the ways in which the parents may have produced or contributed to his/her problem. Despite any possible explanations given by physicians, parents often experience feelings of guilt which may engender stress between husband and wife. Furthermore a congenital or genetic disorder in one family member often involves a risk for relatives and this generates a demand for more extensive carrier testing and counselling.

Table 4. Most frequent reasons for referral for genetic counselling

- Known or suspected hereditary disease in a patient or family
- Birth of a child with a congenital defect
- Unexplained mental retardation
- Advanced maternal age
- Teratogen exposure
- Consanguinity

The process of genetic counselling

The diagnosis

To provide accurate genetic counselling it is usually necessary first to correctly diagnose the condition for which the couple or family is at risk. This means that it is essential to examine the affected patient, whenever possible, to obtain appropriate laboratory analyses and to obtain all relevant medical records.

Laboratory investigations can be very specific and sophisticated. It is important to recognize that because biotechnology is a rapidly evolving field, tests that were not available yesterday might be available today, so knowledge needs to be continually updated.

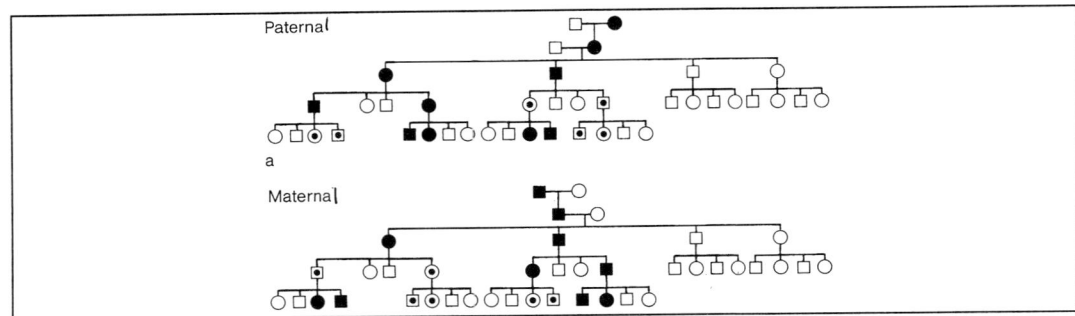

Fig. 1. Hypothetical pedigrees showing maternal and paternal imprinting. The term 'maternal imprinting' is used to imply that there will be no phenotypic effect of the abnormal allele when inherited from the mother and 'paternal imprinting' is used to imply that there will be no phenotypic expression when inherited from the father. For each generation there are equal numbers of non-manifesting male and female carriers (from Duffin Austin & Hall, 1992).

It is well known that genetic heterogeneity and variable expressivity can create problems in diagnosis. Moreover, even the most careful analysis of family pedigree may not always allow the definition of inheritance pattern.

There are four well defined monogenic (or Mendelian) modes of inheritance: autosomal dominant, autosomal recessive, and X-linked recessive or dominant. Dominant traits produce an observable phenotype when inherited from a single parent and recessive traits produce observable effects only when inherited from both parents. X-Linked traits produce an observable effect in hemyzigous males.

However, recent studies have demonstrated that not all heritable traits follow Mendel's law and that genes transmitted by each parent are not always equally expressed in the offspring (Hall, 1990). These 'non-Mendelian' types of transmission include cytoplasmatic inheritance, mosaicism, uniparental disomy and genomic imprinting. These concepts have far-reaching implications for human diseases, ranging from defects in embryonic development to adult cancer. The molecular mechanisms involved are just now beginning to be understood (Duffin Austin & Hall, 1992; Barlow, 1993).

Uniparental disomy involves the inheritance of both members of a chromosome pair from one parent. It has long been assumed that this did not occur in humans. However, genetic markers which allow the parental origin of specific chromosomes to be identified demonstrate that uniparental disomy occurs far more frequently than realized. It may occur through the loss of a chromosome in cases of a trisomy, or through the duplication of a chromosome in cases of monosomy. An interesting corollary of uniparental disomy is that it can result in a child being affected by an autosomal recessive disorder when only one parent is a carrier for that disorder. The son or the daughter inherits two identical copies of the chromosome with the mutation (isodisomy) and so develops the disease. This exact situation has been shown to occur in at least two cases of cystic fibrosis (Spence *et al.*, 1988; Voss, 1989).

Genomic imprinting refers to the concept that certain genes are 'marked' or imprinted in such a way that they are expressed differently depending on their parental origin (Solter, 1988; Marx, 1988). On the basis of classical Mendelian inheritance, it should make no difference which parent transmits a disease gene. Instead, several cases have been described which show that a disorder apparently following autosomal dominant inheritance is only fully expressed when transmitted by one particular sex. Examples of imprinted genes are shown in Table 5 and the pedigrees in Fig. 1 show two hypothetical examples of paternal and maternal imprinting.

Table 5. Some human genes and disorders for which imprinting effects are suspected

Gene or disorder	Chromosomal region
Huntington's disease	4p16
Insulin-dependent diabetes, spinocerebellar atrophy	6pter-p12
Insulin-like growth factor 2 receptor	6q21-7
Cystic fibrosis	7q22-qter
Beckwith–Wiedemann syndrome	11pter-p15
Cerebellar ataxia	11q13- p15
Retinoblastoma, osteosarcoma	13q14-p14.2
Prader–Willi and Angelman's syndrome	15q12-q13
Neurofibromatosis II	22q11-12qter
Fragile X syndrome	Xq28

Modified from Duffin Austin & Hall (1992).

This important and increasingly recognized occurrence is a further example of how our concepts of Mendelian inheritance are becoming more flexible and genetic counselling is becoming more complicated.

Estimation of risk

In order to provide optimal assessment of the risk of recurrence it is important to use all available information, especially when the genotype of the proband is unknown. After having taken a careful pedigree, documented the various details of affected individuals and examined relevant family members, a geneticist is in a position to attempt to estimate the risk of each member, born and unborn, developing the particular disorder. Not all risk estimates are of the same type. They may be based on different sorts of information and may be of greater or lesser reliability. Empirical risks are estimated on observed data rather than theoretical predictions. Empirical risks are available for most of the more common non-Mendelian or chromosomal disorders. Since empirical risks are established from a specific population it is important that the individual receiving genetic counselling comes from an area where this defect has a similar incidence. Mendelian risks can only be given when a clear basis of single gene inheritance can be recognized. They commonly allow a clear differentiation into categories of 'negligible risk' and 'high risk'. Late or variable onset of the disorder, lack of penetrance and variation in expressivity may be major problems in the calculation of risks. As our understanding of gene action and mutations increases, the different mechanisms underlying these phenomena are becoming clearer. It is therefore crucial, once more, to have all the latest information about specific tests available at the biochemical or molecular level for a specific defect.

Communication with the family

Conveying the magnitude of the risk of recurrence of a genetic disease without an understanding of the burden of the disease in question may be almost meaningless. The burden of the disease refers to the clinical prognosis, and the financial, social and emotional problems imposed upon the patient and/or the family. It may vary in severity but will always vary with the individual and family affected.

For a number of genetic diseases it is possible to modify either the burden or the risk. Effective treatment or prevention of secondary effects may affect the way the family look at the diseased child. The availability of prenatal diagnosis may deeply affect the reproductive decisions of couples. Counselling for couples in their early reproductive life should provide information about what might be available in the near future. This aspect is particularly important for diseases that might be recognized prenatally within a few months or years.

It has already been emphasized that genetic counselling goes beyond providing the risk figures. On the other hand it is very difficult to define how much information should be conveyed and at what level.

The information communicated is loaded with emotional content and often contains medical or scientific information that is difficult for patients to understand. For this reason verbal counselling has to be followed by a written report which summarizes the contents of counselling and can be presented to other clinicians.

One should always keep in mind that people might seriously misinterpret or forget information for various reasons and retain risk figures that do not apply to their situation.

Prenatal diagnosis

The objective of prenatal diagnosis is to offer prospective parents the assurance of having unaffected children in the presence of a high (for them!) risk of occurrence. This is not equivalent to an assurance of having normal children. Where prenatal diagnosis is available many couples will prepare to embark on a high-risk pregnancy when they would not have considered doing so in the absence of such diagnostic facilities.

Whenever possible a prenatal diagnosis should be considered, discussed and planned before the pregnancy occurs. It will be inevitable that some cases (maybe most) will be counselled at the beginning of the pregnancy. This has several disadvantages: everything must be done in a hurry. It might be difficult to acquire conclusive data on the factors for or against the prenatal test, and, above all, the woman and her partner may not have a clear vision of the consequences of prenatal diagnosis.

An important development in the approach to prenatal diagnostic services is the multidisciplinary team that deals with each case. The obstetrician, the medical geneticist and other colleagues have the opportunity to meet and discuss the specific aspect of each situation. The clinician giving genetic counselling, whoever he is, must obtain accurate information on the feasibility of prenatal diagnosis before mentioning it to the couple. This is specially relevant when using new molecular advances that might still be undergoing research.

A final point should be considered. Before prenatal diagnosis, the actual risk of recurrence in a particular pregnancy should always be re-evaluated. To be a member of a family where a genetic disease is present is not enough to be automatically at risk of developing or transmitting it. Moreover the situation might have changed in the meanwhile. If the clinician dealing with the woman seeking prenatal diagnosis is not able to evaluate the reality of the risk, then he should ask for advice. Even if prenatal diagnosis were free of risk (which it is not) it should be offered to pregnancies at risk only.

Prenatal diagnostic procedures

Most genetic counselling in relation to prenatal diagnosis is carried out by obstetricians, while specialists in medical genetics are responsible for complex cases.

However it is important to have a knowledge of all technical aspects of procedures and risks involved. In fact it is usual for a woman to ask her doctor for 'personal' advice on which procedure is best in her case.

Current methods for prenatal diagnosis

Table 6 summarizes the current methods for prenatal diagnosis.

Fetal cells sampled with amniocentesis at 16 week of gestation have been one of the major tools of prenatal testing, mainly for cytogenetic and metabolic studies. Examination of the amniotic fluid is mainly used for the confirmation of neural tube defects by measurement of α-foetoprotein.

The development of chorionic villus sampling during the first trimester of gestation has greatly expanded the prenatal diagnosis of genetic disorders by DNA analysis but is also applied to chromosomal and metabolic disorders.

One problem that is worth mentioning is the possibility of a 'discrepancy' between the karyotype of the chorionic tissue and that of the fetus. This has been reported in about 2 per cent of cases (Kalousek, 1988). Moreover, when dealing with chorionic villi to be used for biochemical studies, it is crucial to avoid maternal contamination. The procedure of selection is easy but special accuracy must be used when villi are going to be cultured. Efficient co-ordination between the obstetrical team, the cytogenetic laboratory and the laboratory for biochemical tests is necessary to provide precise results.

Experience with amniocentesis and chorionic villus sampling is now extensive but safety has yet to be agreed on. It is likely that the rate of miscarriage is higher after chorionic villus sampling than after amniocentesis (2–3 per cent *vs* 1 per cent). Some studies have reported an increase in limb reduction defects after chorionic villus sampling at the ninth week or earlier (Firth *et al.*, 1991; Mastroiacovo *et al.*, 1992). A vascular disruptive pathogenesis due to hypoperfusion which interferes with the normal development of the embryo has been suggested. Clearly further studies are necessary to estimate the risk for the embryo exposed to chorionic villus studies but, since it can be postponed later than the tenth week, every patient should be counselled about this potential risk.

Fetal blood, tissue sampling and direct vision of fetus

Direct umbilical cord sampling is now widely used to obtain pure fetal blood. Table 6 shows some of the disorders where diagnosis from fetal blood is useful.

Fetal skin biopsy and liver biopsy have proved to be reliable and safe for a variety of severe conditions, including lethal and dystrophic epidermolysis bullosa, ichthyosiform erythroderma, ornithine carbamyl transferase, etc. The risk of fetal loss is probably around 4 per cent for both procedures.

At present embryoscopy and foetoscopy are used mainly for direct vision of the fetus with the objective of ruling out specific features of genetic syndromes otherwise undiagnosable (polydactily, absence of eyelids, etc.) The fetal loss rate is around 6 per cent.

Table 6. Approaches to prenatal diagnosis

1. Amniocentesis
    Chromosomal disorders (especially where risk is low)
    Open neural tube defects

2. Chorion biopsy
    DNA and enzyme analysis
    Chromosomal disorders (especially when risk is high)

3. Ultrasound scan
    Placental localization, gestational dating, structural malformations (limb, NTD, cardiac, renal...)

4. Fetal blood and tissue sampling
    Haemoglobinopathies and fragile X syndrome when DNA non-feasible, other haematological disorders
    Fetal infections

5. Maternal blood screening
    Triple test
    Fetal cell analysis (under evaluation)

Modified from Harper, 1993.

Future developments in prenatal diagnosis

Prenatal diagnosis is most distressing for couples at high genetic risk, as they suffer great anxiety in every pregnancy and some experience two or three abortions before having a healthy child.

The fast and somewhat unexpected development of '*in vitro* fertilization techniques' and molecular diagnosis of single cells makes pre-implantation diagnosis now realistic. Several approaches are being considered for couples at high risk but the potential impact on the public is still extremely limited. Another possibility to achieve safer and simpler fetal diagnosis is to obtain fetal cells circulating in the maternal blood. Up till now it is not clear yet if any of the methods proposed to isolate foetal from maternal cells will prove successful and every effort has to be considered as still experimental. The new developments in reproductive and genetic technology are not greeted with universal enthusiasm. Many feel that it could be used to the disadvantage of individuals.

I believe that ethical issues are best discussed in the context of practical experience and that every effort should be made to grant everyone the best chance of reaching their personal reproductive goal.

References

Barlow, D.P. (1993): Methylation and imprinting: from host defense to gene regulation? *Science* **260**, 309–310.

Duffin Austin, K. & Hall, J.G. (1992): Non traditional inheritance. *Pediatr. Clin. North Am.* **39**, 335–348.

Firth, H.V., Boyd, P.A., Chamberlain, P., Mackenzie, I.Z. *et al.* (1991): Severe limb abnormalities after chorionic villus sampling at 56–66 days' gestation. *Lancet* **337**, 762–763.

Fletcher, J.C., Berg, K. & Tranoy, K.E. (1985): Ethical aspect of medical genetics. A proposal for guidelines in genetic counselling, prenatal diagnosis and screening. *Clin. Genet.* **25**, 199–205.

Hall, J.G. (1990): Genomic imprinting: review and relevance to human disease. *Am. J. Hum. Genet.* **46**, 857–873.

Harper, P.S. (1993): *Practical genetic counselling*, 4th edn. London: Butterworth–Heinemann.

Kalousek, D.J. (1988): The role of confined chomosomal mosaicism in placental function and human development. *Growth Genet. Horm.* **4 (4)**, 1–3.

Marx, J.P. (1988): A parent's sex may affect gene expression. *Science* **239**, 352–353.

Mastroiacovo, P., Botto, D.L., Cavalcanti, D., Lalatta, F. *et al.* (1992): Limb anomalies following chorionic villus sampling: a registry based case-control study. *Am. J. Med. Genet.* **44**, 856–864.

Modell, B. & Modell, M. (1992): *Towards a healthy baby. Congenital disorders and the new genetics in primary health care*. Oxford: Oxford University Press.

Solter, D. (1988): Differential imprinting and expression of maternal and paternal genomes. *Ann. Rev. Genet.* **22**, 127–146.

Spence, J.E., Perciaccante, R.G., Greig, G.M. *et al.* (1988): Uniparental disomy as a mechanism for human genetic disease. *Am. J. Hum. Genet.* **42**, 217–226.

Voss, R., Ben-Simon, E., Avitai, A. *et al.* (1989): Isodisomy of chromosome 7 in a patient with CF: could uniparental disomy be common in humans? *Am. J. Hum. Genet.* **45**, 373–380.

Weatherall, D.J. (1991): *The new genetics and clinical practice*, 3rd edn. Oxford: Oxford University Press.

Subject Index

A

α-1-antitrypsin deficiency — 73
α-glucosidase deficiency *see* Pompe's disease
acid lipase deficiency — 113
acidaemia
  glutaric — 106, 168
  hyperpipecolic — 132
  isovaleric — 106, 175
  methylmalonic — 103–104, 106, 159
  see also lactic
acidosis, lactic — 30, 75, 80
aciduria
  argininosuccinic — 92, 97
  glutaric — 3–4, 18–20, 134, 150–151
  4-hydroxybutyric — 152
  2-hydroxyglutaric — 142, 150–151
  3-methylglutaconic — 152
  see also methylmalonic; organic; propionic
acute steatosis *see* Reye's syndrome
AcylCoA dehydrogenase deficiency — 13, 14, 17–18
  combined deficiency of β-oxidation enzymes — 18
  3-Hydroxy deficiency (HAD) — 18
  long chain — 17
  medium chain — 17
  short chain — 17–18
  very-long-chain — 18
  see also multiple
AD-CPEO *see* autosomal dominant chronic progressive external ophthalmoplegia
adrenoleucodystrophy — 136, 137, 146, 147, 149
  childhood — 133, 136, 137, 138
  neonatal — 81, 132
  see also X-linked
adrenomyeloneuropathy — 133, 134, 137
adult-onset chronic progressive external ophthalmoplegia — 33
adult-onset muscular presentation in carnitine palmitoyltransferase deficiency — 15–16
ALD *see* adrenoleucodystrophy
Alexander's disease — 146, 148, 149
allopurinol metabolism — 99
alpha-ketoglutarate dehydrogenase deficiency — 44–45
AMN *see* adrenomyeloneuropathy
antitrypsin deficiency — 73
arginase deficiency — 92, 94
argininosuccinate lyase deficiency — 92, 94, 175
argininosuccinate synthetase deficiency — 92, 94
argininosuccinic aciduria — 93, 97
Ashkenazi Jews — 114, 121, 123
Asia — 62
ataxia — 31
autosomal dominant chronic progressive external ophthalmoplegia — 6–7, 33–34

B

β-oxidation, peroxisomal — 130, 131
β-oxidation defects — 11, 13, 14, 16, 18, 106, 149, 152
biotinidase deficiency — 47, 106
bone marrow abnormalities — 85, 86, 88
bone marrow transplantation — 111, 117, 137, 138

C

Canada — 117
Canavan's disease — 146, 147–148, 149, 152
carbamylphosphate deficiency — 92, 94, 98, 99
carbinolamine dehydratase deficiency — 62
carbohydrate deficiency glycoprotein syndrome — 73

METABOLIC ENCEPHALOPATHIES

carbohydrate metabolism disorder	168, 170, 172, 174, 175
carboxylase deficiency	103, 106
see also pyruvate	
cardiomyopathy	4
fatal infantile	26
see also maternally-inherited	
carnitine	56, 106
carnitine acylcarnitine translocase	16
carnitine deficiency, primary	14–15
carnitine palmitoyltransferase deficiency	2–3, 15–16, 17, 46, 153
infantile hepatomuscular phenotype	16
lethal neonatal-early infantile phenotypes	16
type 1	15
type II	13, 14, 15, 16
carnitine palmitoyltransferase II deficiency	13, 14, 16
central nervous system metabolic diseases	145–155
adrenoleucodystrophy	146, 147, 149
Alexander's disease	146, 148, 149
β-oxidation deficiency	149
Canavan's disease	146, 147–148, 149
chronic progressive external ophthalmoplegia	149
chronic progressive external ophthalmoplegia-plus	149
glutaric aciduria	150–151
2-hydroxyglutaric aciduria	142, 150–151
Kearns-Sayre syndrome	145, 149
Krabbe's disease	146–147, 149
Leber's hereditary optic neuropathy	149
Leigh's disease	145, 149
leucodystrophies	146–149
metachromatic leucodystrophy	146, 149
mitochondrial encephalomyopathy, lactic acidosis and stroke-like episodes	145, 149
mitochondrial encephalopathy	152–155
myoclonous epilepsy with ragged-red fibres	149
organic acidopathies	149–152
Pelizaeus-Merbacher disease	146, 149
X-linked adrenoleucodystrophy	147
childhood adrenoleucodystrophy	133, 136, 137, 138
children with chronic disease	187–193
dynamic aspects	191–193
processes of chronic illness	189–190
psychopathology	190–191
children with metabolic diseases	157–164
brain damage, associated factors in determination of	162
central nervous system involvement	160–162
emotional disorders	163
instrumental abilities	160
intelligence quotient	157, 159
maple syrup urine disease	159
methylmalonic acidaemia	159
minimal brain dysfunction	161
parental attitudes	164
psychosocial considerations	162–164
treatment	158
cholesterol	56
chronic disease *see* children	
chronic progressive external ophthalmoplegia	5–6, 149

see also autosomal dominant	
chronic progressive external ophthalmoplegia-plus	4–5, 149
CMD *see* carbohydrate metabolism disorder	
cobalamin F mutation	111, 112, 113, 118
congenital lactic acidosis	75
Conradi-Hünermann disease	133
COX *see* cytochrome-c-oxidase fibres	
CPEO *see* chronic progressive external ophthalmoplegia	
CT *see* carnitine acylcarnitine translocase	
cystinosis	111, 112, 118
cytochrome-c-oxidase deficiency	5–6, 33, 153, 155

D

dehydrogenase deficiency *see* AcylCoA; pyruvate	
DeToni-Fanconi syndrome	34
DHAP-AT *see* dihydroxyacetone phosphate acyltransferase	
DHPR *see* dihydropteridine reductase deficiency	
diet-therapy	
hyperphenylalaninaemia	55–57
maternal phenylketonuria	54–55
organic acidurias	104
dihydropteridine reductase deficiency	62
dihydroxyacetone phosphate acyltransferase	133, 134, 136, 141, 142, 143
Down's syndrome	132

E

electron transfer flavoprotein	13, 19
energy deficiency type	74, 75, 78, 80, 81
epilepsy *see* myoclonous	
ether-phospholipid biosynthesis	131
Europe	62–63, 67

F

Fabry's disease	116
family communication	179–185, 199–200
child's identity	184
diet	183–184
genetic counselling	184
method	181–183
start of school	184
fatal infantile cardiomyopathy	26
fatty acid oxidation disorders	11–20, 74, 76
AcylCoA dehydrogenase deficiency	17–18, 106
carnitine acylcarnitine translocase	16
carnitine palmitoyltransferase deficiency	15–16
classification	13, 14
clinical features	13–14
fatty acid catabolism	11–13
mitochondrial fatty acid oxidation pathway	12

Subject Index

multiple acylCoA dehydrogenation disorder/glutaric aciduria type II	18–20
primary carnitine deficiency	14–15
fatty acids	56–57
FICM *see* fatal infantile cardiomyopathy	
Finland	85, 86
France	42, 71, 73, 133
fructose 1,6-bisphosphatase deficiency	39, 43, 46, 47
fumarase deficiency	3, 44

G

galactosialidosis	112
gangliosidosis	112, 114
Gaucher's disease	81, 88, 112, 114, 115, 116, 117, 121–128
case studies	125
glucocerebrosidase gene	123, 124, 126
neurological symptoms, evolution of	125–127
neuropathology	122–123
non-neurological symptoms, evolution of	125
substitutive enzymatic therapy	125
therapeutic plan	125
type 1	121–122
type 2	122, 127
type 3	122, 126
gene therapy (organ transplant)	108
genetic counselling and prenatal diagnosis	184, 195–202
congenital abnormalities	196
control of genetic disease	196
diagnosis	197–199
family communication	199–200
imprinting	198, 199
risk estimation	199
total load of genetic disease	196
genotype/phenotype relationships	2–5
carnitine palmitoyltransferase deficiency	2–3
chronic progressive ophthalmoplegia-plus with multiple mtDNA and CNS involvement	4–5
fumarase deficiency	3
glutaric aciduria type II	3–4
in vitro studies	2–4
in vivo studies	4–5
myopathy and cardiomyopathy	4
transgenic mice as tools for neurodevelopment pathology	5
globoid cell leucodystrophy *see* Krabbe's disease	
gluconeogenesis defects	41–44, 46, 47
fructose 1,6-bisphosphatase deficiency	43
glucose 6-phosphatase deficiency	43–44
phosphoenolpyruvate carboxykinase deficiency	43
pyruvate carboxylase deficiency	42–43
glucose 6-phosphatase deficiency	39, 43–44, 46, 47
glutaric acidaemia	106
type I	168
glutaric aciduria	134
type I	150–151
type II	3–4, 18–20, 150

glycogen storage disease	88
glycogenosis type I *see* glucose 6-phosphatase deficiency	
glycogenosis type II	113
GM1 gangliosidosis	81
guanosine triphosphate cyclohydrolase deficiency (GTP)	61

H

hepatic presentation	75–76
hepatomegaly	81
hereditary hyperlactacidaemias	75
HHH *see* hyperornithinaemia-hyperammonaemia-homocitrullinuria syndrome	
holocarboxylase synthetase deficiency	106
HPA *see* hyperphenylalaninaemia	
Hunter's disease	116
4-hydroxybutyric aciduria	152
3-hydroxy deficiency (HAD)	18
2-hydroxyglutaric aciduria	142, 150–151
3-hydroxy-3-methyl-glutaryl CoAHMG-CoA lyase deficiency	106
hyperammonaemia	75, 80–81
see also late-onset	
hyperornithinaemia-hyperammonaemia-homocitrullinuria, syndrome	91, 92–93, 94, 95, 98
hyperoxaluria	134
hyperphenylalaninaemia	51–57, 61, 62
clinical phenotypes	51–52
diet-therapy	55–57
maternal phenylketonuria, diet-therapy in	54–55
neurological damage, pathogenesis of	52–53
therapy	53–54
hyperpipecolic acidaemia	132
hypoglycaemia	37, 42, 43
hypoketonic hypoglycaemia	13

I

infantile	
hepatomuscular phenotype in carnitine palmitoyltransferase deficiency	16
Refsum's disease	132
see also neonatal-early infantile	
intelligence quotient	51, 54, 67, 157, 159, 169, 170, 175, 176
intoxication type	73, 74–75, 78, 79–781
IRD *see* infantile Refsum's disease	
isovaleric acidaemia	106, 175
Italy	63–64, 65, 96, 97, 98
see also metabolic disorders	

J

Japan	115

205

K

Kallmann syndrome	5
Kearns-Sayre syndrome	5–6, 25, 28, 29, 145, 149, 152–155
ketoacidosis	79–80
ketosis	78–79
kidney involvement	85, 88, 89
Krabbe's disease	146–147, 149
Krebs cycle defects	37, 42–47
alpha-ketoglutarate dehydrogenase deficiency	44–45
fumarase deficiency	44
KSS *see* Kearns-Sayre syndrome	

L

lactic acidaemia	37–47
gluconeogenesis defects	41–44
Krebs cycle defects	44–45
lactate production by body tissues	38
metabolic fates of pyruvate	39–41, 46
prognosis	47
respiratory chain defects	45–46
treatment options	46–47
lactic acidosis	30, 75, 80
late-onset hyperammonaemias	91–99
allopurinol metabolism and pyrimidine biosynthesis	99
clinical case reports	96–98
diagnosis, tests necessary for	95
history and clinical patterns	93–94
laboratory features	94–96
treatment	98–99
urea cycle	92–93
Leber's hereditary optic neuropathy	26, 149
Leber's hereditary optic neuroretinopathy	25, 31, 32
Leigh's disease	27, 31, 33, 41, 145, 149, 153, 155
maternally inherited	26
leucodystrophies	146–149
see also metachromatic	
LHON *see* Leber's hereditary optic neuroretinopathy	
lipofuscinosis	113
lipoprotein metabolism	56
liver dysfunction	81
liver transplantation	107–108
long-chain AcylCoA dehydrogenase deficiency	17, 18
Lowe's syndrome	75
LPI *see* lysinuric protein intolerance	
lung involvement	85, 88, 89
lysinuric protein intolerance	85–89, 91, 92, 95, 98
atypical features	86, 88
clinical presentation	86
complications	88–89
diagnosis	86
geographic origin	86, 87
initial misdiagnoses	88
therapy	89
lysosomal disorders	71, 73, 75
lysosomal storage diseases	88, 111–118
acid lipase deficiency	113
bone marrow transplantation	111, 117
cobalamin F mutation	111, 112, 113, 118
cystinosis	111, 112, 118
definition and classification	111–113
diagnosis	113
Fabry's disease	116
galactosialidosis	112
gangliosidosis	112, 114
Gaucher's disease	112, 114, 115, 116, 117
glycogenosis type II	113
heterogeneity	114
Hunter's disease	116
lipofuscinosis	113
metachromatic leucodystrophy	112, 114, 115, 116
molecular analysis	114–115
mucolipidosis	112
Niemann-Pick disease	111, 112
post-diagnosis	115–117
pseudodeficiency	114
sialic acid storage disease	111, 112
skeletal dysostosis	118
sphingolipid activator proteins or saposins	112
sphingolipidosis	112
Tay-Sachs disease	116
visceromegaly	118
lyssencephaly	5

M

maple syrup urine disease	71, 73, 75, 77, 78, 104, 106, 159, 175
maternal phenylketonuria	54–55
maternally-inherited Leigh's disease	26
maternally-inherited myopathy and cardiomyopathy (Mimyca)	25, 30–31, 32
Mediterranean	63, 67
medium-chain AcylCoA dehydrogenase deficiency	17, 19, 20
MELAS *see* mitochondrial encephalomyopathy, lactic acidosis and stroke-like episodes	
MERRF *see* myoclonous epilepsy with ragged-red fibres	
metabolic disorders	1–7
autosomal dominant chronic progressive opthalmoplegia	6–7
genotype/phenotype relationships	2–5
local expression of mutation in cells directly involved in pathology	5–6
new genes, search for	6–7
see also children	
metabolic disorders with acute neonatal onset	71–82
biological approach	77–78
cardiac presentation	76
clinical approach	78–81
hepatic presentation	75–76
hepatomegaly and liver dysfunction	81
hypotonia	75

Subject Index

lactic acidosis with neurological distress of energy deficient type	80
neonates at risk, identification of	74
neurological deterioration	74–75
neurological deterioration of energy deficient type without ketoacidosis and without hyperammonaemia	81
neurological distress of intoxication type with hyperammonaemia and without ketoacidosis	80–81
neurological distress of intoxication type with ketoacidosis	79–80
neurological distress of intoxication type with ketosis	78, 79
pathophysiological considerations	73–74
seizures	75
storage disorders without metabolic disturbances	81
metabolic disorders in Italy	167–176
behavioural area	169, 170, 172
cognitive area	169, 170, 172
linguistic area	169, 170, 172
methods	168–170
neurological area	169, 170, 172
results	170–174
statistical analysis	170
metachromatic leucodystrophy	112, 114, 115, 116, 146, 149
3-methylglutaconic aciduria	152
methylmalonic acidaemia	103–104, 106, 159
methylmalonic aciduria	105, 106, 107, 108, 152, 168, 175
metronidazole	107
MILS *see* maternally-inherited Leigh's disease	
Mimyca *see* maternally-inherited myopathy with cardiomyopathy	
minerals	55–56
mit-point mutations	31
mitochondrial encephalomyopathies	25–34, 149, 152–155
biochemical classification	29
clinical considerations	27–28
diagnostic considerations	34
DNA defects	28–30
genetic classification	27
genome, molecular and genetic features	26–27
mit-point mutations	31
mitochondrial DNA communication	33–34
mitochondrial protein importation defects	33
nuclear DNA defects	32–34
respiratory chain	32–33
syn-point mutations	30–32
mitochondrial encephalomyopathy, lactic acidosis and stroke-like episodes	25, 30–32, 145, 149, 153–155
mitochondrial fatty acid oxidation pathway	12
mitochondrial myopathy	88
and cardiopathy	26
MLD *see* metachromatic leucodystrophy	
MMA *see* methylmalonic acidaemia	
MMC *see* mitochondrial myopathy and cardiopathy	
MSUD *see* maple syrup urine disease	
mucolipidosis	112
multiple acylCoA dehydrogenase disorder	18–20
electron transfer flavoprotein deficiencies	19
riboflavin-responsive glutaric aciduria type II	19–20
myoclonous epilepsy with ragged-red fibres	6, 25, 30, 31, 149
myopathy	4
mitochondrial	26, 88
see also maternally-inherited	

N

NALD *see* neonatal adrenoleucodystrophy	
NARP *see* neuropathy, ataxia and retinitis pigmentosa complex	
Near East	63
neonatal	
adrenoleucodystrophy	81, 132
see also metabolic disorders	
Netherlands	133
neurological distress	
of intoxication type with hyperammonaemia and without ketoacidosis	80–81
of intoxication type with ketoacidosis	79–80
of intoxication type with ketosis	78, 79
neuropathy, ataxia and retinitis pigmentosa complex	25, 31, 33
Niemann-Pick disease	111, 112
type C	81, 88
non-ketotic hyperglycinaemia (NKH)	75
North America	42–43
nuclear DNA defects	32–34

O

OA *see* organic acidurias	
ophthalmoplegia *see* adult-onset; autosomal dominant; progressive; sporadic	
organic acidopathies	149–152
organic acidurias	73, 75, 78, 103–106, 168, 170, 172, 174, 175
cofactor replacement	105–106
dietary treatment	104
gene therapy (organ transplant)	108
overtreatment and insufficient treatment	105
therapeutic strategies	104
toxic metabolites excretion or enhancing alternative pathways	106–107
ornithine transcarbamylase (OTC) deficiency	81, 92, 93, 94, 95, 96, 97, 98, 99

P

pancreatitis	85, 88
PD *see* pseudodeficiency	
Pearson's syndrome	28–29
Pelizaeus-Merbacher disease	146, 149

PEO *see* progressive external ophthalmoplegia
peroxisomal b-oxidation 130, 131
peroxisomal disorders 73, 75, 129–138
  adrenoleucodystrophy 136, 137
  adrenomyeloneuropathy 133, 134, 137
  biochemical characteristics 134–137
  childhood adrenoleucodystrophy 133, 136, 137, 138
  classification 130
  clinical characteristics with neurological involvement 132–134
    Conradi-Hünermann disease 133
  dihydroxyacetone phosphate acyltransferase 133, 134, 136
  ether-phospholipid biosynthesis 131
  glutaric aciduria 134
  hyperoxaluria 134
  hyperpipecolic acidaemia 132
  infantile Refsum's disease 132
  neonatal adrenoleucodystrophy 132
  peroxisomal β-oxidation 130, 131
  rhizomelic chondrodysplasia punctata 132–133, 134, 136
  treatment 137
  X-linked adrenoleucodystrophy 133, 134, 136, 137, 138
  X-linked dominant and recessive chondrodysplasia 133
  Zellweger-like syndrome 132
  Zellweger's syndrome 129, 132, 134, 135–136, 137
peroxisomal oxidation and respiration 130–131
phenotype *see* genotype; phenylketonuria
phenylketonuria 51, 52, 57
  genotype/phenotype correlation 61–67
  maternal 54–55
  mutations, geographic distribution of 62–64, 65, 66
  phenylalanine hydroxylase deficiency 62
phosphoenolpyruvate carboxykinase deficiency 43
phosphorylase β-kinase deficiency 76
pigmentary retinopathy 28
PKU *see* phenylketonuria
Pompe's disease 75, 76
prenatal diagnosis *see under* genetic counselling
primary carnitine deficiency 14–15
progressive external ophthalmoplegia 28, 29, 30, 32
propionic acidaemia 106
propionic aciduria 105, 107, 108, 168, 175
pseudodeficiency 114
PTPS *see* pyruvoyl tetrahydropterin synthase deficiency
pyrimidine biosynthesis 99
pyruvate 38
  carboxylase deficiency 42–43, 46, 47, 74
  dehydrogenase deficiency 37, 40–41, 44, 47, 74
  metabolism 39–41, 45, 46
pyruvoyl tetrahydropterin synthase deficiency 61
PZO *see* peroxisomal disorders

R

RCDP *see* rhizomelic chondrodysplasia punctata

respiratory chain defects 37, 45–46, 47, 74, 75, 76, 80
retinitis pigmentosa complex 31
Reye's syndrome 76
rhizomelic chondrodysplasia punctata 132–133, 134, 136, 141–143
riboflavin-responsive glutaric aciduria type II 19–20

S

SAP *see* sphingolipid activator proteins
saposins 112
seizures 75, 174
short-chain AcylCoA dehydrogenase deficiency 17–18, 19, 20
sialic acid storage disease 111, 112
skeletal dysostosis 118
SO *see* sulphite oxidase deficiency
sphingolipid activator proteins 112
sphingolipidosis 112, 121
sporadic progressive external ophthalmoplegia 25, 28
storage disorders 75, 81, 88, 111, 112
  see also lysosomal
subacute necrotizing encephalopathy *see* Leigh's disease
sulphite oxidase deficiency 75
syn-point mutations 30–32

T

taurine 56
Tay-Sachs disease 116
tetrahydrobiopterin (BH4) deficiency 52–53, 61, 62
trace elements 55–56
Turkey 86
tyrosinaemia type I 73, 108

U

UCD *see* urea cycle defects
United States 117, 133
urea cycle defects 73, 75–76, 78, 80–81, 92–93, 100, 168, 170, 172, 175

V

very-long-chain polyunsaturated fatty acids (VLCP) 55, 56–57
Von Gierke's disease *see* glucose 6-phosphatase deficiency

X

X-linked adrenoleucodystrophy (X-ALD) 133, 134, 136, 137, 138, 147

X-linked dominant and recessive chondrodysplasia 133

Z
Zellweger-like syndrome 132

Zellweger's syndrome 13, 75, 81, 129, 132, 134, 135–136, 137

QUERY
Pelizaeus-Merbacher and Merzbacher also under central nervous system